GYNAECOLOGY ILLUSTRATED

David McKay Hart MD FRCS(Glas) FRCOG

Consultant Gynaecologist, North Glasgow University NHS Trust and
Honorary Senior Research Fellow, Department of Obstetrics and Gynaecology, University of Glasgow,
Glasgow, UK

Jane Norman MD MRCOG

Senior Lecturer, Department of Obstetrics and Gynaecology, University of Glasgow,
Glasgow, UK

Illustrated by

Robin Callander FFPh FMAA AIMBI

Medical Illustrator, Formerly Director of Medical Illustrations, University of Glasgow,
Glasgow, UK

Ian Ramsden

Head of Medical Illustration Unit, University of Glasgow,
Glasgow, UK

FIFTH EDITION

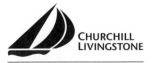 CHURCHILL
LIVINGSTONE

EDINBURGH LONDON NEW YORK PHILADELPHIA ST LOUIS SYDNEY TORONTO 2000

CHURCHILL LIVINGSTONE
An imprint of Harcourt Publishers Limited

© Harcourt Publishers Limited 2000

✍ is a registered trademark of Harcourt Publishers Limited

The right of David McKay Hart and Jane Norman to be identified
as authors of this work has been asserted by them in accordance with
the Copyright, Designs and Patents Act 1988

First edition 1972
Second edition 1978
Third edition 1985
Fourth edition 1993
Fifth edition 2000

Standard edition ISBN 0 443 06198 X

International Student Edition ISBN 0 443 06199 8

British Library Cataloguing in Publication Data
A catalogue record for this book is available from the British Library

Library of Congress Cataloging in Publication Data
A catalog record for this book is available from the Library of
Congress

Note

Medical knowledge is constantly changing. As new information
becomes available, changes in treatment, procedures, equipment and
the use of drugs become necessary. The authors and the publishers
have, as far as it is possible, taken care to ensure that the information
given in this text is accurate and up to date. However, readers are
strongly advised to confirm that the information, especially with
regard to drug usage, complies with the latest legislation and
standards of practice.

The
publisher's
policy is to use
**paper manufactured
from sustainable forests**

Printed in China

GYNAECOLOGY ILLUSTRATED

Commissioning Editor: Timothy Horne
Project Development Manager: Janice Urquhart
Project Manager: Frances Affleck
Design: Jim Farley

Developments in gynaecological practice, including advances in medical treatment and increasing use of day-care surgery, have made it necessary to rewrite and update this book. Evidence-based practice has challenged some long-held beliefs and there have been particular advances in the management of infertility and malignant disease.

A new, younger, academic author has become involved to ensure that the book meets the requirements of the medical student and the primary care doctor. We have attempted to stress what is important and relevant in contemporary gynaecology and the emphasis on visual presentation, where possible, has been maintained.

David McKay Hart
Jane Norman

CONTENTS

CHAPTER 1

EMBRYOLOGY OF THE REPRODUCTIVE TRACT

DEVELOPMENT OF THE OVARY

The germ cells which will eventually inhabit the gonads originate from the primitive hind gut. They appear around the 25th day.

By 30 days the gut complete with mesentery is formed. The germ cells now migrate from the gut to the root of the mesentery. About 1 to 2 million remain at birth and about 300,000 at puberty, of the original 6 or 7 million. A smaller number may be a factor in leading to premature menopause.

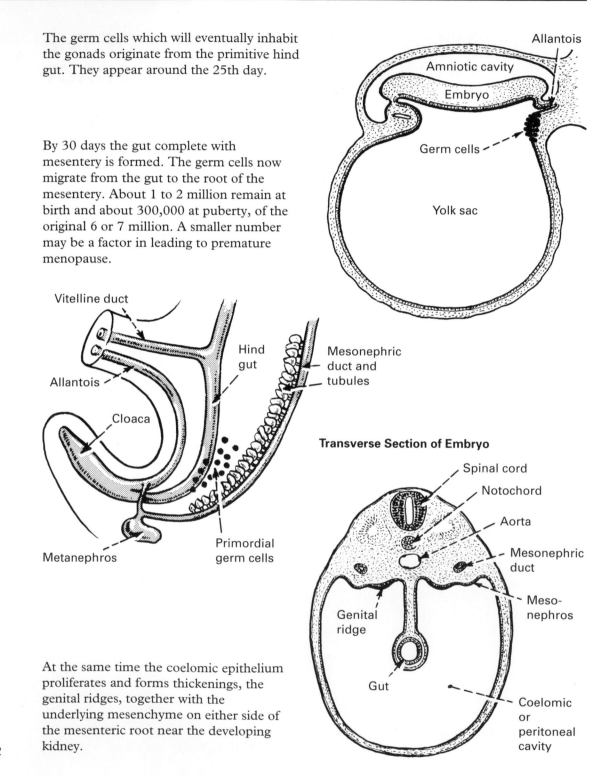

Transverse Section of Embryo

At the same time the coelomic epithelium proliferates and forms thickenings, the genital ridges, together with the underlying mesenchyme on either side of the mesenteric root near the developing kidney.

DEVELOPMENT OF THE OVARY

At this stage the primitive gonad (genital ridge) consists of mesoderm (coelomic epithelium plus mesenchyme) covered by coelomic epithelium. The germ cells now migrate from the root of the mesentery to the genital ridge.

The coelomic epithelium growing into the genital ridge forms so-called sex cords which enclose each germ cell.

Up to this time, around the 7th week, the gonad is of indifferent type, male being indistinguishable from female.

The germ cells and most of the sex cord cells remain in the superficial part, the future cortex of the ovary. The cords lose contact with the surface epithelium and form small groups of cells each with its germ cell, a primitive follicle. Some of the sex cord cells grow into the medulla. These tend to regress and form rudimentary tubules, the rete.

As the ovary grows it projects increasingly into the peritoneal (coelomic) cavity, thus forming a mesentery.

3

DEVELOPMENT OF THE OVARY

At the same time the ovary descends extraperitoneally in the abdominal cavity. Two ligaments develop and these may help to control its descent, guiding it to its final position and preventing its complete descent through the inguinal ring in contrast to the testes. The first structure is the suspensory ligament attached to the anterior (cephalic) pole of the ovary and connecting it with its site of origin, the genital ridge.

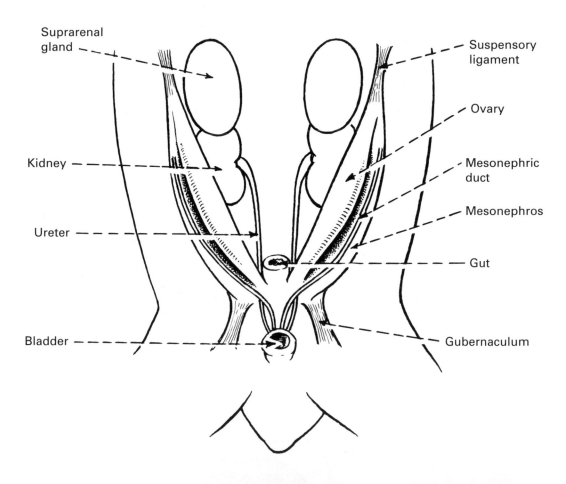

Another ligament or gubernaculum develops at the posterior or caudal end of the ovary. At first attached to the genital ridge it later becomes attached to the developing uterus and becomes the ovarian ligament.

DEVELOPMENT OF UTERUS AND FALLOPIAN TUBES

When the embryo reaches a size of 10 mm at 35–36 days a longitudinal groove appears on the dorsal aspect of the coelomic cavity lateral to the Wolffian (mesonephric) ridge.

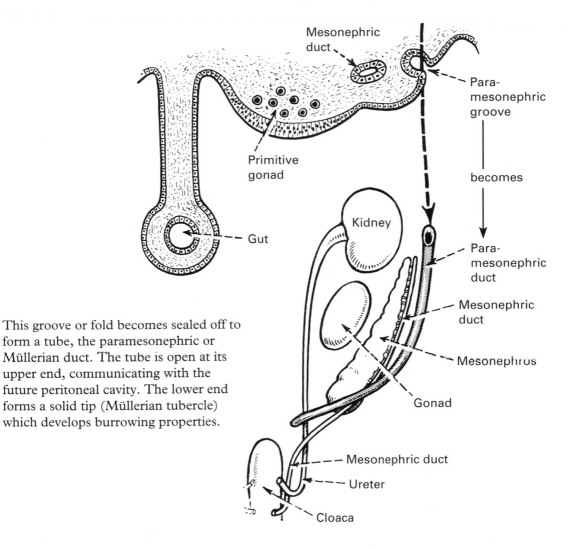

This groove or fold becomes sealed off to form a tube, the paramesonephric or Müllerian duct. The tube is open at its upper end, communicating with the future peritoneal cavity. The lower end forms a solid tip (Müllerian tubercle) which develops burrowing properties.

DEVELOPMENT OF UTERUS AND FALLOPIAN TUBES

The Müllerian ducts from either side grow in a caudal direction, extraperitoneally. They also bend medially and anteriorly and ultimately fuse in front of the hind gut. The mesonephric duct becomes involved in the walls of the paramesonephric ducts.

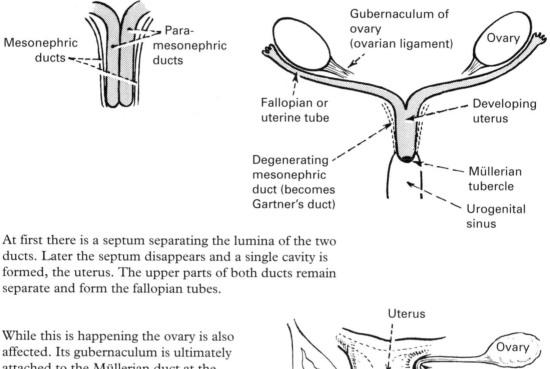

At first there is a septum separating the lumina of the two ducts. Later the septum disappears and a single cavity is formed, the uterus. The upper parts of both ducts remain separate and form the fallopian tubes.

While this is happening the ovary is also affected. Its gubernaculum is ultimately attached to the Müllerian duct at the cornu of the developing uterus. Its effect is to pull the ovary medially so that its long axis becomes horizontal.

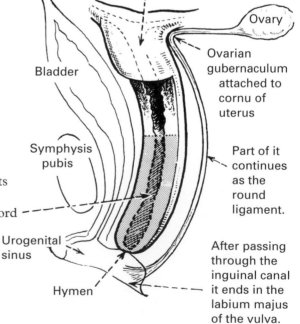

The lower end of the fused Müllerian ducts beyond the uterine lumen remains solid, proliferates and forms a solid cord. This cord will canalise to form the vagina which opens into the urogenital sinus.

At the point of entry into the urogenital sinus, part of the Müllerian tubercle persists and forms the hymen.

DEVELOPMENT OF EXTERNAL GENITALIA

At an early stage the hind gut and the various urogenital ducts open into a common cloaca.

A septum (urorectal) grows down between the allantois and the hind gut during the 5th week.

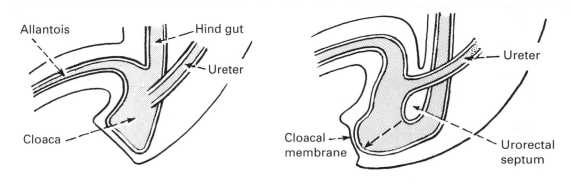

Eventually this septum fuses with the cloacal membrane dividing the cloaca into two compartments — the rectum dorsally and the urogenital sinus ventrally. At the same time the developing uterus grows down and makes contact with the urogenital sinus.

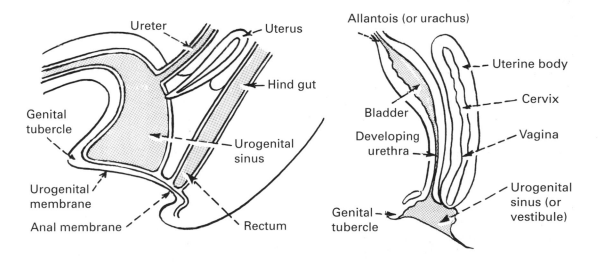

At the end of the 7th week the urogenital membrane breaks down so that the urogenital sinus opens on to the surface.

The developing uterus and vagina push downwards and cause an elongation and narrowing of the upper part of the urogenital sinus. This will form the urethra.

DEVELOPMENT OF EXTERNAL GENITALIA

Meanwhile on the surface of the embryo around the urogenital sinus five swellings appear. At the cephalic end a midline swelling grows, the genital tubercle, which will become the clitoris. Posterior to the genital tubercle and on either side of the urogenital membrane a fold is formed — urethral folds. Lateral to each of these a further swelling appears — the genital or labial swelling. These swellings approach each other at their posterior ends, fuse and form the posterior commissure. The remaining swellings become the labia minora.

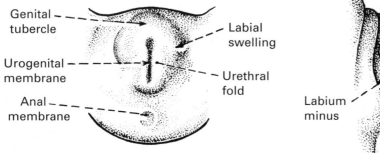

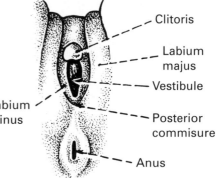

Certain small but clinically important glands are formed in and around the urogenital sinus.

In the embryo epithelial buds arise from the urethra and also from the epithelium of the urogenital sinus. In the male these two sets of buds grow together and give rise to the glands of the prostate. They remain separate in the female, the urethral buds forming the urethral glands and the urogenital buds giving rise to the para-urethral glands of Skene. The ducts of the latter open into the vestibule on either side of the urethra.

Two other small glands arise by budding from the epithelium of the posterior part of the vestibule, one on either side of the vaginal opening. These are the greater vestibular or Bartholin's glands. Similar smaller glands also arise in the anterior portion of the vestibule.

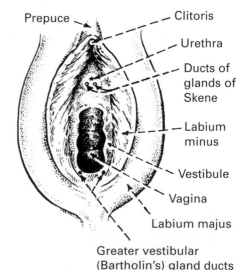

DEVELOPMENT OF MALE EXTERNAL GENITALIA

As in the female a mesodermal mass, the urorectal septum, grows downwards and separates the urogenital sinus from the rectum and anus. The urogenital portion of the cloacal membrane disintegrates so that an open gutter is formed through which the urine drains. This gutter is continuous anteriorly with the primitive urethral groove on the phallus.

The ectoderm on the under surface of the phallus disappears, exposing the underlying endodermal plate.

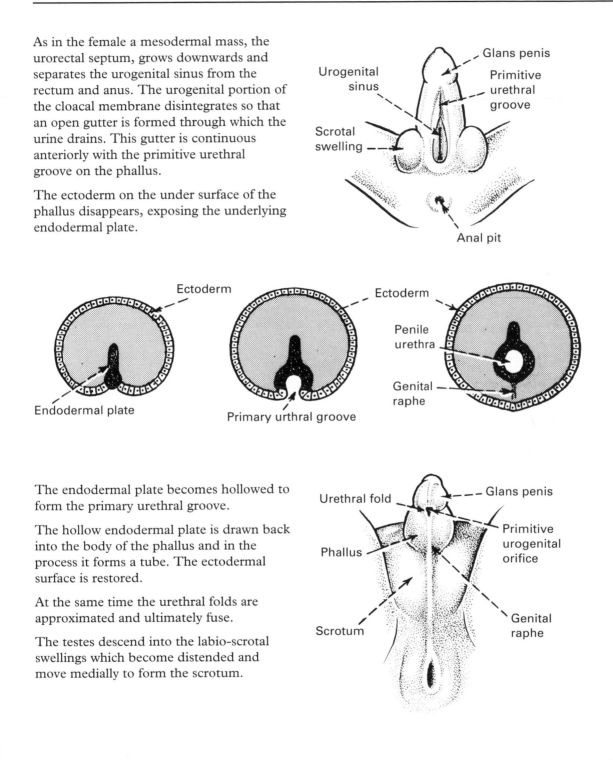

The endodermal plate becomes hollowed to form the primary urethral groove.

The hollow endodermal plate is drawn back into the body of the phallus and in the process it forms a tube. The ectodermal surface is restored.

At the same time the urethral folds are approximated and ultimately fuse.

The testes descend into the labio-scrotal swellings which become distended and move medially to form the scrotum.

CHAPTER 2

ANATOMY OF THE REPRODUCTIVE TRACT

THE PERINEUM

The **PERINEUM** (Gk. 'around the natal area')

The **anatomical** or true perineum is the diamond-shaped outlet of the pelvis and the soft tissues which cover it.

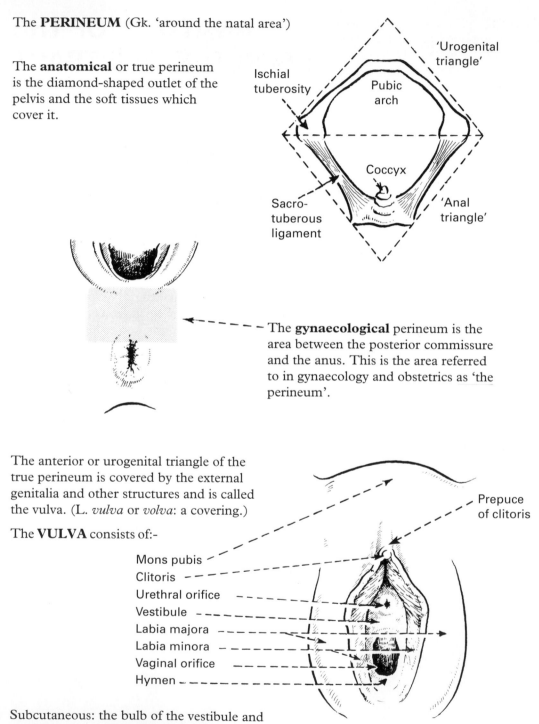

The **gynaecological** perineum is the area between the posterior commissure and the anus. This is the area referred to in gynaecology and obstetrics as 'the perineum'.

The anterior or urogenital triangle of the true perineum is covered by the external genitalia and other structures and is called the vulva. (L. *vulva* or *volva*: a covering.)

The **VULVA** consists of:-

Mons pubis
Clitoris
Urethral orifice
Vestibule
Labia majora
Labia minora
Vaginal orifice
Hymen

Prepuce
of clitoris

Subcutaneous: the bulb of the vestibule and the greater vestibular (Bartholin's) glands.

THE VULVA

MONS PUBIS and LABIA MAJORA

The mons pubis is a pad of fatty tissue overlying the symphysis pubis and covered by skin and pubic hair. The labia are folds of skin and fat which pass from the mons back to the perineum. The lateral labial surfaces are pigmented and hairy, the inner smooth and containing many sebaceous, sweat and apocrine glands which give off the odour peculiar to the vulva.

The substance of the labia consists of vascular fatty tissue with many lymphatics, and also vestigial remnants of the dartos muscle. (The labium is the homologue of the scrotum.)

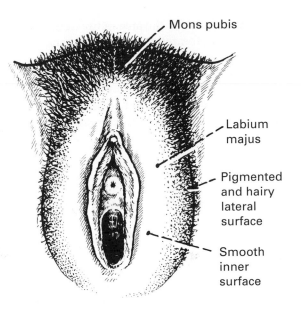

CLITORIS and LABIA MINORA

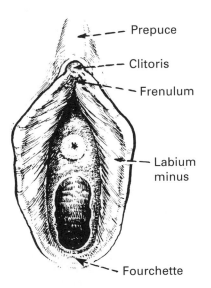

The clitoris is the vestigial homologue of the penis and is formed the same way from two corpora cavernosa and a glans of spongy erectile tissue which has a copious blood supply from the clitoral artery. The clitoris is highly innervated.

The labia minora are two cutaneous folds enclosing the urethral and vaginal orifices. Anteriorly each divides to form a hood or prepuce, and a frenulum for the clitoris. Posteriorly they unite in a frenulum or fourchette which is obliterated by the delivery of a baby. The labia minora contain no fat but many sebaceous glands.

13

THE VULVA

The **VESTIBULE** is the area between the labia minora. It is perforated by the urethral and vaginal orifices and the ducts of Bartholin's and Skene's glands. The fossa navicularis between the vagina and the fourchette is, like the fourchette, obliterated by childbirth. The lesser vestibular glands are mucosal glands discharging on to the surface of the vestibule.

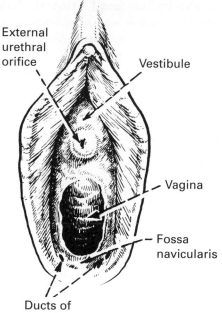

The **EXTERNAL URETHRAL ORIFICE** is in the healthy state a small protuberance with a vertical cleft. The tiny orifices of the paraurethral (Skene's) ducts lie just inside or outside the meatus. The paraurethral glands are homologues of the prostate and form a system of tubular glands surrounding most of the urethra.

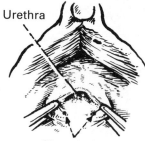

The **VAGINAL ORIFICE** is a midline aperture incompletely closed by the **HYMEN**. The hymen is a thin septum of tissue lined by squamous epithelium with a small hole (sometimes several) for the passage of menstrual blood. It is ruptured by coitus and more or less obliterated by childbirth. A few tags of skin are left called carunculae myrtiformes. The appearances of the hymen are unreliable as medicolegal evidence, whether of virginity or childbirth.

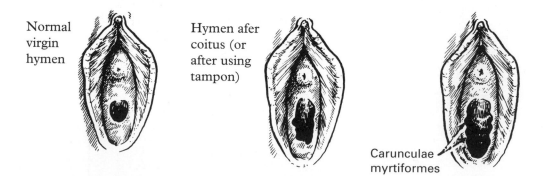

BARTHOLIN'S GLAND

The **BULB of the VESTIBULE** consists of two masses of erectile tissue on either side of the vagina, lying beneath the skin and bulbospongiosus muscle but superficial to the perineal membrane. They are connected anteriorly by a narrow transverse strip and are the homologue of the bulb of the penis.

BARTHOLIN'S (Greater vestibular) glands are the homologues of the bulbo-urethral (Cowper's) glands in the male but lie superficial instead of deep to the perineal membrane. Each gland is partly covered by the erectile tissue of the bulb and drains by a duct about 2cm long which opens into the vaginal orifice lateral to the hymen. Bartholin's gland is not palpable in the healthy state.

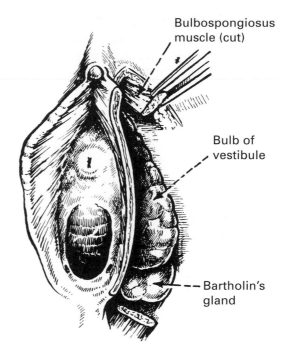

Bulbospongiosus muscle (cut)

Bulb of vestibule

Bartholin's gland

The erectile tissue of the bulb becomes tumescent during sexual excitement and the glands secrete a mucoid discharge which acts as a lubricant.

Histology of Bartholin's Gland

The gland is formed of racemose glands lined with columnar or cuboid epithelium. The duct demonstrates the very intimate embryological connection between genital and urinary tracts by being lined with transitional epithelium.

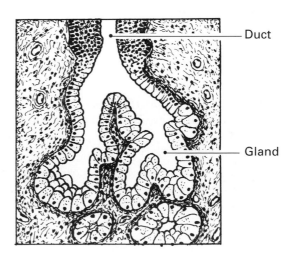

Duct

Gland

MUSCLES OF THE PERINEUM

Ischiocavernosus
This muscle compresses the root of the clitoris during sexual excitement, to produce erection by venous congestion.

Bulbospongiosus
This muscle conceals the vestibular bulb and Bartholin's glands. Its function is to diminish the vaginal orifice during coitus.

Transversus perinei superficialis
A feeble muscle which helps to fix the perineal body.

Sphincter ani externus
Normally in a state of contraction to keep the anus closed. It also helps to fix the perineal body.

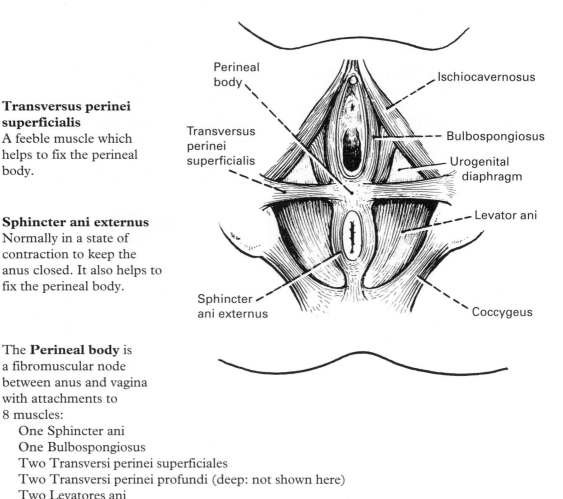

The **Perineal body** is a fibromuscular node between anus and vagina with attachments to 8 muscles:
    One Sphincter ani
    One Bulbospongiosus
    Two Transversi perinei superficiales
    Two Transversi perinei profundi (deep: not shown here)
    Two Levatores ani

The whole mass is what gynaecologists mean when they talk about 'the perineum'. If it is damaged during parturition and not properly repaired and healed it will not function properly and the efficiency of the whole pelvic diaphragm may suffer.

THE UROGENITAL DIAPHRAGM

The UROGENITAL DIAPHRAGM (Triangular ligament)

This area of the perineum is more developed and surgically more important in the male. It consists of two sheets of fascia with a layer of muscle in between. It covers the pubic arch and is pierced by the urethra and, in the female, by the vagina.

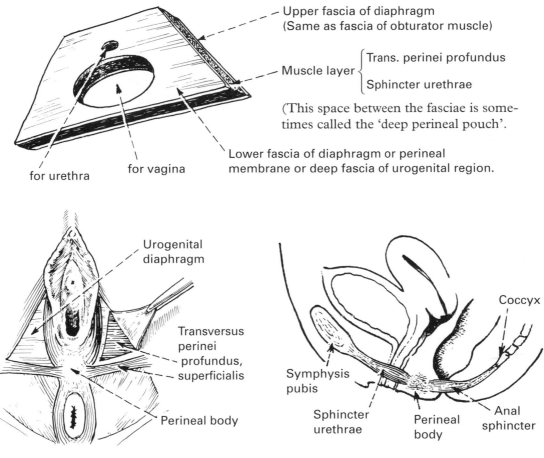

Upper fascia of diaphragm
(Same as fascia of obturator muscle)

Muscle layer { Trans. perinei profundus
Sphincter urethrae

(This space between the fasciae is sometimes called the 'deep perineal pouch'.

Lower fascia of diaphragm or perineal membrane or deep fascia of urogenital region.

for urethra   for vagina

Urogenital diaphragm

Transversus perinei profundus, superficialis

Perineal body

Coccyx

Symphysis pubis

Sphincter urethrae   Perineal body   Anal sphincter

All the perineal muscles lie superficial to the perineal membrane except the transversus perinei profundus which helps to fix the perineal body.

(See page 309 on the function of the sphincter.)

The 'sphincter urethrae' is the system of musculature which assists the bladder muscle in closing the urethra. It is made up of the transversus perinei, the bulbospongiosus and the levator ani; the anchoring bony points are the lower border of the symphysis pubis and the coccyx.

ANATOMY OF THE PELVIS

ISCHIORECTAL FOSSA
A wedge-shaped space between the ischial tuberosity and the anus, filled with fat and crossed by vessels and nerves.

Boundaries:-
Laterally, the obturator fascia and ischial tuberosity.
Posteriorly, the sacrotuberous ligament.
Anteriorly, the urogenital diaphragm.
Medially, the sphincter ani and levator (anal) fascia.

The ischiorectal fat is traversed by the pudendal vessels and nerves and some small perineal branches of sacral nerves.

This pad of fat supports the anal canal and pelvic diaphragm.

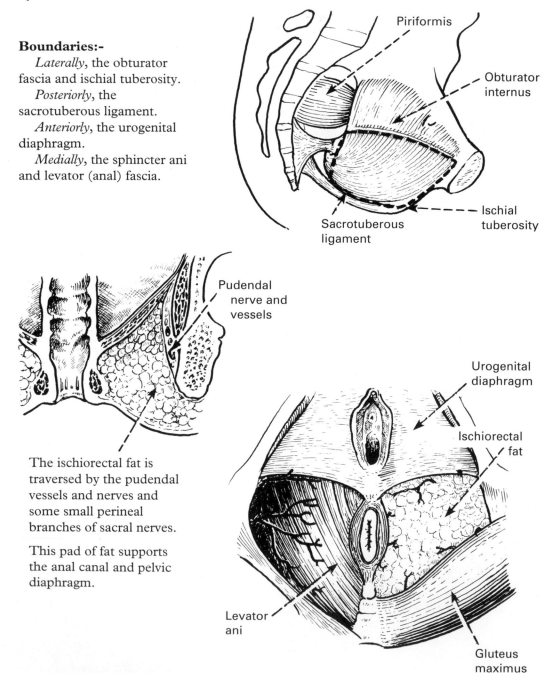

MUSCLES OF THE PELVIS

Levator ani ⎫
Coccygeus ⎬ Pelvic diaphragm
Obturator internus
Piriformis

The **Levator ani** arises from the back of the pubis, the obturator fascia (by a 'tendinous arch' or 'white line') and the ischial spine.

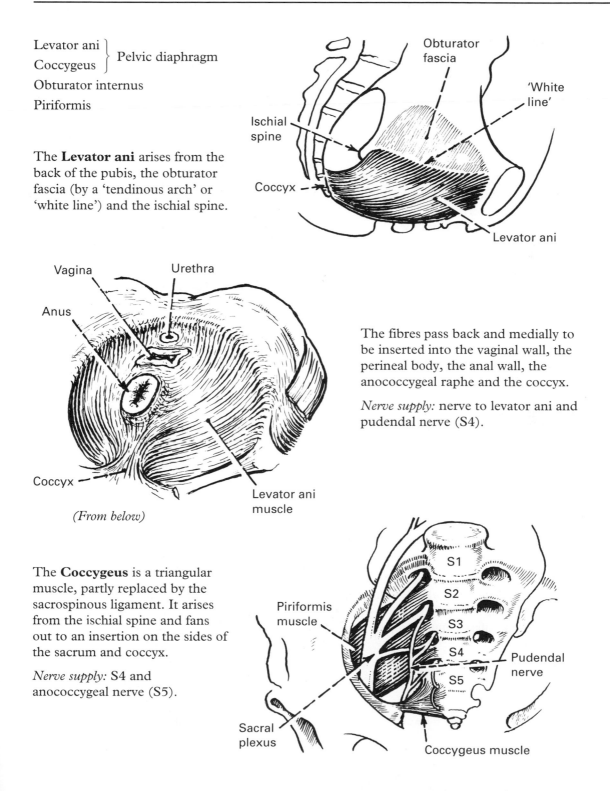

(From below)

The fibres pass back and medially to be inserted into the vaginal wall, the perineal body, the anal wall, the anococcygeal raphe and the coccyx.

Nerve supply: nerve to levator ani and pudendal nerve (S4).

The **Coccygeus** is a triangular muscle, partly replaced by the sacrospinous ligament. It arises from the ischial spine and fans out to an insertion on the sides of the sacrum and coccyx.

Nerve supply: S4 and anococcygeal nerve (S5).

19

PELVIC DIAPHRAGM

The **Obturator internus** arises from the anterolateral wall of the pelvis (and obturator membrane) and passes backwards through the lesser sciatic foramen to be inserted into the trochanter of the femur. (L5, S1 and S2)

The **Piriformis** arises from the front of the sacrum and passes through the greater sciatic foramen to be inserted into the trochanter of the femur. (S1 and 2)

These muscles are primarily lateral rotators of the hip and postural muscles.

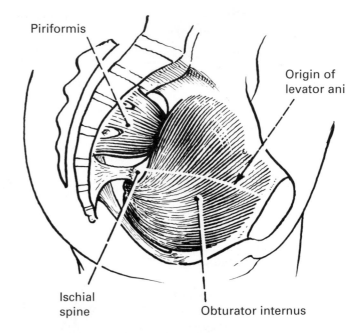

Piriformis

Origin of levator ani

Ischial spine

Obturator internus

FUNCTIONS of the PELVIC DIAPHRAGM

Apart from helping to fix the perineal body and assist the vaginal and anal sphincters, the main function of the pelvic diaphragm is to support the pelvic viscera.

The muscles used to be named:

$$\left.\begin{array}{l} \text{pubococcygeus} \\ \text{iliococcygeus} \end{array}\right\} = \text{levator ani}$$

ischiococcygeus = coccygeus

and in the lower animals their function is to move the tail (the coccyx). In man they have to meet the requirements of the erect position and resist the strain imposed by any increase in intra-abdominal pressure such as laughing, coughing, straining at stool, etc. In addition a complete relaxation of the muscles should be possible during parturition so that the vaginal foramen may enlarge almost to the size of the bony pelvic outlet.

PELVIC FASCIA

The PELVIC FASCIA

Parietal layer
The aponeuroses and fascial sheaths of the pelvic muscles (the 'wallpaper' of the pelvis).

Visceral layer
The fascial sheaths of the organs and the fatty tissue filling the space between them (the 'stuffing' of the pelvis).

In certain areas this stuffing is condensed and strengthened by plain muscle fibres and elastic tissue to form the ligaments of the uterus (pages 28, 29, 30, 31).

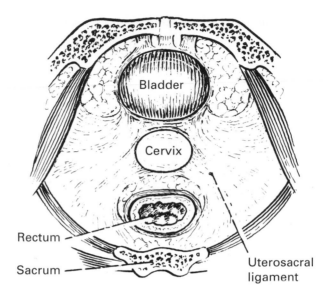

Relations of the Fascia
The nerve trunks, which leave the pelvis may be described as 'outside' the fascia which gives them fascial sheaths. The vessels are 'inside' and lie between fascia and peritoneum.

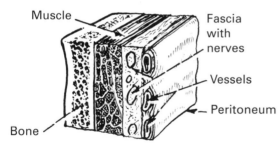

These fascial prolongations on structures leaving the pelvis form points at which pus may track from a pelvic abscess to a point in the buttock or groin or above the inguinal ligament.

(The greater sciatic notch is not shown.)

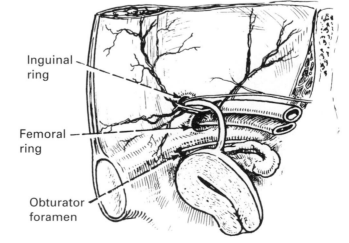

THE VAGINA

A canal of plain muscle extending from the vestibule to the uterus.

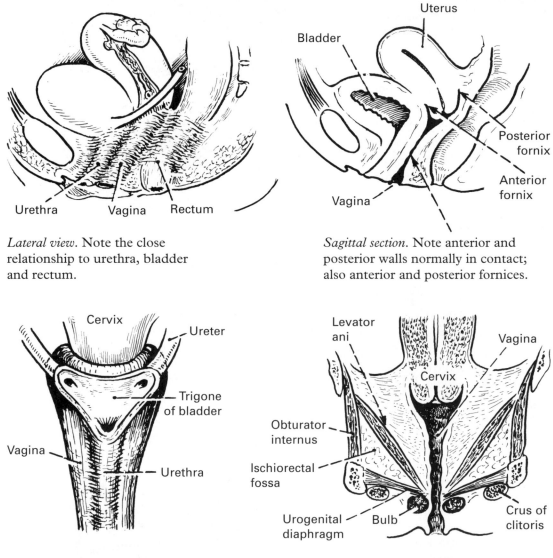

Lateral view. Note the close relationship to urethra, bladder and rectum.

Sagittal section. Note anterior and posterior walls normally in contact; also anterior and posterior fornices.

Anterior view shows the very intimate relationship with the bladder base and ureters.

Coronal section shows the relationship of vagina and pelvic floor.

THE VAGINA

In the nulliparous adult the vagina is H-shaped in section and marked by longitudinal furrows — the columns of the vagina — and numerous transverse ridges or rugae. This configuration permits great distension during parturition; and is much less marked in the parous woman.

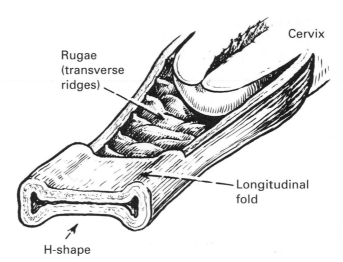

Vaginal Fornices
These are gutters at the top of the vagina, surrounding the cervix.

Anterior Fornix — related to the bladder base and the utero-vesical fossa.

Posterior Fornix — related to peritoneum of the Pouch of Douglas. This fornix is deeper than the anterior one because of the angle the cervix makes with the vagina. The male's ejaculate is deposited in the posterior fornix during coitus, where it is in close contact with the cervical os.

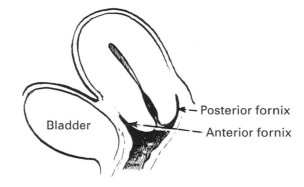

Lateral Fornices — related to the ureters and the uterine vessels.

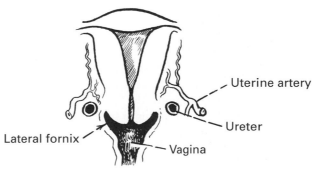

THE VAGINA

HISTOLOGY

Its length is about 9cm along the posterior wall and 7.5cm along the anterior. The width gradually increases from below upwards.

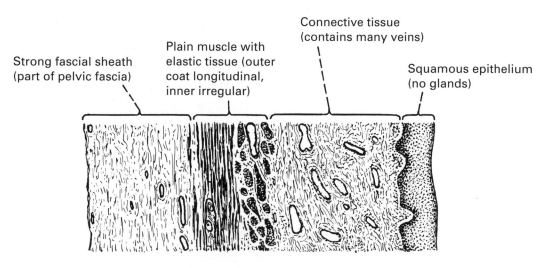

Strong fascial sheath (part of pelvic fascia)

Plain muscle with elastic tissue (outer coat longitudinal, inner irregular)

Connective tissue (contains many veins)

Squamous epithelium (no glands)

The vagina pierces the urogenital diaphragm and is encircled at its lower end by the voluntary bulbospongiosus which has some sphincteric action, although the levator ani muscle is more effective.

Vaginal secretion

This is composed of alkaline cervical secretion, desquamated epithelial cells and bacteria. The epithelium is rich in glycogen which is converted by Doderlein's bacillus into lactic acid. The vaginal pH is about 4.5 and provides a fairly effective barrier against infection.

The vaginal epithelium

This is composed of several layers of squamous cells with no keratinisation. It develops papillae which dip into the fibrous corium. It is much thinner in the child and the rugae are absent. This appearance recurs in old age. Cyclic changes are discussed on page 52.

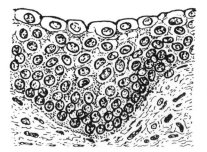

UTERUS

The uterus is a hollow viscus composed of smooth muscle whose sole function is gestation.

It lies between the rectum and the bladder and is continuous with the vagina.

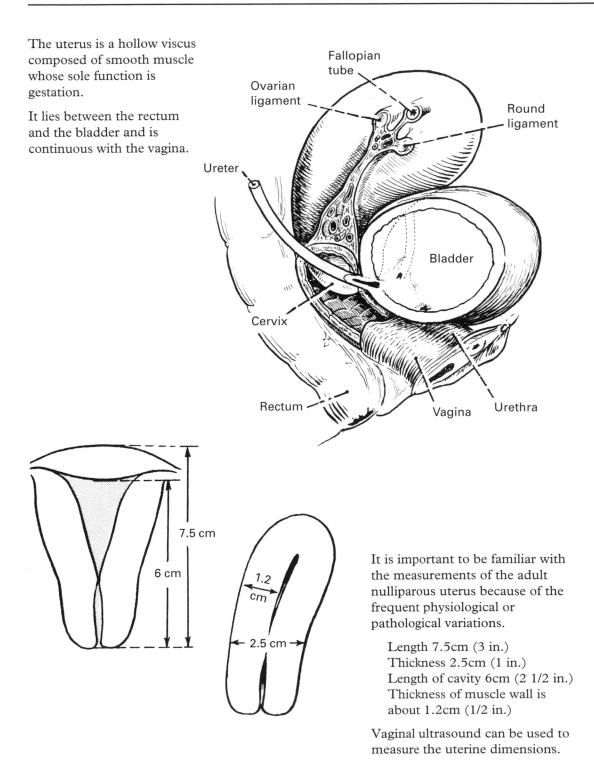

It is important to be familiar with the measurements of the adult nulliparous uterus because of the frequent physiological or pathological variations.

> Length 7.5cm (3 in.)
> Thickness 2.5cm (1 in.)
> Length of cavity 6cm (2 1/2 in.)
> Thickness of muscle wall is about 1.2cm (1/2 in.)

Vaginal ultrasound can be used to measure the uterine dimensions.

25

UTERUS

CORPUS and CERVIX

The upper two-thirds of the uterus are called the corpus or body, and the lower third the cervix or neck. They are quite distinct in function and therefore in structure as well, although the transition from muscle to fibrous tissue is gradual.

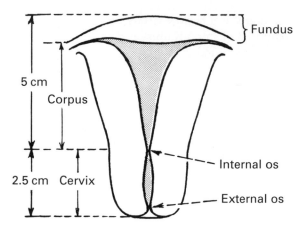

CORPUS

Its function is to provide a mucous membrane (endometrium) suitable for implantation, and thereafter to contain the growing fetus until it is mature. It is composed mainly of unstriped muscle.

CERVIX

Its function is to provide an alkaline secretion favourable to sperm penetration, and once the uterus is gravid, to act as a sphincter. It is composed mainly of fibro-elastic tissue.

ISTHMUS UTERI This name is sometimes given to the upper few millimetres of the cervical canal below the internal os, an area to which the specific function of developing into the lower segment has been ascribed. The epithelium is intermediate between corpus and cervix; but if it were not for the importance of the lower segment in the modern theory of the physiology of pregnancy, it is unlikely that anatomists would have provided either an identity or a name for the isthmus uteri.

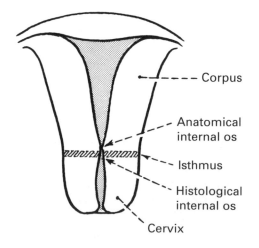

UTERUS

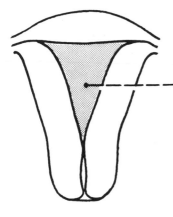

CAVITY of the CORPUS

The anterior and posterior walls are almost in contact but in coronal plane the cavity is triangular.

The muscle wall at each cornu is pierced by the very narrow interstitial portion of the fallopian tube.

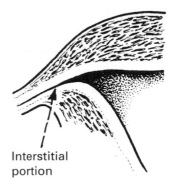

Interstitial portion

CERVIX

The external os is small before parturition and is sometimes called the os tincae (mouth of a small fish). After the birth of a child it becomes a transverse slit — 'the parous os'.

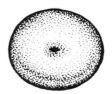

Nulliparous os

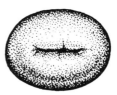

Parous os

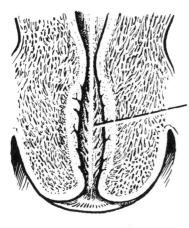

The cervical canal is fusiform and marked by curious folds called the 'arbor vitae'.

The cervix is divided into supra- and infravaginal portions by the attachments of the vagina. The infravaginal part is also called the 'portio vaginalis'.

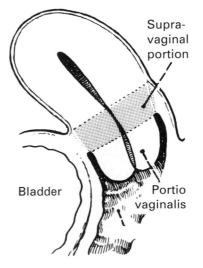

Supra-vaginal portion

Bladder

Portio vaginalis

UTERUS

RELATIONSHIP of UTERUS and URETER

The ureter is directly related to the uterine artery and the vaginal vault but is not in direct contact with the uterus.

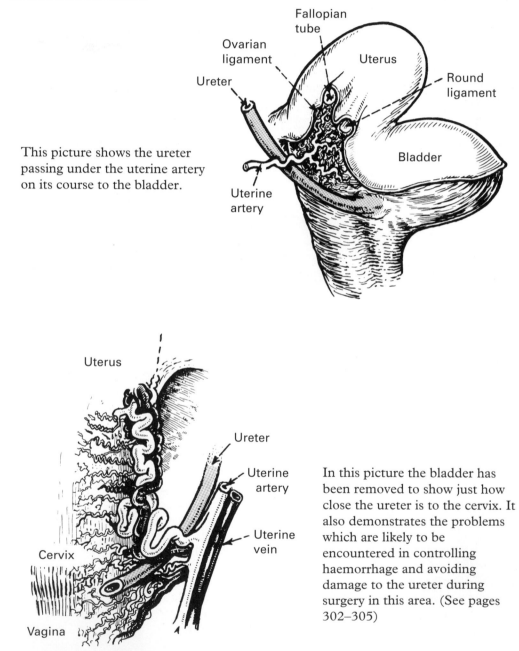

This picture shows the ureter passing under the uterine artery on its course to the bladder.

In this picture the bladder has been removed to show just how close the ureter is to the cervix. It also demonstrates the problems which are likely to be encountered in controlling haemorrhage and avoiding damage to the ureter during surgery in this area. (See pages 302–305)

UTERUS

LIGAMENTS of the UTERUS

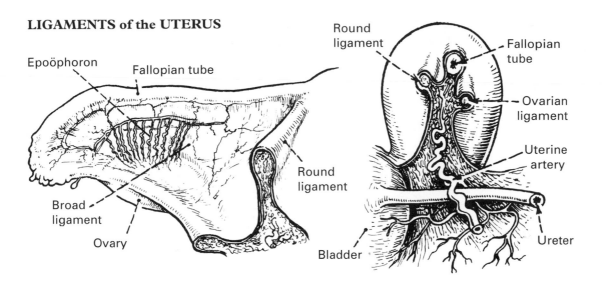

The **Broad ligament** is a fold of peritoneum passing from the uterus to the side wall of the pelvis. It contains the fallopian tube, the round and ovarian ligaments, the mesonephric remnants, the ovario-uterine anastomosis and, in its base, the ureter.

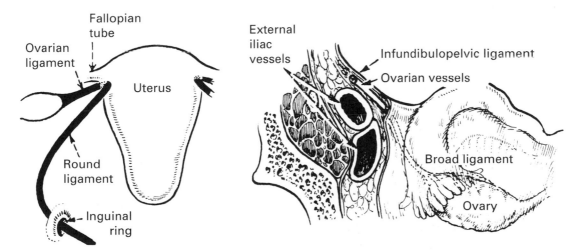

The ovarian and round ligaments are the vestigial gubernaculum. The round ligament ends in the inguinal canal and its fibres disperse in the labium majus.

The part of the broad ligament between the infundibulum and pelvic wall is called the infundibulopelvic ligament and contains the ovarian vessels and nerves. Note proximity of external iliac vessels.

UTERUS

LIGAMENTS of the UTERUS — (*contd*)

The main supports of the uterus are the fibromuscular condensations of tissue in the pelvic fascia (page 21).

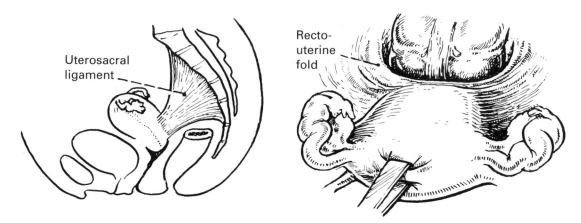

The **Uterosacral Ligaments** pass from the back of the uterus to the front of the sacrum and are easily identified by the covering recto-uterine fold of peritoneum. These ligaments maintain the anteverted position of the uterus, and they are accompanied by uterine vessels and nerves.

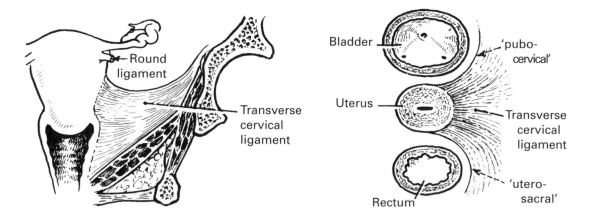

The **Transverse Cervical Ligaments** (Mackenrodt's, cardinal ligaments) pass from uterus and vagina to a wide insertion in the lateral pelvic wall. They lie below the broad ligament and contain vessels and nerves. The uterosacral ligament may be regarded as the posterior edge of the transverse cervical; its anterior edge is sometimes called the pubocervical but this is not well defined.

UTERUS

HISTOLOGY

The uterus has an incomplete peritoneal coat which is very adherent. The anterior bare area is to allow movement of the bladder. There is a complete fascial sheath continuous with the vagina and the body is made of smooth muscle interspersed with fibro-elastic tissue. There is a reversion of the ratio of muscle to connective tissue as the cervix is approached; and the cervix is nearly all fibrous.

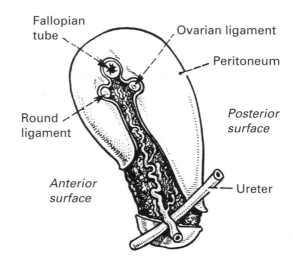

The epithelium of the cavity is called the endometrium and consists of a single layer of cuboid or columnar ciliated cells on a cellular stroma. The stroma is deeply pierced by invaginations of the epithelium called uterine glands which secrete a small amount of mucus to maintain moistness.

For cyclical changes in the endometrium see page 52.

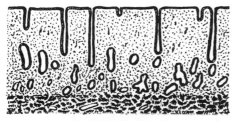

Endometrium (low power)

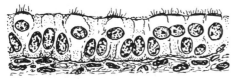

Uterine gland (high power)

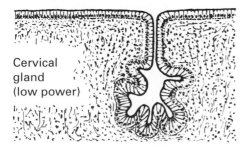

Cervical gland (low power)

The cervix is lined by a single layer of high columnar ciliated epithelium which covers the folds of the arbor vitae (page 27) and lines the cervical glands. The glands secrete an alkaline mucus which is favourable to the activity of spermatozoa.

FALLOPIAN TUBE

The tube extends from the cornu of the uterus into the peritoneal cavity and is about 10cm long. The two tubes are twice the width of the pelvis and they do more than just provide a passage for the ovum into the uterus. They must be sufficiently mobile to assist the ovum onwards by peristalsis; and sufficiently long to allow the ovum time for maturation after it has been fertilised in the ampulla and before it is ready for implantation in the uterus. The tube and ovary together are called the adnexa ('viscera adnexa' — organs next to) of the uterus.

Interstitial part

1 cm long and very narrow (less than 1 mm).

Isthmus

2 cm long, straight and cord-like. 1 mm diameter.

Ampulla

5 cm long, thin walled and convoluted.

Infundibulum

2 cm long. The terminal expansion, with fimbrial processes which help to attract the ovum.

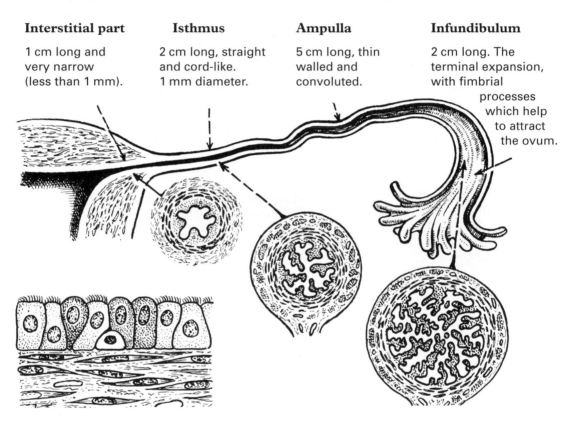

The tube has a lining of ciliated cells interspersed with non-ciliated secretory cells ('peg' cells). There is little or no submucosa. The epithelium is arranged in a complex pattern of plications which becomes more marked as the outer end is approached. (For cyclical changes see page 52.)

BROAD LIGAMENT

Blood Vessels

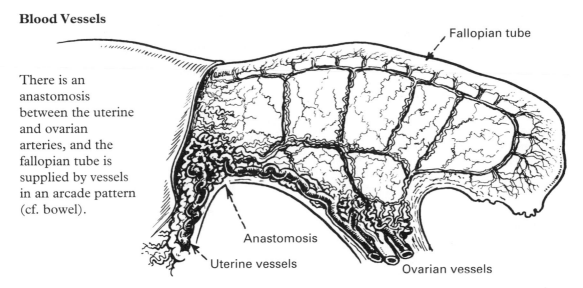

There is an anastomosis between the uterine and ovarian arteries, and the fallopian tube is supplied by vessels in an arcade pattern (cf. bowel).

Fallopian tube

Anastomosis

Uterine vessels

Ovarian vessels

Vestigial Structures

The epoophoron and the paroophoron are remnants of the mesonephros, and the duct (Gartner's duct) is the vestige of the mesonephric duct which passes into the uterine muscle about the level of the internal os and continues downwards in the vaginal wall.

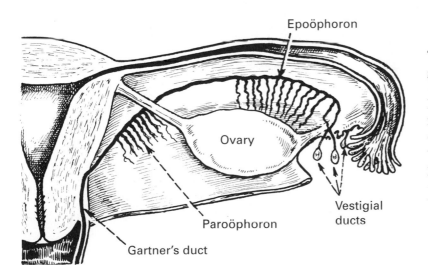

Epoöphoron

Ovary

Paroöphoron

Gartner's duct

Vestigial ducts

These structures may give rise to cysts (Hydatids of Morgagni, Kobelt's tubules, fimbrial cysts) whose embryonic derivation is uncertain. They are probably mesonephric and can be grouped together as 'vestigial cysts'.

OVARY

The ovary is about 3 cm long and 1.5 cm wide, roughly the size and shape of a date. It has its own mesentery, the mesovarium, from the posterior leaf of the broad ligament and is attached to the cornu of the uterus by the ovarian ligament which is continuous with the round ligament, the vestigial gubernaculum.

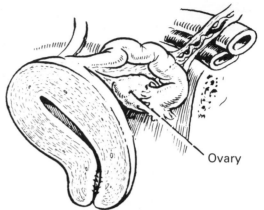

Ovary

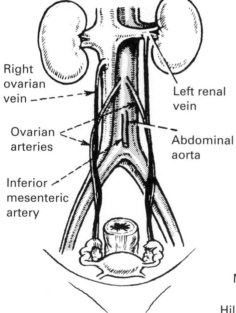

Right ovarian vein

Ovarian arteries

Inferior mesenteric artery

Left renal vein

Abdominal aorta

The ovary is developmentally an abdominal organ and its blood supply is from the abdominal aorta. The ovarian vessels lie in the infundibulopelvic ligaments.

Note: The left ovarian vein empties into the left renal vein.

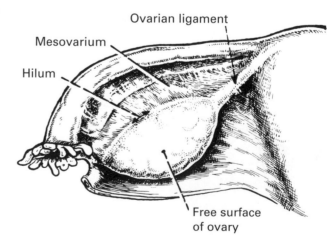

Ovarian ligament

Mesovarium

Hilum

Free surface of ovary

The free surface of the ovary has no peritoneal covering, only a surface epithelium. The part attached to the mesovarium through which all vessels and nerves pass, is called the hilum.

OVARY

HISTOLOGY

Cross-section shows the ovary to be roughly divided into a vascular medulla and a cortex.

The cortex is composed of a specialised ovarian stroma with a cuboidal surface epithelium which, like the tubal ostium, is intraperitoneal.

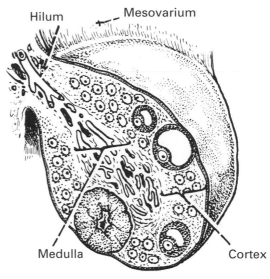

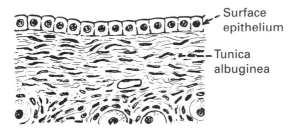

Note the condensed layer of stroma under the surface epithelium, called the tunica albuginea.

Ova are very numerous in the infant and child (at least over 100,000) but much less so in the adult.

The hilum is characterised by the presence of paroöphoron tubules which are of smooth muscle lined with ciliated epithelium; and by vestigial remnants of the sex cords called the rete ovarii, the analogue of the seminiferous tubules. These tissues are one reason for the extraordinary variety of ovarian tumours which can develop.

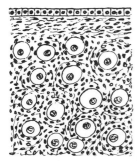

Cortex in an infant   Cortex in an adult

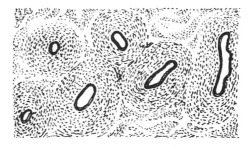

The hilum, showing cross-section of paroöphoron tubules.

OVARY

The **CORPUS LUTEUM** ('yellow body': carotene gives the mature corpus luteum a yellow colour.) During growth the Graafian follicle gradually approaches the surface of the ovary and eventually extrudes the ovum through the stigma, into the waiting fimbriae of the tube. The follicle cells then quickly become luteinised by the retention of fluid to form the corpus luteum whose function is to secrete progestins and prepare the endometrium for implantation of the fertilised ovum.

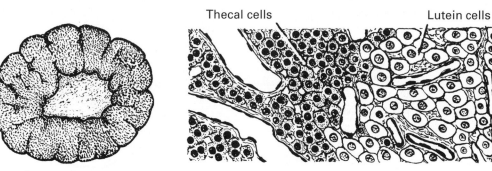

Thecal cells   Lutein cells

Corpus luteum (low power)   Corpus luteum (high power)

The growing corpus luteum is supplied with capillaries from the ovarian stromal vessels, and both theca and granulosa lutein cells secrete all the hormones — oestrogens, progestins (predominantly) and androgens.

Corpus albicans

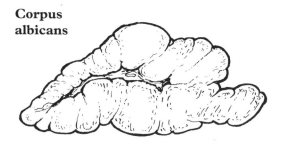

As the physiological cycle proceeds degeneration gradually occurs, and eventually the corpus luteum is hyalinised — a corpus albicans — and is absorbed in about a year. Consequent scarring accounts for the irregular surface of the ovary in the more mature woman.

Follicular atresia

More than half the oocytes present at birth are absorbed before puberty and all are gone at the menopause. Only about 400 can ever become mature follicles, but at each cycle and probably during childhood several follicles may start to develop and for a time produce hormones. This abortive attempt ends in atresia and the atretic follicle is absorbed; but the process may account for anovular cycles and for the oestrogens produced by young pre-pubertal girls whose breasts are beginning to develop.

CHANGES IN THE GENITAL TRACT WITH AGE

Apart from normal growth the appearances of the genital tract depend entirely on the supply of oestrogens.

The Vulva
This is only a cleft in the perineum before puberty. Then the labia minora become more prominent and the fat of the mons and the labia majora is increased. Apart from the effects of coitus and parturition (page 14) the most obvious sign of ageing is the gradual increase in size of the labia minora compared with the labia majora.

The Vagina
The rugae are absent before puberty and gradually (over several years) disappear after the menopause. In old women the vagina is thin, atrophic and completely smooth.

The Ovary
This is at its largest during the reproductive stage and shrinks thereafter. All the oocytes are gone by the time of the menopause and the cortex consists of fibrous tissue.

The Uterus

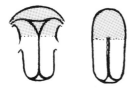

Infantile: the cervix is longer than the corpus and there is no flexion.

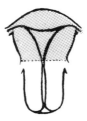

Pubertal: with the gradual increase in oestrogens the corpus grows in relation to the cervix.

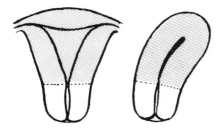

Adult: the corpus is now twice as long as the cervix and the normal degree of flexion has appeared.

After the menopause the uterus gradually atrophies and in an old woman the cavity may be less than 5cm and the cervix simply an aperture in the senile vaginal vault.

BLOOD SUPPLY OF THE PELVIS

The common iliac artery bifurcates at the level of the sacrovertebral junction into external and internal iliac arteries. The internal iliac runs for about 4cm and divides into an anterior and posterior trunk which are the main pelvic supply. The branches are subject to great variation.

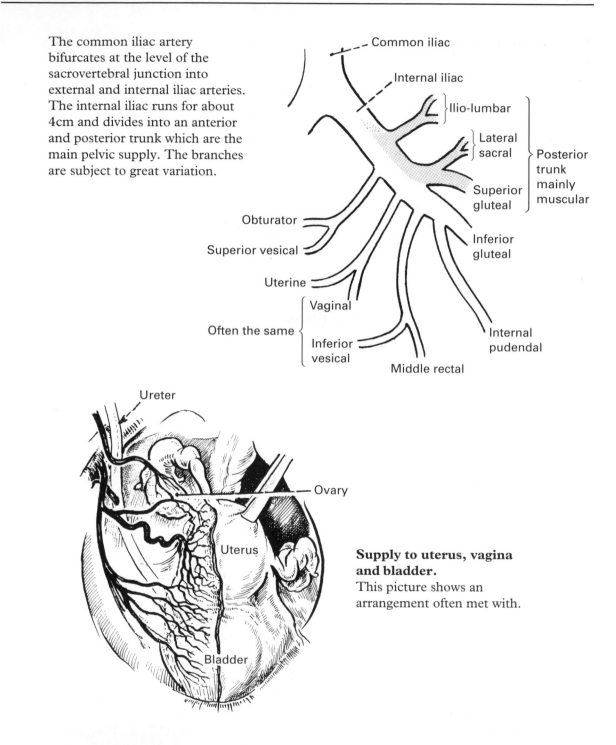

Supply to uterus, vagina and bladder.
This picture shows an arrangement often met with.

BLOOD SUPPLY OF THE PELVIS

The vessels of the uterus and vagina are much coiled to provide extra length during pregnancy. Note the nearness of the ureter.

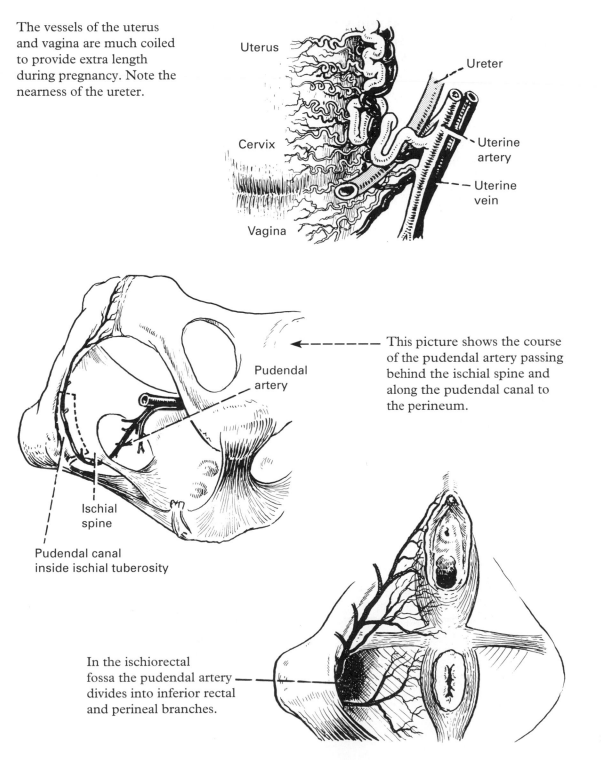

Uterus

Ureter

Cervix

Uterine artery

Uterine vein

Vagina

Pudendal artery

This picture shows the course of the pudendal artery passing behind the ischial spine and along the pudendal canal to the perineum.

Ischial spine

Pudendal canal inside ischial tuberosity

In the ischiorectal fossa the pudendal artery divides into inferior rectal and perineal branches.

BLOOD SUPPLY OF THE PELVIS

COLLATERAL BLOOD SUPPLY

If the internal iliac artery has to be ligated, the collateral circulation should be adequate. It depends on anastomoses with the abdominal aorta, external iliac and femoral arteries.

Abdominal aorta

1. Ovarian artery → uterine artery.

2. Inferior mesenteric → superior rectal → inferior rectal (pudendal).

3. Median sacral → lateral sacral.

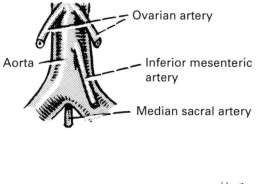

External iliac artery

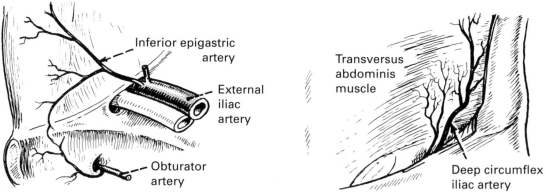

The inferior epigastric anastomoses with the obturator; the deep circumflex iliac with the iliolumbar and lumbar arteries.

The Femoral artery

The deep external pudendal anastomoses with the internal pudendal.

The superior and inferior gluteal arteries anastomose with the perforating and circumflex branches of the femoral and profunda femoris. (This is the 'cruciate' anastomosis.)

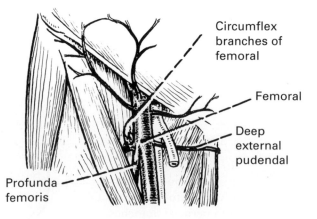

LYMPHATIC DRAINAGE OF THE GENITAL TRACT

The lymphatic plexuses accompany the blood vessels and drain into groups of glands which are constant in position and are given names.

It will be seen that while the uterus is likely to drain into the external iliac group on the lateral wall of the pelvis, the vagina drains into the internal iliac group and the ovary drains direct to the aortic glands.

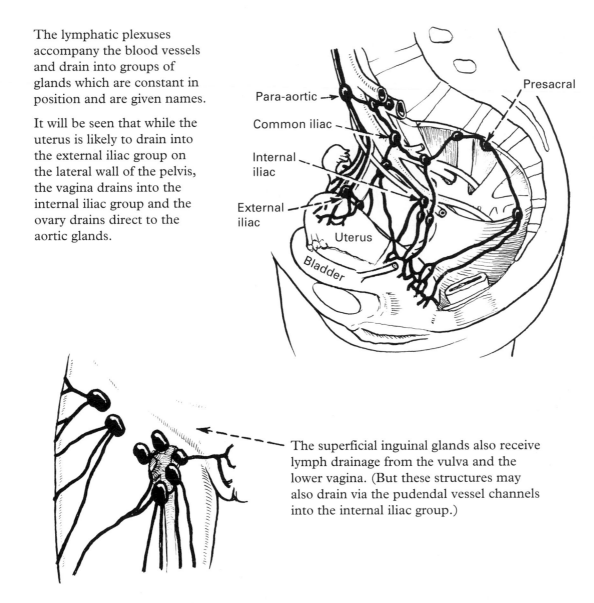

The superficial inguinal glands also receive lymph drainage from the vulva and the lower vagina. (But these structures may also drain via the pudendal vessel channels into the internal iliac group.)

Because lymphatic plexuses and glands are a path of metastatic spread of cancer, treatment either by irradiation or surgery must involve an attack on the area of lymphatic drainage of the organs concerned. The lymphatic network is so widespread and the metastatic paths are not always the same; and it is now recognised that the chance of cure is much reduced once the spread to the glands has occurred, whatever treatment is given.

NERVES OF THE PELVIS

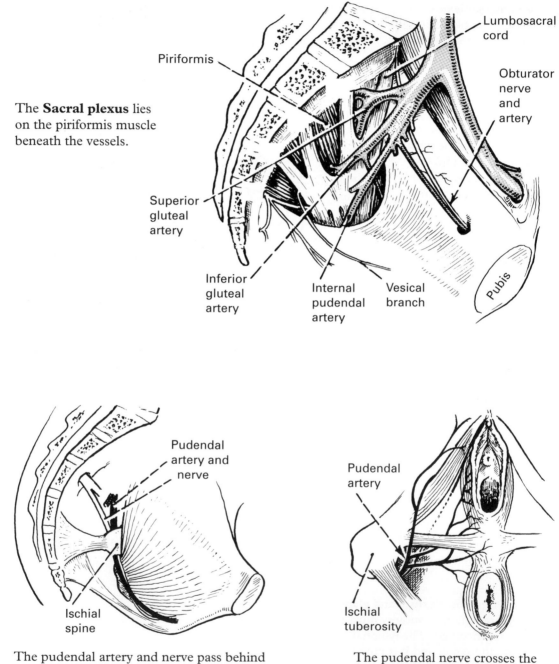

Piriformis

Lumbosacral cord

The **Sacral plexus** lies on the piriformis muscle beneath the vessels.

Obturator nerve and artery

Superior gluteal artery

Inferior gluteal artery

Internal pudendal artery

Vesical branch

Pubis

Pudendal artery and nerve

Ischial spine

The pudendal artery and nerve pass behind the ischial spine to gain the ischiorectal fossa.

Pudendal artery

Ischial tuberosity

The pudendal nerve crosses the ischiorectal fossa to supply the vulva and perineum.

AUTONOMIC NERVE SUPPLY OF THE PELVIS

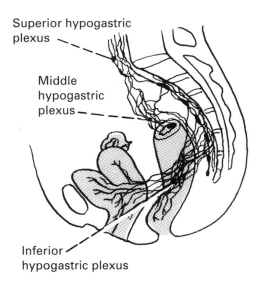

Superior hypogastric plexus

Middle hypogastric plexus

Inferior hypogastric plexus

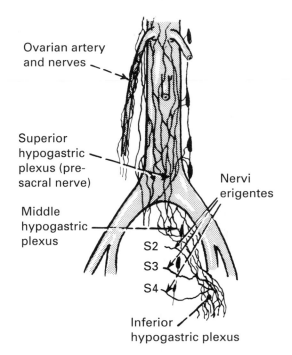

Ovarian artery and nerves

Superior hypogastric plexus (pre-sacral nerve)

Middle hypogastric plexus

Nervi erigentes

S2
S3
S4

Inferior hypogastric plexus

Sympathetic fibres enter via the lumbosacral chain and the mesenteric nerves. These are called the presacral nerve at the bifurcation of the aorta. They pass forward in the uterosacral ligaments to reach the viscera and are known there as the hypogastric plexus or plexus of Frankenhauser.

Parasympathetic nerves (nervi erigentes) join the hypogastric plexuses from sacral roots 2, 3, 4.

There is an additional sympathetic supply by the nerves accompanying the ovarian vessels.

Function of the autonomic nerves is not understood. In practice it is possible to cauterise the cervix causing only a sensation of heat. The cervix or vagina may be grasped by forceps in some subjects with only a momentary pricking sensation, and a sound in the uterine cavity causes a vague 'visceral' discomfort, yet cervical dilatation must be done under anaesthesia, and even then it has been known to cause a severe vasovagal collapse. The relief of pelvic pain by partial cordotomy has to be done well above the pelvis to be effective, and the level of choice is T.2.

CHAPTER 3

PHYSIOLOGY OF THE REPRODUCTIVE TRACT

OVULATION

FEMALE REPRODUCTIVE PHYSIOLOGY

The dominant process which appears to govern the physiology of the female genital organs during reproductive life is the cyclical growth and maturation of ovarian follicles.

The ovary is covered by a cuboidal 'germinal' epithelium which at the hilum is continuous with that lining the peritoneal cavity. This is supported by a thin layer of fibrous tissue, beneath which is the true cortex. The latter consists of a specialised stroma or parenchyma embedded in which are the primordial follicles.

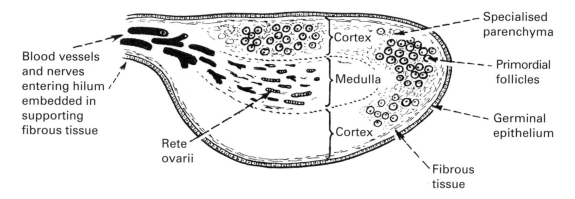

The primordial follicle consists of a primary oocyte surrounded by a single layer of flattened cells, the pre-granulosa, said to be derived from the cells of the sex cords.

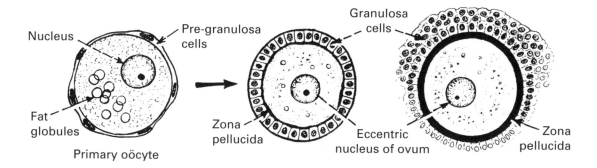

The pre-granulosa cells become cuboidal and proliferate to form a shell several layers thick. At this stage a hyaline membrane is formed immediately around the ovum — the zona pellucida.

OVULATION

The granulosa cells continue to proliferate until the follicle is approximately 200 µm in diameter. Fluid spaces now appear between the granulosa cells. They coalesce to form a cavity, the antrum, pushing the ovum to one side. The granulosa cells immediately surrounding the ovum are now known as the corona radiata and the whole mass of cells in this situation is termed the cumulus oophorus.

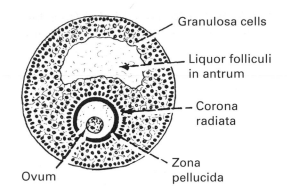

At the same time the surrounding parenchymal cells arrange themselves concentrically around the follicle and, opposite the site of the ovum, some become smaller and epithelial in appearance. As the follicle increases in size this epithelial change spreads to the parenchymal cells around the circumference of the follicle. This band of cells constitutes the theca interna. The cells are surrounded by sinusoidal capillaries thus making a structure like an endocrine gland. External to this band the parenchymal cells are also arranged concentrically but retain their fusiform shape.

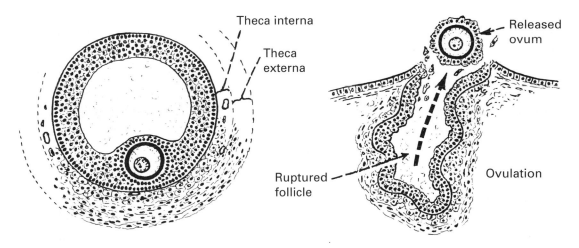

The follicle, which is called the Graafian follicle, continues to grow to a size of more than 1.0 cm. Approximately 4–5 follicles may attain this size and project on the surface of one ovary. One of these follicles ruptures on the surface, releasing the ovum surrounded by some of the granulosa cells. Ovulation is initiated by the gonadotrophin surge occurring in response to the long loop oestradiol positive feedback. Vascular changes occur in the follicle within minutes of the LH (luteinising hormone) surge, possibly due to release of histamine or other kinins. Proteolytic enzymes are released and collagen disintegrates. It is likely that insulin-like growth factors such as IGF-1 regulate granulosa differentiation. It is not known whether ovarian adrenergic nerve fibres or smooth muscle cells are involved. Prostaglandins may play a role.

OVULATION

From fetal life to the menopause follicular growth is continuous. Oestrogen initiates the process. Three phases can be distinguished:–

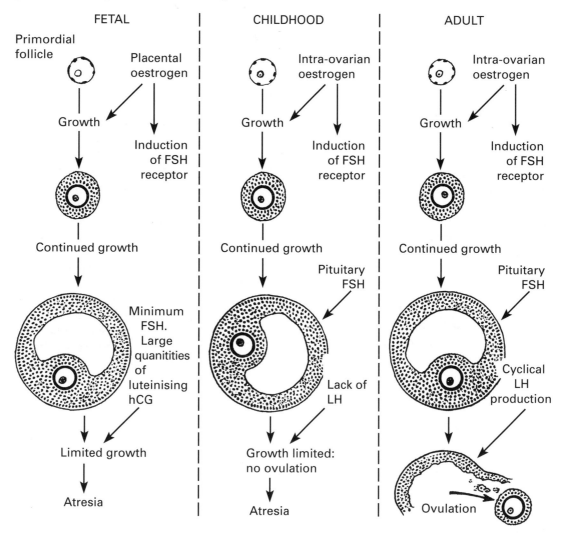

hCG = Human Chorionic Gonadotrophin.
FSH = Follicle Stimulating Hormone.
LH = Luteinising Hormone.

Normally only one follicle ovulates. Cohorts of follicles enter the growth phase in succession, thus follicles of various sizes are usually found. The follicle destined to ovulate is in a cohort stimulated to grow by FSH secreted by the pituitary during the last few days of the cycle.

There is continuous wastage of follicles from fetal life onwards and only about 400 of the original 2 million follicles will reach the ovulatory stage.

OVULATION

Ovulation is the final event in a step-wise stimulatory mechanism starting in the hypothalamus which contains gonadotrophin releasing cells. These produce a gonadotrophin releasing hormone (GnRH).

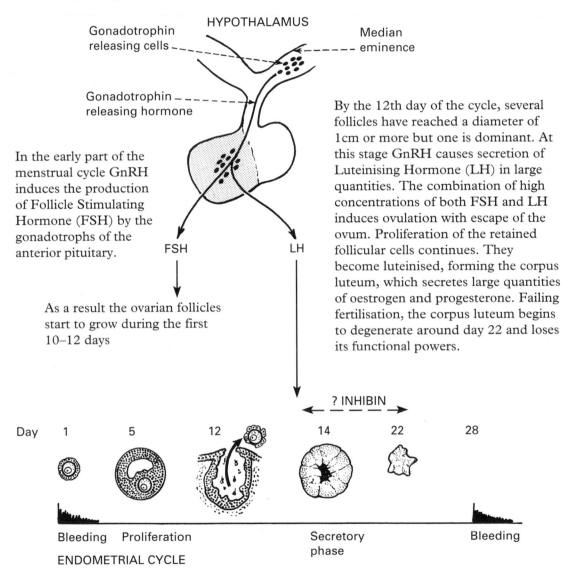

In the early part of the menstrual cycle GnRH induces the production of Follicle Stimulating Hormone (FSH) by the gonadotrophs of the anterior pituitary.

As a result the ovarian follicles start to grow during the first 10–12 days

By the 12th day of the cycle, several follicles have reached a diameter of 1cm or more but one is dominant. At this stage GnRH causes secretion of Luteinising Hormone (LH) in large quantities. The combination of high concentrations of both FSH and LH induces ovulation with escape of the ovum. Proliferation of the retained follicular cells continues. They become luteinised, forming the corpus luteum, which secretes large quantities of oestrogen and progesterone. Failing fertilisation, the corpus luteum begins to degenerate around day 22 and loses its functional powers.

GONADOTROPHIN RELEASING HORMONE (GnRH)

This substance begins to be secreted just before puberty in pulses every hour and continues in this fashion for the rest of life. There is only a single releasing hormone responsible for the production of both FSH and LH. The type of gonadotrophin secreted by the pituitary appears to be determined by other factors related to the phase of the menstrual cycle.

OVULATION

FSH

Inhibin, which inhibits the secretion of FSH, is produced by the corpus luteum while it is active. As a result follicular growth ceases. After the 22nd day, when the corpus luteum becomes inactive, FSH secretion and growth of follicles are resumed. Oestrogen levels begin to increase. A peak of FSH is reached by the 6th day of the succeeding menstrual cycle. At this point the rising oestrogen has a negative feedback effect and the FSH curve languishes for a day or two and then resumes its upward trend to achieve a second peak at the time of ovulation on day 12. Very low levels of LH are recorded in the early part of the cycle but a sudden surge, coinciding with the second peak of FSH induces ovulation and formation of the corpus luteum. Shortly thereafter the level of LH returns to pre-ovulatory values.

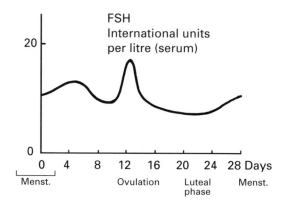

Gonadotrophin Secretion (International Units per Litre)

	Menstruation		Follicular phase		Ovulation		Luteal phase	
	Mean	Range	Mean	Range	Mean	Range	Mean	Range
FSH	10	3–13	8	3–15	20	4–32	5	2–0
LH	8	3–12	8	6–14	65	43–88	8	2–13

Control Mechanisms in Ovulation

Two forms of control operate during follicle maturation. These act in concert to produce the histological changes associated with ovulation. The first of these is indicated by a comparison of the blood concentrations of FSH and oestrogens. These show an inverse relationship. As stated above, after the 22nd day of one cycle FSH is rising and continues to do so until the 6th day of the succeeding cycle while the curve of oestrogen only shows a significant increase a day or two before this point. FSH then declines. This is due to the negative feedback effect of rising oestrogen. The upward curve of oestrogen indicating continuing follicular growth proceeds smoothly.

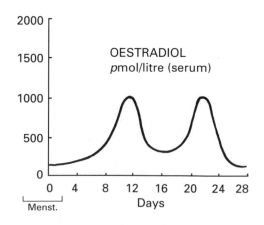

OVULATION

Control Mechanism (*contd*)

The apparent anomaly of increasing oestrogen in the face of FSH inhibition is related to the second system of control, which involves the dominant follicle about to ovulate. At each stage of gonadotrophin production and follicular growth specific proteins are formed which are involved in the transport and reception of the various hormones from the releasing hormone onward, e.g.:

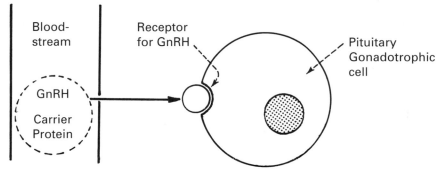

Having accepted GnRH the pituitary cell will then secrete the appropriate hormone. The same mechanism will then operate in regard to the carriage of the pituitary hormone and the reception by the ovarian follicle. The key to the continuing growth of the follicle and production of oestrogen is the amount of receptor protein in the follicular cell. The larger the follicle the greater the concentration of receptor protein and therefore the greater the amount of pituitary hormone the ovarian cell is able to accept and store. Thus although the blood FSH is temporarily reduced after the 6th day the larger follicles have accumulated sufficient FSH to maintain growth and oestrogen production.

As the blood concentration of oestrogen continues to increase it appears to reach a critical level at the 12th day, and in place of its usual negative feedback effect on the pituitary it suddenly exerts a positive feedback effect with consequent rise in FSH (the second peak) and secretion of LH.

Luteinising Hormone
LH is present throughout the menstrual cycle but, apart from a short period at ovulation, it remains at a low level. The rapid increase at ovulation coincides with the second peak of FSH secretion.

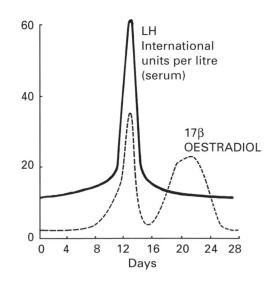

ENDOMETRIAL CYCLE

By the 5th day of the menstrual cycle the endometrium shows proliferation of its stroma and glands, the latter elongating. The cells lining the glands are cuboidal with definite limiting membranes and the stromal cells are thin and spindly — early proliferative phase.

In a week's time (12th day) the glands are very large and are now dilated — late proliferative phase. The blood vessels are also more prominent and capillaries are dilated.

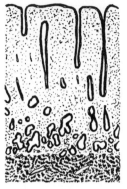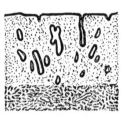

Early proliferative phase   Late proliferative phase

These proliferative changes are due to the influence of oestrogen secreted by the ovary at this time.

Following ovulation the corpus luteum produces large quantities of progesterone which induce secretory changes in the glands and swelling of the stromal cells. There is a rich blood supply and the capillaries become sinusoidal.

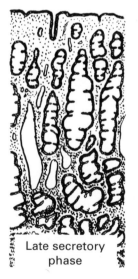

Late secretory phase

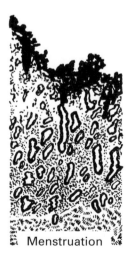

Menstruation

Towards the end of the 28-day cycle the stroma becomes even more vascular and oedematous, small haemorrhages and thrombi appear and the endometrium ultimately breaks down due to withdrawal of the hormonal support. Vessel necrosis is preceded by intense vasospasm possibly stimulated by prostaglandin F2-α.

The superficial layers of endometrium together with blood and leucocytes are shed and discharged — menstruation. Within a day or two the raw surface is healed over by epithelium proliferating from the basal portions of glands.

CYCLICAL OVARIAN HORMONAL CHANGES

OESTROGENS

The plasma values of the three main oestrogens, oestradiol, oestrone and oestriol, are almost parallel throughout the cycle. Oestrone and oestradiol show a ratio of 2:1 but oestriol output has no strict mathematical relationship to the others. The levels are low during menstruation and very gradually increase. Significant changes are noted around the 7th–8th day of the cycle, rising to a maximum around the 12th day — ovulation peak. A fall occurs 24 hours later followed by a further increase a week later — the maximum phase of corpus luteum activity.

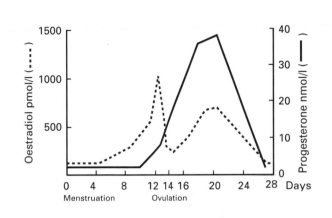

PROGESTERONE

Progesterone is almost absent from the plasma in the early stages of the menstrual cycle. At the time of ovulation there is a steep rise and a maximum value is achieved around the 20th–22nd day. Thereafter a steep fall occurs.

ACTION OF OVARIAN HORMONES

OESTROGEN

Oestrogens have multiple effects including stimulation of growth and development of secondary sex features in the female.

PROGESTERONE

This hormone prepares the endometrium for implantation of the fertilised ovum and has no homologue in the male. In a clinical sense, it has an anti-oestrogen action.

TARGET TISSUES

HYPOTHALAMUS
BREASTS
GENITAL TRACT

Tissues of these structures are particularly sensitive to oestrogen stimulation. The cytoplasm of their cells contains a specific oestrogen receptor molecule which has an affinity for oestrogen 100,000 times greater than the carrier protein which retains the hormone in the bloodstream. Oestrogen also acts at the cell membrane, regulating ligand-gated ion channels.

Progesterone receptors appear in the cytoplasm only after the cell has been primed by oestrogen.

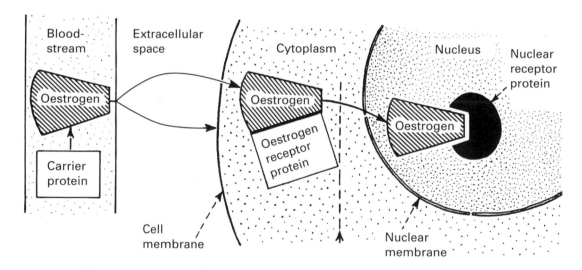

Transfer of the oestrogen molecule to the cell nucleus occurs more readily during the FSH phase of the cycle than during the LH phase, when progesterone levels are highest. The number of oestrogen receptors is reduced after the menopause, but they never disappear.

The steroids, being lipids, are transported by quite separate lipophilic proteins and the tissues stimulated by the steroids have their receptors in the cell cytoplasm instead of on the cell surface as in the preceding steps of the ovulatory process.

EFFECTS OF OVARIAN HORMONES

GENITAL TRACT

Oestrogen stimulates growth and vascularisation, while progesterone increases endometrial gland secretion. In the cervix, secretion is considerably increased by oestrogen (to produce a favourable medium for spermatozoa) while progesterone reduces this. In the vagina, oestrogen causes cornification of cells and enlargement of nuclei with increased deposits of glycogen.

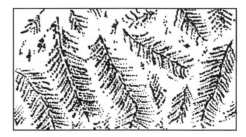

'Ferning' pattern in vaginal smear due to oestrogen stimulation.

BREAST

Oestrogen stimulates growth of the stroma, duct system and pigmentation, while cyclical progesterone stimulates growth of gland alveoli. Secondary sex characteristics are controlled by oestrogen.

HYPOTHALAMUS

The hypothalamic–pituitary axis mediates the effects of ovarian hormones and through FSH and LH controls the menstrual cycle.

CARDIOVASCULAR SYSTEM

Oestrogen relaxes smooth muscle of the vascular tree and causes vasodilatation, tending to improve circulation and prevent hypertension. Oestrogen and progesterone cause water and salt retention.

SKELETON

Oestrogen is an anti-resorptive agent which helps to retain calcium in the bones and at puberty produces the growth spurt and then closure of long bone epiphyses.

PSYCHOLOGICAL CHARACTERISTICS

Mood may fluctuate with the menstrual cycle. Some women experience adverse psychological and physical symptoms premenstrually, termed premenstrual syndrome (PMS) or premenstrual tension (PMT).

PUBERTY

Puberty is the period of rapid growth when the child develops the physical characteristics of the adult. In addition to growth in stature, enlargement and changes in function of internal organs occur. Sexual changes are the most obvious. The mechanisms are poorly understood but the main feature is an awakening of centres in the hypothalamus, with an increase in the pulsatile release of GnRH leading to secretion of gonadotrophins. The reason for the absence of pulsatile GnRH secretion in infancy is not known.

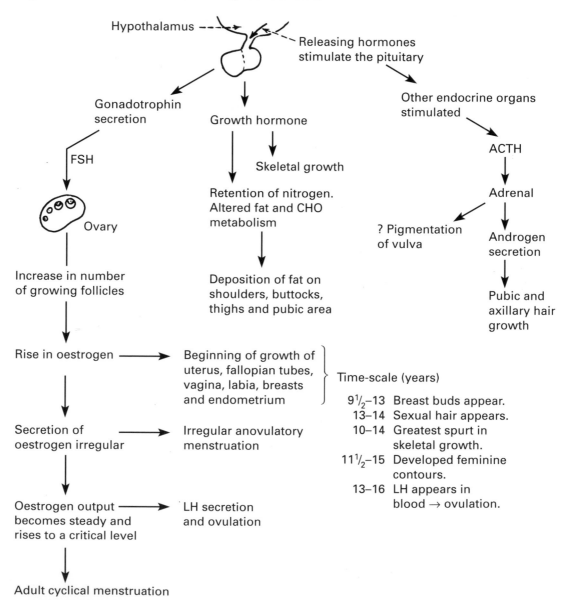

Hypothalamus

Releasing hormones stimulate the pituitary

Gonadotrophin secretion

Growth hormone

Other endocrine organs stimulated

ACTH

FSH

Skeletal growth

Ovary

Retention of nitrogen. Altered fat and CHO metabolism

Adrenal

? Pigmentation of vulva

Androgen secretion

Increase in number of growing follicles

Deposition of fat on shoulders, buttocks, thighs and pubic area

Pubic and axillary hair growth

Rise in oestrogen ⟶ Beginning of growth of uterus, fallopian tubes, vagina, labia, breasts and endometrium

Time-scale (years)

9½–13 Breast buds appear.
13–14 Sexual hair appears.
10–14 Greatest spurt in skeletal growth.
11½–15 Developed feminine contours.
13–16 LH appears in blood → ovulation.

Secretion of oestrogen irregular ⟶ Irregular anovulatory menstruation

Oestrogen output becomes steady and rises to a critical level ⟶ LH secretion and ovulation

Adult cyclical menstruation

THE MENOPAUSE

Menopause is the name given to the stage in life when the woman gradually loses her cyclical ovarian activity. In many ways it is a reversal of the changes occurring at puberty. It usually takes place between the ages of 47 and 52 and is termed premature if it occurs before 45.

Menstruation rarely ceases abruptly but tends to become somewhat irregular and less frequent over a year or a little longer. The cessation does not appear to be due to a complete disappearance of ovarian follicles. Primordial follicles have been found in the ovaries of old women. It would appear that there has to be a critical number of actively growing follicles before the menstrual cycle can operate.

For details of the patho-physiology and clinical features etc. of the menopause, see pages 411 et seq.

CHAPTER 4

GENETIC AND CONGENITAL ABNORMALITIES

MATURATION OF GERM CELLS

Before fertilisation of the ovum can occur there has to be a rearrangement of the genetic material within the nuclei of the germ cells of both male and female. In the female this occurs during fetal life but in the male it is delayed until puberty.

Every cell in the adult contains 46 chromosomes, two of which are of sex type, XX in the female, XY in the male.

Prior to fertilisation the chromosomes must be reduced from 46 to 23 in both ovum and sperm, and each will possess one sex chromosome. This reduction division process is termed MEIOSIS.

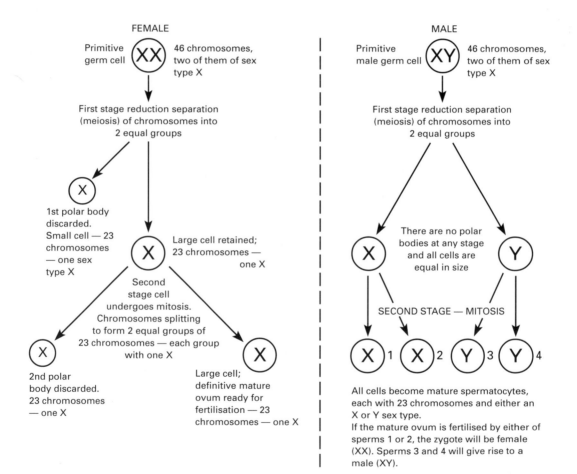

GENETIC ABNORMALITIES

Clinical syndromes

The clinical results of these chromosomal abnormalities are not quite as straightforward as one might expect. The X chromosome favours development of female characteristics but full development is only possible if there are two such chromosomes. Any alteration in this number leads to abnormalities. Development of the testis is entirely dependent on the presence of a Y chromosome. The testis, in addition to forming testosterone which aids the development of male characteristics, also produces a Müllerian inhibitory factor. In the absence of a testis the whole Müllerian tract will develop but curiously this does not depend on the presence of ovaries. These inter-relationships result in syndromes with variations in individual cases.

Investigations of genetic defects

In all cases it is important to obtain a family history as complete as possible. Siblings and relatives of patients frequently give a history of amenorrhoea and infertility.

Laboratory studies

Examination of cells, e.g. a buccal smear, from a normal female, stained suitably will show a small pyramidal mass of chromatin at the edge of the nuclear membrane. The cells are stated to be 'chromatin positive' and the mass of chromatin is called a 'Barr body'.

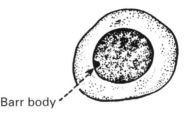

Barr body

The presence of such a chromatin mass indicates that the individual possesses two X chromosomes, but this is no guarantee that the patient is genetically normal. The sex chromosome pattern could well be XXY or some other variant. It merely indicates the presence of two X chromosomes. If the individual possesses more than two X chromosomes, e.g. XXX, there will be two Barr bodies, i.e. there is always one Barr body less than the number of X chromosomes.

Absence of the Barr body indicates that the patient has only one X chromosome. This is the situation in the normal male (XY) but if it is associated with some malformation of the genitalia the individual may be an incomplete female (XO).

Another cellular feature of females is to be found in polymorphonuclear leucocytes. These cells commonly have a small mass of chromatin projecting from the nucleus in the form of a drumstick.

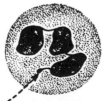

'Drumstick'

Chromosome analysis

While tests for Barr bodies can be useful, in many instances it may be necessary to establish the complete chromosome pattern. This is done by culturing cells from the patient, either lymphocytes separated from a blood sample or fibrocytes from a biopsy of fibrous tissue. The cells are grown in the presence of colchicine which terminates the mitotic process at the metaphase. The resulting chromosomes are separated, counted, arranged in their groups and studied.

GENETIC ABNORMALITIES

TURNER'S SYNDROME — Sex chromosome deletion (X)

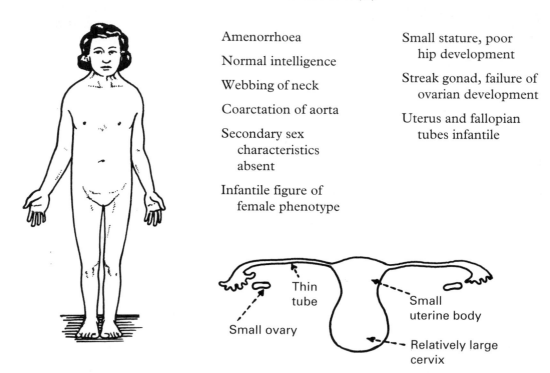

Amenorrhoea

Normal intelligence

Webbing of neck

Coarctation of aorta

Secondary sex characteristics absent

Infantile figure of female phenotype

Small stature, poor hip development

Streak gonad, failure of ovarian development

Uterus and fallopian tubes infantile

Thin tube

Small ovary

Small uterine body

Relatively large cervix

In 'typical' Turner's syndrome the chromosomal pattern is 45XO. Some patients may exhibit a few of the stigmata — so-called atypical cases, and in these subjects there is usually partial deletion of an X chromosome giving an Xx pattern. Mosaicism, e.g. XO/XX, may result in the appearance of some of the features of Turner's syndrome but the presence of cells with an XX configuration can be associated with perfectly formed ovaries and menstruation may occur.

In males some of the somatic stigmata of Turner's may appear. This may be due to partial deletion of the Y chromosome — Xy, or to mosaicism — XO/XY.

Treatment

It is essential that diagnosis should be established as early as possible. Blood should be sent for chromosome analysis in any female child of exceptionally small stature. At the age of 11 or 12 years, ethinyl oestradiol 0.025 to 0.05 mg should be given daily for 3 to 6 months to stimulate growth of uterus and breasts. Following this, oestrogen may be given daily with cyclical progestogen in the form of a standard sequential HRT preparation. This results in a 'menstrual' cycle. Occasionally it may be necessary to give anabolic steroids to help breast development.

GENETIC ABNORMALITIES

KLINEFELTER'S SYNDROME (Sex chromosome acquisition — X)

This clinical condition is associated with an increase in the number of X chromosomes. The pattern may be XXY, XXXY, XXXYY or XXXXXY. Despite the X chromosomes which cause the cells of the individual to be chromatin positive usually associated with female sex, the influence of the X chromosomes is nullified by the Y chromosome. Physically, the appearance is that of a male. At puberty, however, the testes fail to enlarge. Facial hair is scanty and pubic hair has a female distribution and there may be some breast development. There is infertility. Increase in the number of X chromosomes is associated with increasing mental retardation.

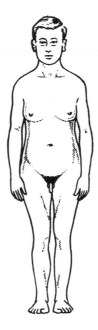

SUPER-FEMALE (Sex chromosome acquisition — X, sometimes at both stages of meiosis)

This is a term sometimes used when the subject possesses extra X chromosomes but no Y chromosome. The pattern may be XXX, XXXX or even XXXXX. Physically these individuals are normal females, but the important point is that there is usually some mental retardation and the degree of this increases with each extra X chromosome. Diagnosis is made by examination of a buccal smear, which will reveal multiple Barr bodies, the number being equal to the number of X chromosomes minus 1.

CONGENITAL ABNORMALITIES

TESTICULAR FEMINISATION (Total androgen insensitivity)

This is a condition which may be mistaken for a sex chromosome abnormality. It is due to the insensitivity of the fetal tissues to hormones. The chromosomal pattern is 46XY but although the individual possesses testes he is an apparent female. Androgens are secreted but tissues appear to be insensitive and develop along female lines. Usually the diagnosis is made in early adult life when the patient complains of amenorrhoea.

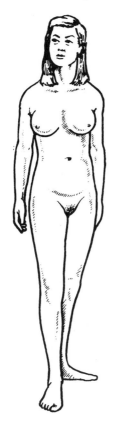

Female phenotype with tendency to eunuchoid proportions.

Normal or large breasts with small nipples.

Absent or scanty (sometimes normal) pubic hair.

Absent or scanty axillary hair.

Female external genitalia with blind vagina.

Absent or rudimentary internal genitalia.

Undescended testes anywhere along course of normal descent (20% become malignant in 4th decade).

Testes secrete oestrogens and androgens. Probably Leydig cells produce feminising hormones.

Hereditary from mother:
One quarter of female offspring are carriers.
One quarter of male offspring are feminised.
The remainder are normal.
Carriers may show scanty pubic and axillary hair and may have delayed menarche.

The almost complete absence of Müllerian structures would suggest that the testes are still producing the Müllerian inhibitory factor.

Until full growth is achieved no therapy should be attempted. When the epiphyses have fused the gonads should be excised. This is a precautionary measure in view of the increased incidence of tumours in such gonads. Following this treatment the patient is liable to have menopausal symptoms and should be given hormone replacement therapy, ideally combined continuous oestrogen/progestogen for symptom control and for skeletal and cardiovascular prophylaxis until age 50 years at least.

All of these foregoing syndromes, whether genetic or not, can pose social, psychological and sexual problems. The patient may have to make a great deal of mental adjustment and in such cases sensitive counselling will be required.

CONGENITAL ABNORMALITIES

A number of other developmental abnormalities of the female sex organs occasionally arise, some of which may suggest sex chromosome abnormalities. It is essential to diagnose these conditions as early as possible since treatment can often allow the infant to develop normally.

ADRENOGENITAL SYNDROME

Adrenal dysfunction due to congenital deficiency of the enzyme 21-hydroxylase. It should be detected and treated at birth.

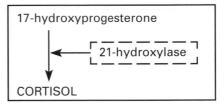

17-hydroxyprogesterone

21-hydroxylase

CORTISOL

1. Deficiency of 21-hydroxylase leads to low cortisol secretion.
2. Low cortisol leads to unopposed high ACTH secretion.
3. High ACTH secretion leads to adrenal hypertrophy.
4. Adrenal hypertrophy leads to high 17-hydroxyprogesterone secretion.
5. Since the pathway to cortisol is blocked the alternative pathway to androgen formation is taken.
6. The fetus and neonate show signs of virilism, and if the baby survives she will suffer from primary amenorrhoea.

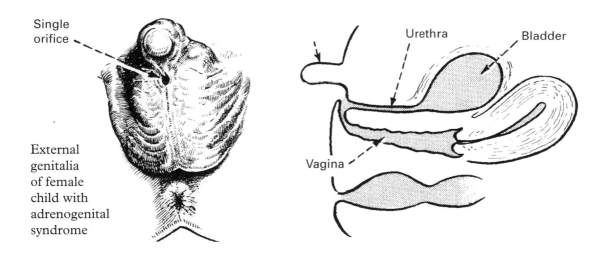

Single orifice

External genitalia of female child with adrenogenital syndrome

Urethra   Bladder

Vagina

Treatment

Chromosome analysis will reveal XX karyotype. Addisonian crisis may develop at any time and may be fatal. The diagnosis must be recognised as soon as possible and treatment given immediately with corticosteroids which will reverse the changes in the endocrine organs, reducing the ACTH level and ultimately the adrenal hypertrophy. Virilisation will regress. Prompt recognition and treatment will allow the infant to grow into a normal female. The abnormal genitalia should alert the attendant at the birth and help should be sought from a paediatrician.

ABNORMALITIES OF OVARY AND TUBE

Congenital abnormalities arise from:-

1. Incomplete development of the Müllerian ducts.
2. Imperfect development of the gonad.
3. Imperfect development of the cloacal region.
4. Sex chromosome abnormalities.

Many abnormalities in many combinations may be met with, but only those compatible with life and growth are of interest to the gynaecologist. Because of the close relationship between the genital and urinary tracts, intravenous pyelography should always be carried out when a genital abnormality is found.

ABNORMALITIES of the OVARY

1. Absence of one ovary may occur in an otherwise normal woman. Before operating on one ovary, always look at the other.

2. This is seen in cases of ovarian dysgenesis. In place of the ovary there is a strip of whitish connective tissue continuous with the ovarian ligament. It may contain vestiges of a rete, and occasional cells which may be of germ cell type, but no follicles. These 'streak' ovaries are sometimes the seat of tumour growth such as gonadoblastoma and dysgerminoma and should always be removed.

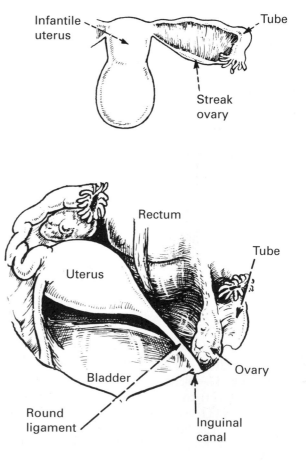

ABNORMALITIES of the FALLOPIAN TUBE

Absence is rare. The tube may be imperfectly developed.

This illustration shows a condition in which the proximal half of the left tube has failed to develop. The right adnexa are normal. All of these conditions are rare but their importance lies in their association with infertility.

ABNORMALITIES OF THE UTERUS

1. Absent or rudimentary uterus

The uterus consists of two nodules connected by a membrane ('ribbon' uterus). The other structures are normal. The patient may be asymptomatic apart from infertility. If a cavity exists in a nodule, cryptomenorrhoea and dysmenorrhoea may arise and retrograde flow lead to pelvic endometriosis.

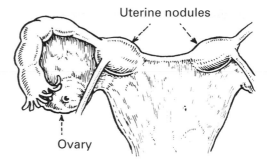

Uterine nodules

Ovary

2. Double uterus (Bicornuate uterus)

One or other variant of this condition is the commonest abnormality. It is due to failure of fusion of the Müllerian ducts, or failure of one to develop. Examples:

(a) Uterus Didelphys

Double uterus and cervix, usually with double vagina. Some writers call this 'pseudodidelphys' unless there is also a double vulva.

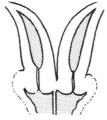

(b) Uterus Bicornis

Note the ligament which usually passes from rectum to bladder

(c) Uterus Bicornis Bicollis

Twocorpora withfused cervices.

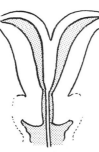

(d) Uterus with accessory horn

The accessory horn has no cervix. If it menstruates, cryptomenorrhoea will follow. Spermatozoa can reach the horn by crossing the peritoneal cavity.

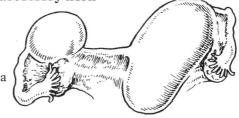

3. Uterus Unicornis

Oneduct hasfailed todevelop.

These abnormalities may be associated with infertility. If pregnancy occurs in 2(a), (b) and (c), the non-pregnant horn may continue to menstruate, simulating abortion. More frequently abortion does occur. In 2(d) cryptomenorrhoea may arise in the accessory horn. Endometriosis and dysmenorrhoea may follow due to retrograde flow.

ABNORMALITIES OF THE VAGINA

Gynatresia (Occlusion of the genital canal) may be due to complete absence of the vagina, or incomplete development, or the presence of a transverse septum producing the same effect as an imperforate hymen. There may also be a longitudinal septum producing a double vagina, usually in association with a double uterus. A few examples are shown.

a. Absence of the whole genital tract except for the lower one third of the vagina. Coitus is possible but there is no possibility of pregnancy.

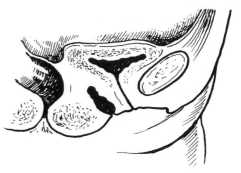

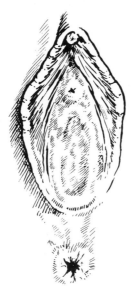

b. Complete absence of vagina. There is a slight depression over the hymen. Normal coitus is not possible.

c. Septate (double) vagina showing also two cervices.

Normal pregnancy and delivery are possible.

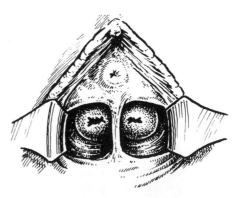

Vaginal abnormalities can occur alone, but are usually associated with abnormal internal genitalia, and inspection by laparoscopy or laparotomy with gonadal biopsy is called for. If the internal genitalia are relatively normal cryptomenorrhoea with dysmenorrhoea and possibly endometriosis will occur in (a) and (b).

ABNORMALITIES OF THE VULVA

1. Complete absence of the vulva has never been found in a liveborn child. Double vulva is exceedingly rare, but cases have been reported of complete duplication of the whole genital tract and bladder with normal function.

2. Ectopia Vesicae

This is an extreme defect seen in the newborn, but one which is susceptible to surgical treatment. There is failure of development of the symphysis pubis, mons, lower abdominal wall and anterior wall of bladder. The tissues exposed are the posterior wall of the bladder, the ureteric orifices and the floor of the urethra.

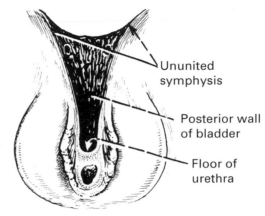

Ununited symphysis

Posterior wall of bladder

Floor of urethra

CONGENITAL ABNORMALITIES of CLOACAL ORIGIN

These are due to failure of the cloacal septum to divide the cloaca perfectly into hindgut and urogenital sinus. The less serious degrees may persist unnoticed in adults as some form of ectopic anus.

Patients with these abnormalities can defaecate through vestibule or vagina apparently without suffering from incontinence.

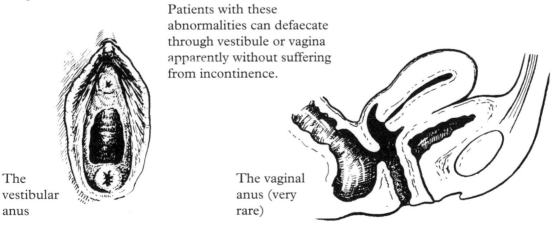

The vestibular anus

The vaginal anus (very rare)

In all of these vulval abnormalities infection is a problem - of the urinary tract in ectopia vesicae and of the genital tract in the other two.

GENITAL ABNORMALITIES

The results of these conditions as they relate to gynaecological practice have already been mentioned in the section dealing with amenorrhoea.

CHAPTER 5

EXAMINATION OF THE PATIENT

TAKING THE HISTORY

An accurate and complete history is most important. An inaccurate or incomplete history may lead to inappropriate investigation or treatment. Do not assume that a referral letter to a clinic is accurate or complete. Ask what the *main problem* is — it may be hidden away among a list of relatively unimportant or misleading complaints. Gynaecological patients may be shy or embarrassed and require . . .

. . . Privacy
The consultation should be held in a room with adequate facilities and privacy. Permission should be sought for the presence of a nurse or student. Ideally a chaperone should be present with both male and female doctors.

. . . Time
She should be allowed to tell her own story before any attempt is made to elicit specific symptoms.

. . . Sympathy
The doctor's manner must be one of interest and understanding.

Once a rapport is established, enquire about age, parity, menstrual history and past history with special reference to previous gynaecological treatment.

GYNAECOLOGICAL HISTORY
Previous gynaecological treatment is best learnt about from clinical records if obtainable. Patients' recollections may be incorrect or misleading.

Enquire about vaginal discharge (see page 138 et seq.).

GENERAL HISTORY
The gynaecologist should know if his patient has ever suffered from tuberculosis, cardiac or endocrine disease or psychiatric illness. Previous surgical procedures should be noted especially if they may make a gynaecological procedure more hazardous.

OBSTETRIC HISTORY
Record the number of pregnancies followed by the number of abortions e.g. 5^{+2}.

Note the year of each pregnancy, the type of delivery, any history of trauma, excessively long labour or any other complication.

Puerperal infection? This may be the origin of a chronic pelvic inflammation.

Infertility? If so, is it voluntary or involuntary? Methods of contraception should be asked about.

Abortions? The degree of haemorrhage should be established, and whether ultrasound or curettage was done. There is a tendency to attribute any irregular and unexpected bleeding to a 'very early miscarriage'. Distinguish between spontaneous and therapeutic abortion.

MENSTRUAL HISTORY

This can vary very much from patient to patient and still be within normal limits. Vague complaints are unlikely to be due to gynaecological disease.

Menarche

This is the age of onset of menstruation, normally between 10 and 16 years.

Rhythm of cycle and duration of flow

These are conveniently expressed together as a numerical fraction. Thus 5/28 means that the patient menstruates for 5 days every 28 days. The normal cycle lasts between 21 and 30 days and the bleeding lasts for between 3 and 9 days. Make sure that you are told the number of days of bleeding and the number of days from day one of a period to day one of the next. Ask if a menstrual diary is kept. Poor memory or irregular cycles may produce fractions such as 5–10/21–35.

Irregular bleeding

This can be caused by ovulation, hormonal fluctuation or organic disease, and the history is in fact often misleading.

Bleeding after intercourse (post-coital bleeding) and post-menopausal bleeding are always taken to suggest the possibility of malignant disease: yet the cause is more often benign.

Menopause

The cessation of menstruation.

It usually occurs between 48 and 53 years. Menorrhagia at this time is not normal. The patient should be asked about the extent of vasomotor disturbance ('hot flushes') and other symptoms and whether she is taking, or has taken, HRT.

Volume of blood loss

This can vary between 30 and 200ml. Blood should be liquid, but parous women may pass small clots. Large clots mean that the loss is abnormal and the fibrinolytic system cannot break down all the clot.

15g haemoglobin represents 50mg elemental iron, so a menstrual loss of 80ml would mean a loss of about 40mg iron. About a dozen internal tampons might be used for one menstruation. The patient's estimate of loss may be unreliable, especially if she uses phrases like 'torrential' or 'welling up'.

Menstrual molimina
(Lat: *molimen*, great exertion)

These are the secondary effects of the menstrual cycle. Some discomfort is normal, and there may be irritability, depression, breast discomfort, backache, pelvic pain. These symptoms should stop short of premenstrual tension and the pain should not be so severe as to keep the patient from undertaking her normal activities.

COMPLAINTS OF PAIN

PAIN

The patient is asked where pain is felt, and whether it is intermittent, related to menstruation or continuous. The 'ordinary' period pain is felt in the back, lower abdomen and down the thighs. It must be distinguished from other abdominal causes of pain such as appendicitis.

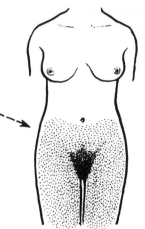

Areas of referred pain during menstruation

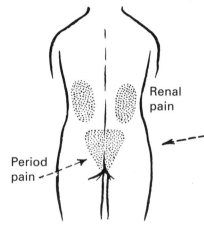

Renal pain

Period pain

The backache of period pain ('like a steel plate pressing inwards') is referred to the sacral area and should be distinguished from the loin pain of renal disease which can be exacerbated by the congestion of menstruation.

Pain associated with intercourse (dyspareunia) may not be mentioned spontaneously, and the doctor should ask if pain is caused or worsened by intercourse.

The severity of pain can be judged to some extent by its effect on the patient's behaviour. She should not have to go off her work for 'normal' dysmenorrhoea: if it is so severe as to cause fainting or nausea, tubal pregnancy must be considered. Torsion of an ovarian cyst produces intense, continuous pain.

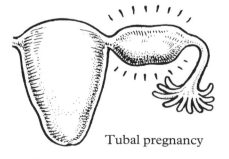

Tubal pregnancy

EXAMINATION OF THE BREASTS

A gynaecological examination provides a suitable opportunity for examining the breasts. Signs of pregnancy or lactation may be observed or a lump may be palpated. The breast is a much commoner site of cancer than the genital tract.

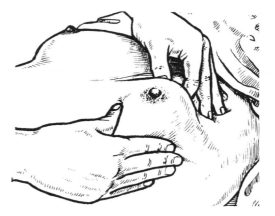

The examination should be made with the patient seated and also lying on her back. The breast is gently but thoroughly palpated with the fingers, and the axilla is also palpated.

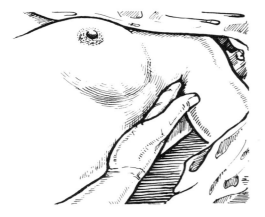

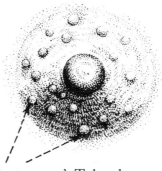

Montgomery's Tubercles, seen in early pregnancy.

Method of testing for colostrum or milk. The hands gently squeeze the whole breast. - - - ->

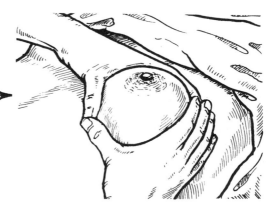

Routine X-ray mammography is offered by the NHS every 3 years between 50 and 65 years of age. In women with a first degree relative diagnosed with breast cancer before 50 years, mammography may be appropriate and referral to a breast cancer family history clinic is ideal.

ABDOMINAL EXAMINATION

This must never be omitted, whatever the patient's complaint. Many gynaecological tumours form large swellings which leave the pelvis altogether; and an undisclosed pregnancy may be present. Always examine the upper abdomen. Be certain that the bladder is empty. Instruct the patient to tell you if you are hurting her.

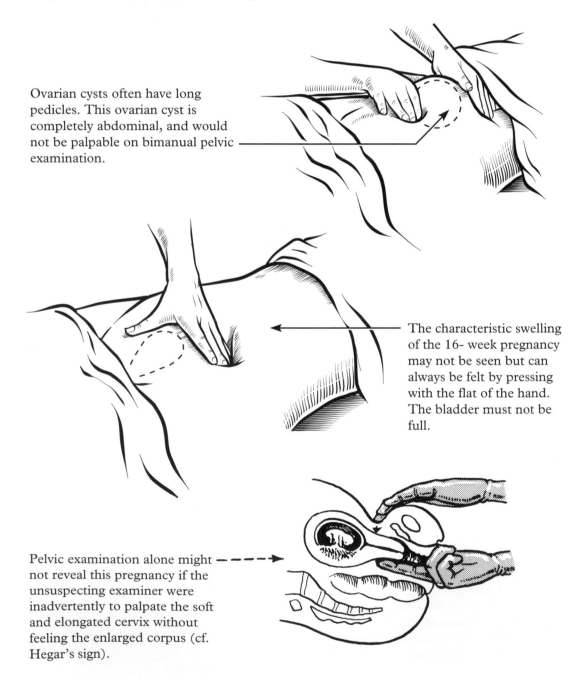

Ovarian cysts often have long pedicles. This ovarian cyst is completely abdominal, and would not be palpable on bimanual pelvic examination.

The characteristic swelling of the 16- week pregnancy may not be seen but can always be felt by pressing with the flat of the hand. The bladder must not be full.

Pelvic examination alone might not reveal this pregnancy if the unsuspecting examiner were inadvertently to palpate the soft and elongated cervix without feeling the enlarged corpus (cf. Hegar's sign).

ABDOMINAL EXAMINATION

All the classical techniques of inspection, palpation, percussion and auscultation (for a fetal heart) are advised, but the most important is gentle palpation with the flat of the hand to detect solid or semi-solid tumours.

The examiner must bear in mind the various intra-abdominal structures which may give rise to swellings.

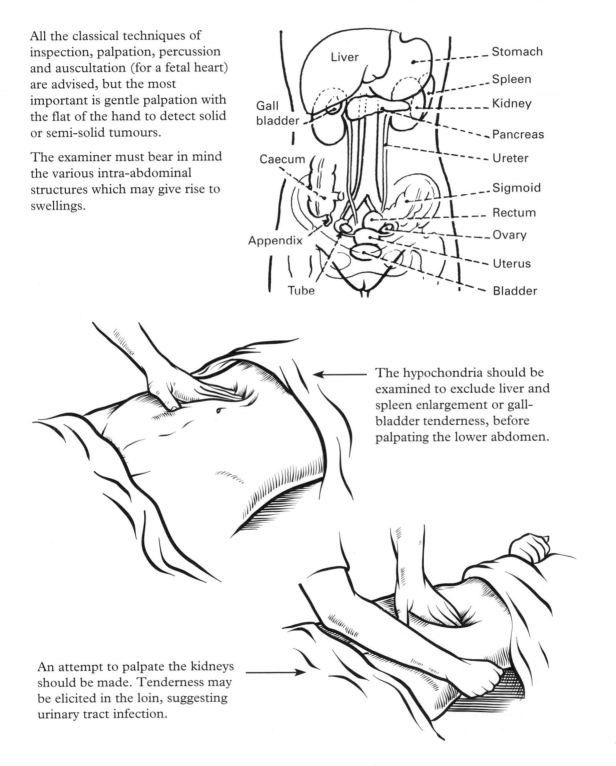

The hypochondria should be examined to exclude liver and spleen enlargement or gall-bladder tenderness, before palpating the lower abdomen.

An attempt to palpate the kidneys should be made. Tenderness may be elicited in the loin, suggesting urinary tract infection.

ABDOMINAL EXAMINATION

Inspection may show the characteristic shape of a large ovarian cyst. The outline is rounded and uniform, the skin is stretched and a fluid thrill may be elicited.

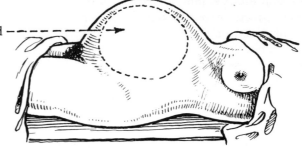

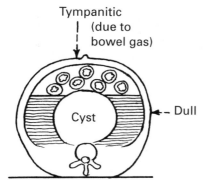

If ascites is present (and this means that the cyst is probably malignant) the outline tends to be cylindrical, with some flattening at the top. The umbilicus is everted and the percussion note is dull in the flanks but tympanitic above because of the upward floating of the intestines.

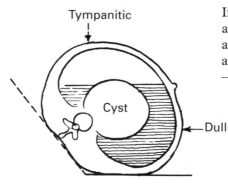

If the patient is turned on her side and the percussion is repeated after about 30 seconds the dull and tympanitic areas are reversed — 'shifting dullness'.

The very fat abdomen is not uncommon in gynaecology. Palpation is extremely difficult and examination under anaesthesia and more elaborate investigations will be necessary (ultrasonography, X-rays, laparoscopy if feasible). With an 'abdominal apron' of fat, the symphysis pubis may be mistaken for a hard lower abdominal mass on palpation.

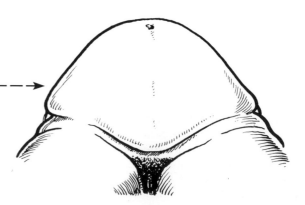

EXAMINATION OF THE VULVA

The dorsal position is most convenient for patient and doctor although some prefer the patient to be in the lateral position. During palpation, the condition of the labia, clitoris, anus and surrounding skin should be noted. Thus excoriation suggests irritant discharge and pruritus; purplish discoloration might be a sign of diabetes. Skin conditions, such as eczema, may occur on the vulva. Excessive use of lubricants on gloves should be avoided.

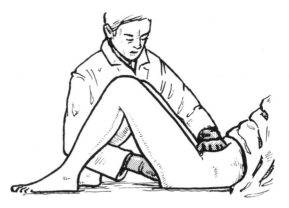

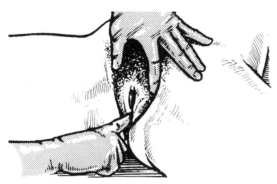

1. A single finger presses on the perineum, avoiding the sensitive vestibule, and accustoming the patient to the examiner's touch.

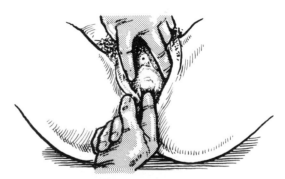

2. Urethral meatus and vestibule are exposed. Pressure from the finger will squeeze any pus from the peri-urethral glands.

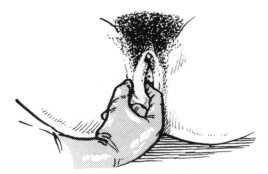

3. Bartholin's gland is palpated (on both sides). It is difficult to feel the normal gland.

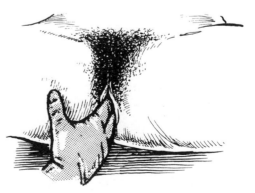

4. If there is room, a second finger is inserted and the perineal floor is palpated by stretching.

79

BIMANUAL PELVIC EXAMINATION

This technique needs practice. Formal consent is essential before examination of a patient by a student. The external hand is the more important and supplies more information. It is customary to use two fingers in the vagina, but an adequate outpatient examination may be made with only one finger. Very little information is gained if the patient finds the examination painful. In a virgin or a child only rectal examination should be carried out.

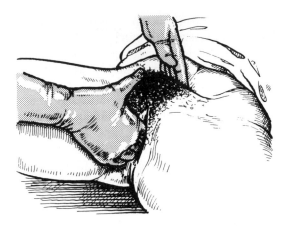

Pelvic models are available, with interchangeable uterine and adnexal components to simulate normal and pathological conditions, for practice examination.

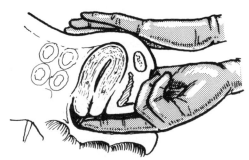

1. The cervix is palpated and any hardness or irregularity noted.

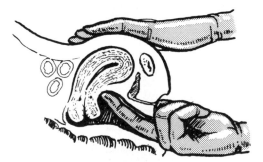

2. The whole uterus is identified, and size, shape, position, mobility and tenderness are noted.

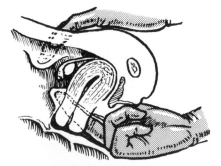

3. The lateral pelvis is palpated and any swelling noted. Normal adnexa are difficult to feel unless the ovary contains a corpus luteum.

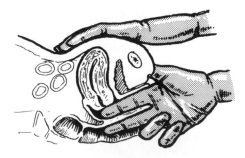

4. Sometimes rectovaginal examination is helpful, if the vagina admits only one finger or if the rectovaginal septum is to be examined.

SPECULUM EXAMINATION

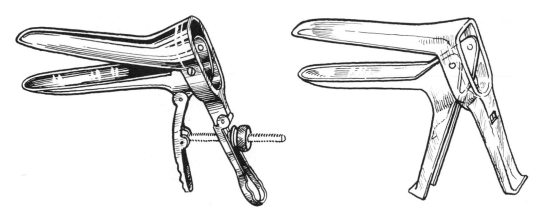

The bi-valve speculum is the most useful (Cusco's pattern is shown here). It is made either of steel or perspex (disposable) and is designed to open after insertion so that the cervix can be seen and a cytological smear or bacteriological swab taken as required. The steel speculum has a screw for maintaining it in the open position. Plastic specula are available with a ratchet device for the same purpose. Excessive amounts of lubricant should be avoided.

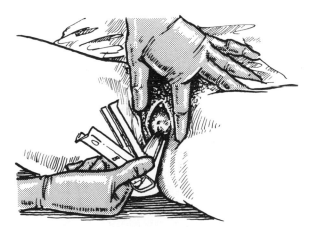

1. The speculum is applied to the vulva at an angle of 45 degrees from the vertical. This allows the easiest insertion.

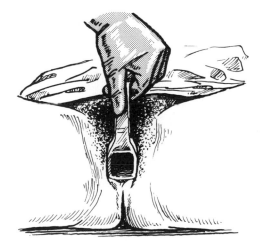

2. When fully inserted it is gently opened out and held in position with the cervix between the blades. A good light is needed for inspection.

SPECULUM EXAMINATION

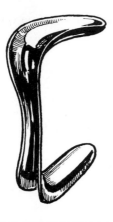

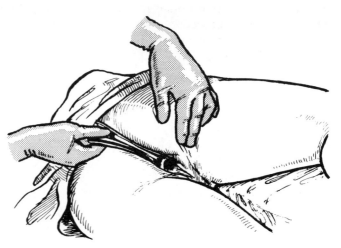

SIMS' SPECULUM (the duckbill speculum) is designed to hold back the posterior vaginal wall so that air enters the vagina, due to negative intra-abdominal pressure, and the anterior wall and cervix are exposed.

In this picture the patient is in Sims' position (semi-prone) which is useful if the anterior wall is to be studied (e.g. if fistula is suspected).

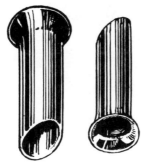

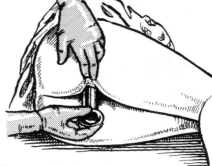

FERGUSON'S SPECULUM is essentially a metal tube and, although obsolescent, can prove useful in cases of marked vaginal prolapse when the bi-valve speculum cannot hold back the vaginal wall sufficiently to allow a view of the cervix. In this picture the patient is in the lateral position, which is sometimes used if the cervix cannot be seen in the dorsal position.

LAPAROSCOPY

Inspection of the pelvic organs through an endoscope passed through the abdominal wall. This is a common procedure, frequently performed in day surgery units, but it does carry risks which must be taken into account.

Technique
The patient is anaesthetised, the bladder emptied, the uterus sounded and often curetted and a cannula and forceps fixed to the cervix. This allows the uterus to be moved about once the endoscope is passed, and dye can be injected through the cannula to test the patency of the tubes.

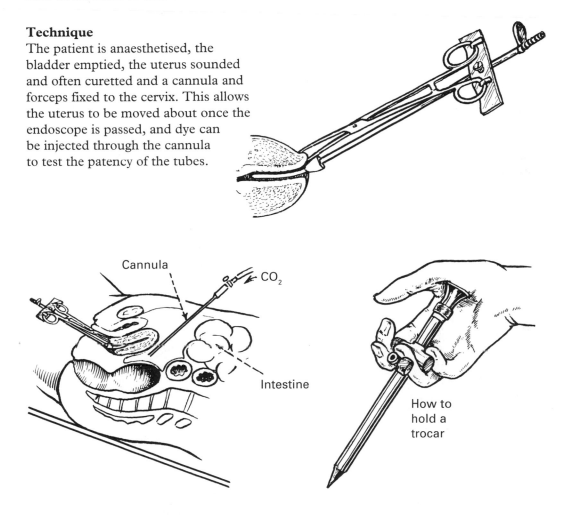

Cannula

CO_2

Intestine

How to hold a trocar

The table is tilted head down, to encourage the intestines to fall away from the pelvis and about 2 litres of CO_2 injected through a Verre's needle, or a disposable device with a safety indicator. A small incision is made through skin, fat and sometimes rectus sheath just below the umbilicus and a trocar and cannula large enough to accommodate the endoscope are forced through the abdominal wall which should by now be elevated away from the viscera. Many instruments for laparoscopy are now disposable and incorporate retractable safety features to help avoid perforation of viscera.

LAPAROSCOPY

The coldlight endoscope is passed through the cannula and the inspection made. An assistant or the operator himself can move the uterus about by means of the forceps on the cervix and a dilator or Spackman's cannula in the uterus. A camera attached to the eyepiece of the laparoscope permits assistants and observers to share the surgeon's view on a video screen and permits video recording of the findings or procedure.

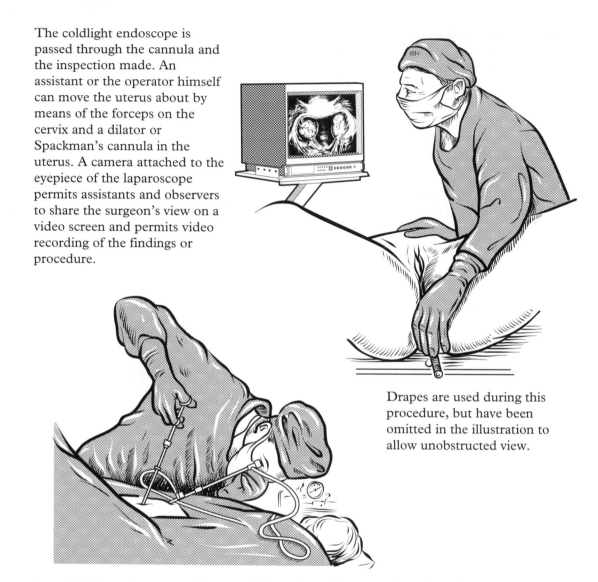

Drapes are used during this procedure, but have been omitted in the illustration to allow unobstructed view.

A special biopsy forceps can be passed through another cannula and used to lift up any tissue that may be obstructing the view or to take ovarian biopsies. Some adhesions may be divided using laparoscopy scissors. Many procedures are now performed entirely by laparoscopy or assisted by laparoscopy.

LAPAROSCOPY

Complications

1. Perforation of a viscus, especially bowel. An adequate amount of CO_2 must be instilled to raise the abdominal wall, and the table must be acutely tilted so that the bowel falls back from the pelvis.

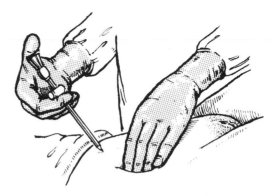

2. Haemorrhage from damage to vessels, or from a trocar puncture.

3. Infection is very rare and nearly always the result of unnoticed bowel damage. Complications are more frequent with operative laparoscopy than with purely diagnostic laparoscopy.

Indications

1. Diagnostic. Such conditions as salpingitis, early tubal pregnancy and ovarian pathology can be identified or excluded. Laparoscopy is particularly important in investigating complaints of vague abdominal pain.
2. Infertility investigation. Besides inspection, the patency of fallopian tubes can be demonstrated by observing the passage of dye injected through the cervix (hydrotubation). In specialised units the endosalpinx can be inspected by passing a fine endoscope along the tube (salpingoscopy).
3. Sterilisation. See page 290.
4. Other applications of laparoscopy include:
   Division of adhesions.
   Oophorectomy.
   Ovarian cystectomy (small).
   Salpingectomy and salpingostomy.
   Laparoscopically assisted vaginal hysterectomy.
   Colposuspension.
   Vaginal vault suspension for vault prolapse.

Special care required

1. Previous abdominal surgery. Bowel or omentum may be adherent to the scar or to pelvic structures.

2. Very obese subjects.

CHAPTER 6

ABNORMALITIES OF
MENSTRUATION

AMENORRHOEA

Normal menstrual cycles have a length of 21–35 days (mean 28 days). A normal period lasts for 3–7 days. Menstrual blood loss of 30–50 ml/month is normal. Menstrual blood loss is considered as excessive when it is greater than 80 ml/month.

Amenorrhoea is the absence of menstruation for six months in a woman who has previously menstruated normally (sometimes called 2^0 amenorrhoea)

or:

Amenorrhoea is the term given when a girl has failed to menstruate by the age of 16 (sometimes called 1^0 amenorrhoea).

In practice, the distinction between 1^0 and 2^0 amenorrhoea is not generally helpful in making a diagnosis. A similar process of investigation should be carried out whether or not the patient has previously menstruated. Amenorrhoea occurs in a number of physiological conditions, and these should be borne in mind when initiating investigation.

Menarche

Menarche is the onset of menstruation at puberty. The median age at which menarche occurs (13y) is relatively late in the events occurring around puberty. The growth spurt and secondary sexual characteristics such as breast development and the growth of pubic and axillary hair often precede the onset of menstruation.

It should be borne in mind that absent or late puberty may present with amenorrhoea. If a girl over the age of 14 presents with amenorrhoea, investigation may be delayed only if signs of puberty such as growth spurt or secondary sexual characteristics are present.

Pregnancy

During pregnancy, the levels of oestrogen and progesterone remain high, thus ensuring the integrity of the endometrium and therefore amenorrhoea. Initially, the corpus luteum is the source of oestrogen and progesterone. Later in pregnancy, the production of oestrogen and progesterone is taken over by the placenta. Pregnancy should be considered in the differential diagnosis of all women who present with amenorrhoea.

AMENORRHOEA

Lactation

Soon after delivery prolactin is secreted in large quantities by the anterior pituitary. There is partial suppression of LH production so that ovarian follicles may grow, but ovulation does not occur and amenorrhoea is the result. If the mother does not breast feed, menstruation will return in 2 to 3 months, but if she does breast feed the period of amenorrhoea will be prolonged.

Menopause

The menopause is the cessation of menstruation (mean age 51y) due to exhaustion of the supply of ovarian follicles. Oestrogen production therefore falls. This fall in oestrogen production is accompanied by a progressive rise in FSH levels which continues for a considerable time. In a proportion of women menstruation ceases abruptly, but in many the menstrual cycles alter. Frequently they become shorter initially but later they lengthen and tend to be irregular before ceasing entirely.

Causes of amenorrhoea

Amenorrhoea may be classified in a number of ways. One of the most helpful classifications is shown below:

1. Uterine causes
2. Ovarian causes
3. Pituitary causes
4. Hypothalamic causes

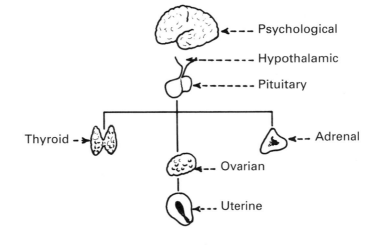

UTERINE DISORDERS

1. IMPERFORATE HYMEN OR TRANSVERSE VAGINAL SEPTUM

Usually presents with primary amenorrhoea. There is no visible bleeding although the usual cyclical molimina are present. In that there is no flow of blood the term amenorrhoea can be used, but the cause is an obstruction by a vaginal septum or an imperforate hymen rather than a functional abnormality.

Three degrees are recognised.

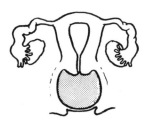 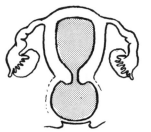 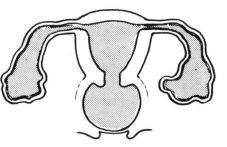

Haematocolpos. Only the vagina is distended by altered blood.

Haematometra. The uterus is also distended.

Haematosalpinx. In longstanding cases the tubes are also involved.

Clinical features
The patient is usually a girl of 17 or so, complaining of primary amenorrhoea and pelvic pain of increasing severity. In longstanding cases the pressure of the distended vagina may cause urinary retention. Pregnancy must be excluded.

Examination
A pelvic mass is palpated and may even be visible. The vaginal membrane or hymen is bulging.

Treatment
Incision and drainage. Very large amounts of inspissated blood may be released, and if the septum is particularly thick, some form of plastic operation may subsequently be required.

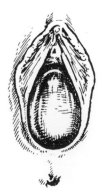 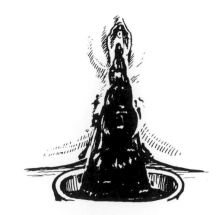

UTERINE DISORDERS

2. ASHERMAN'S SYNDROME

In Asherman's syndrome, the uterine cavity is obliterated by adhesions. The condition is usually caused by overzealous curettage, e.g. during termination of pregnancy. In developing countries, infections such as tuberculosis and schistosomiasis are commoner causes of Asherman's syndrome.

The adhesions should be broken down using a hysteroscope. High dose oestrogens are used to stimulate endometrial proliferation. Some authorities advocate the use of a Foley catheter placed in the uterus for a short time after adhesiolysis to prevent recurrence. Pregnancy rates following treatment are in the order of 80%. Such pregnancies are often complicated, e.g. by placenta accreta.

3. MULLERIAN AGENESIS

The Müllerian ducts fuse by the 10th week of gestation to form the fallopian tubes, uterus and upper portion of the vagina. Agenesis or lack of development of the Müllerian ducts (the Mayer-Rokitansky-Kuster-Hauser syndrome) leads to absence of these structures. Absence or hypoplasia of the vagina is a constant feature, but the uterine abnormalities vary. Provided there is a cavity lined by endometrium, menstruation can be normal.

The diagnosis of Müllerian agenesis is made in women with primary amenorrhoea, an absent vagina but normal female chromosomes. Ovarian function is normal. Müllerian agenesis is the second commonest cause of primary amenorrhoea after gonadal dysgenesis.

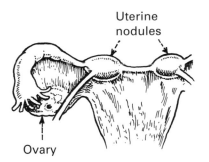

Uterine nodules

Ovary

4. TESTICULAR FEMINISATION SYNDROME

Testicular feminisation syndrome (androgen insensitivity) is the third commonest cause of primary amenorrhoea. The individual is phenotypically female, but chromosomally male (see p.64).

OVARIAN DISORDERS

Ovarian disorders

1. Gonadal dysgenesis
2. Premature ovarian failure
3. Resistant ovary syndrome
4. Disorders of ovulation such as polycystic ovarian syndrome
5. Hormone producing tumours such as granulosa cell tumours (oestrogen producing) or Leydig cell tumours (androgen producing)

1. GONADAL DYSGENESIS

Women with gonadal dysgenesis have abnormal ovarian development leading to absent or streak ovaries. The number of germ cells which migrated to the ovary during intrauterine life is reduced. These woman present with primary or secondary amenorrhoea, and have persistently elevated gonadotrophins on testing.

In women under 30 years of age at the time of presentation, a karyotype should be performed. Turner's syndrome (p.62) is the classic form of gonadal dysgenesis, but other karyotypes, including 46XX are also found. If a Y chromosome is present, consideration should be given to gonadectomy because of the risk of neoplasia.

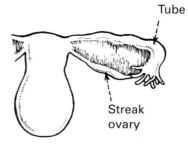

OVARIAN DISORDERS

2. PREMATURE OVARIAN FAILURE

In this condition, ovarian follicles are depleted from the ovary before the normal age of the menopause, and a premature menopause ensues. In addition to amenorrhoea, the patient may complain of menopausal symptoms such as hot flushes, loss of libido, etc. This condition is not uncommon: 1% of women will have ovarian failure by the age of 40. Premature ovarian failure is found in around 10% of women with amenorrhoea.

Cause

The majority of women with premature ovarian failure have no obvious cause for their condition. It is associated with chromosomal abnormalities such as Turner's syndrome (XO). It may occur in association with autoimmune disease, following infections such as mumps, or following chemotherapy or pelvic radiotherapy.

Diagnosis

The diagnosis is made by finding elevated serum FSH levels (> 20IU/L). Since FSH levels are elevated physiologically mid-cycle, at least two FSH levels should be obtained at six weekly intervals. If a high FSH level is followed two weeks later by menstruation, the cause of the elevated FSH is likely to be physiological rather than pathological.

Ovarian biopsy

Premature ovarian failure can only be distinguished from the resistant ovary syndrome by taking an ovarian biopsy. In practice, ovarian biopsy is usually not helpful: it may stimulate adhesion formation and the absence of follicles can only reliably be determined once the entire ovary has been examined.

Treatment

Women with premature ovarian failure should be advised that they are likely to be infertile, although spontaneous pregnancies have been reported. Pregnancy can be achieved by IVF with donor oocytes. Oestrogen replacement is essential to reduce the risk of osteoporosis and cardiovascular disease.

3. RESISTANT OVARY SYNDROME

In this condition, the ovarian follicles fail to develop, despite high circulating levels of gonadotrophins. The clinical and biochemical features are that of premature ovarian failure. An ovarian biopsy will reveal ovarian follicles, and thus distinguish the condition from premature ovarian failure. In practice this is not helpful (see above) and treatment is as for premature ovarian failure.

OVARIAN DISORDERS

4. POLYCYSTIC OVARIAN SYNDROME (PCOS)

Polycystic ovarian syndrome is a functional derangement of the hypothalamo-pituitary ovarian axis associated with anovulation. A relatively 'steady state' of gonadotrophins and sex steroids exists. In this steady state, LH levels are relatively high and FSH levels are relatively low, leading to an elevated LH:FSH ratio. Oestradiol levels are similar to those in the early follicular phase. In response to the elevated levels of LH, increased levels of testosterone, androstendione and DHA are secreted by the ovary. Some of these androgens are converted to oestrone in peripheral tissues. In response to high androgen levels, sex hormone binding globulin (SHBG) is reduced by about 50%, leading to an increase in the proportion of unbound, active, androgens. Hence, androgenic side effects are common, despite only a modest rise in serum total testosterone levels.

The syndrome is complex and other compartments become involved. The adrenal gland produces elevated levels of DHAS (dehydroepiandrosterone sulphate). Insulin resistance (resistance to insulin-stimulated glucose uptake) is also common.

Pathophysiology

The pathophysiology of polycystic ovarian syndrome is unknown. There is no defect in hypothalamic-pituitary-ovarian axis function. A genetic element to the disorder has been proposed and may account for the condition in a number of women.

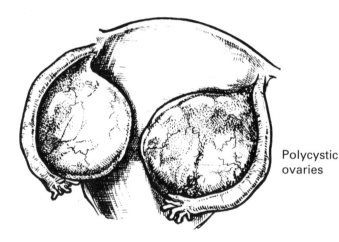

Polycystic ovaries

Clinical features

The clinical feature of PCOS are variable. In the classic 'Stein Leventhal' syndrome, described in 1935, the presenting features are oligomenorrhoea, hirsutism and obesity. Other manifestations are common however, and include:

      menstrual disorders ranging from amenorrhoea to menorrhagia
      signs of androgen excess such as hirsutism and acne
      infertility

OVARIAN DISORDERS

Polycystic ovarian syndrome (PCOS) *(cont.)*

Diagnosis

No specific features of polycystic ovarian syndrome are diagnostic of the condition. The diagnosis is normally made on clinical grounds, supported by some or all of the following:

1. *Ultrasound.*
   Ultrasound will show multiple follicular cysts up to 6–8 mm diameter within the ovary. The volume of the ovarian subcortical stroma is increased. Such findings on ultrasound support rather than confirm a diagnosis of PCOS, since 25% of normal women will demonstrate these features on ultrasound.

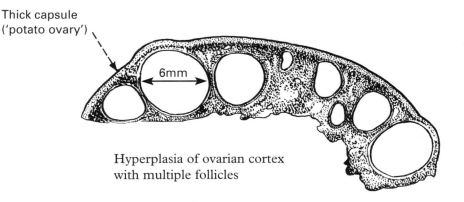

Thick capsule ('potato ovary')

6mm

Hyperplasia of ovarian cortex with multiple follicles

2. *Elevated LH:FSH ratio.*
   Again, an LH:FSH ratio of around 3:1 supports rather than confirms the diagnosis.

3. *Elevated free testosterone levels.*
   A modest increase in total testosterone is accompanied by an decrease in SHBG resulting in a doubling of free testosterone levels.

OVARIAN DISORDERS

Polycystic ovarian syndrome (PCOS) *(cont.)*

Long-term effects of PCOS

1. Women with PCOS who are anovulatory are at increased risk of endometrial cancer (×3), due to the high oestrogen and low progesterone levels.
2. The hyperinsulinaemia associated with insulin resistance leads to an increased risk of diabetes mellitus.
3. Women with PCOS who are obese and insulin resistant have an increased risk of hypertension and cardiovascular disease.

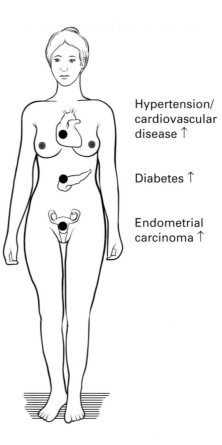

Hypertension/ cardiovascular disease ↑

Diabetes ↑

Endometrial carcinoma ↑

Treatment of PCOS

The treatment for PCOS is aimed at relieving symptoms and preventing adverse long term effects.

1. *Infertility.*
   Anovulatory women with infertility should be treated with clomiphene in the first instance. Women who fail to respond may require gonadotrophins ± GNRH analogues (see p.403).
2. *Amenorrhoea.*
   Women with amenorrhoea may be treated with the combined oral contraceptive pill if contraception is required, or cyclical gestogens (e.g. medroxyprogesterone acetate 10 mg daily from d15–25) if contraception is not required. The prevention of amenorrhoea is important in PCOS to reduce the risk of endometrial carcinoma.
3. *Hirsutism.*
   See p.106–108.

PITUITARY DISORDERS

PITUITARY DISORDERS
1. Hyperprolactinaemia
2. Pituitary adenoma
3. Craniopharyngioma
4. Other tumours such as meningioma
5. Pituitary necrosis (Sheehan's syndrome/Simmond's disease)

Pituitary tumours are normally benign. However, since they grow in a confined space, they may cause symptoms by compressing surrounding tissue and structures. Functioning pituitary tumours may exert effects because of the hormones they release. The commonest or these are prolactin secreting pituitary tumours, accounting for 50% of all pituitary adenomas.

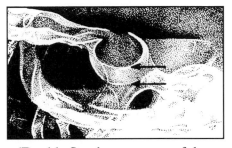

'Double floor' appearance of the pituitary fossa due to tumour

HYPERPROLACTINAEMIA
Prolactin is secreted from the anterior pituitary, and the normal blood level is between 150 and 400 mU/L depending on the laboratory. During pregnancy there is a tenfold increase in serum prolactin levels. 'Inappropriate' hyperprolactinaemia, occurring when the woman is non-pregnant, can cause amenorrhoea or galactorrhoea (inappropriate lactation) or both. Hyperlactinaemia is the principal cause of amenorrhoea in around 20% of women with this condition.

97

PITUITARY DISORDERS

Hyperprolactinaemia *(cont.)*

Aetiology

1. *Pituitary tumour*
   microadenoma < 10 mm diameter
   macroadenoma > 10 mm diameter

2. *Hypothyroidism*
   Thyroid function tests should be
   performed on all women with
   hyperprolactinaemia. In primary
   hypothyroidism, TRH is increased.
   Since TRH stimulates pituitary
   prolactin production,
   hyperprolactinaemia results.
   Treatment with L-thyroxine should
   restore prolactin levels to normal.

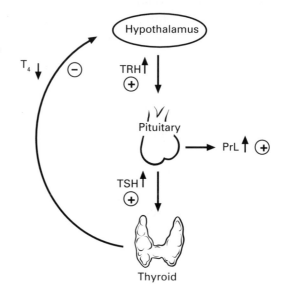

3. *Drugs*
   Drugs with dopamine agonistic activity cause hyperprolactinaemia by attenuating the
   inhibitory action of dopamine on pituitary prolactin production.

   Commonly used dopamine agonists
       Phenothiazines
       e.g. chlorpromazine
            thioridazine
            prochlorperazine
       Butyrephenones
       e.g. haloperidol
       Benzamides
       e.g. metoclopramide
       Cimetidine
       Methyldopa
   Other drugs which may cause hyperprolactinaemia
       tricyclic antidepressants
       monoamine oxidase inhibitors
       opiates★
       cocaine★
   ★especially during chronic abuse

4. *Idiopathic*

PITUITARY DISORDERS

Hyperprolactinaemia *(cont.)*

Diagnosis of hyperprolactinaemia

The diagnosis of hyperprolactinaemia can be made on a single serum measurement. In the presence of oligo- or amenorrhoea, a serum prolactin of 800 mU/L or greater is likely to be of pathological significance. In the absence of an obvious alternative cause, radiological examination such as computerised tomography (CT) scanning or magnetic resonance imaging (MRI) should be performed to exclude a pituitary tumour.

Mechanism of amenorrhoea

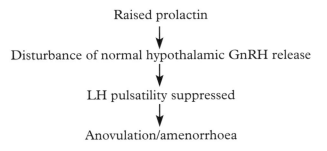

Raised prolactin

↓

Disturbance of normal hypothalamic GnRH release

↓

LH pulsatility suppressed

↓

Anovulation/amenorrhoea

Control of prolactin release

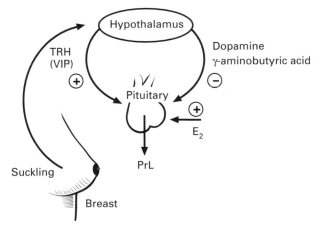

PITUITARY DISORDERS

Hyperprolactinaemia *(cont.)*

TREATMENT

Medication

1. *Bromocriptine*
    This is a semi-synthetic ergot alkaloid which directly opposes prolactin secretion probably by acting in the same manner as dopamine which is believed to be the hypothalamic prolactin-release-inhibiting factor (PRIF). [The serotonin antagonist, metergoline, has the same effect.] The dose is up to 2.5mg up to three times daily, taken with meals. Side effects include nausea and giddiness with fainting (syncope). Side effects may be minimised by commencing with a small dose (e.g. 1.25mg daily) and increasing gradually. Vaginal administration has been shown to reduce side effects.

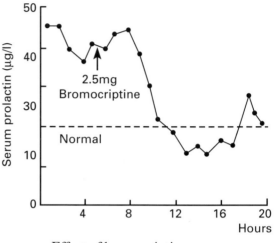

Effect of bromocriptine on serum prolactin. Duration 12–16 hours.

2. *Quinagolide*
    Quinagolide, a new dopamine agonist is given daily and may be tolerated better than bromocriptine.

3. *Cabergoline*
    Cabergoline is a new dopamine agonist with a long half-life. It is administered weekly.

Surgery

Transnasal

Trans-sphenoidal surgery can be used to resect both micro- and macroadenomas. The long term cure rate is around 50% for microadenomas, and less than 50% for macroadenomas. Symptoms of hypopituitarism, particularly diabetes insipidus, may be a long term consequence of surgery. The results of treatment vary greatly between centres. A knowledge of local data can be used to determine whether surgery or medical treatment is most appropriate for each patient.

Radiotherapy

Radiotherapy is rarely indicated as a first line treatment for hyperprolactinaemia and should be reserved for patients who fail to respond to medical therapy or surgery.

PITUITARY DISORDERS

PITUITARY ADENOMA

Pituitary adenomas secreting hormones other than prolactin may also affect menstrual function. An example is an ACTH secreting tumour (Cushing's disease). The increase in ACTH secretion leads to increased cortisol production and the clinical manifestations of the disease. Increased cortisol production (Cushing's syndrome) may also be caused by an adenoma or carcinoma of the adrenal cortex, or ectopic production of ACTH by other tumours such as bronchial carcinoma or carcinoid tumours.

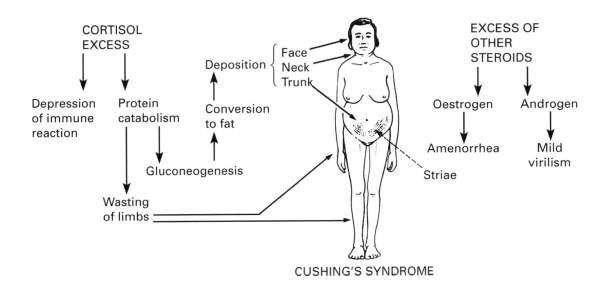

CUSHING'S SYNDROME

HYPOTHALAMIC DISORDERS

Disorders of the hypothalamus result in hypogonoadotrophic hypogonadism, and hence amenorrhoea.

Diagnosis

The diagnosis is made by exclusion. These patients have low gonadotrophins, normal prolactin levels, a normal pituitary gland on radiological evaluation, and they fail to bleed in response to progesterones.

The pathophysiology is dopaminergic inhibition of GnRH pulse frequency in response to increased concentration of endogenous opioids and dopamine. Since GnRH pulse frequency is attenuated, gonadotrophin production is reduced.

Causes

1. *Anorexia*

    This condition is thought to relate to the inability to cope with the onset of adult sexuality. It is most common in women between the ages of 10 and 30. The patient's weight is more than 15% below normal for her age and height.

    In moderate to severe disease it is important to treat the psychological cause of the condition and this is best done by referral to a psychiatrist. Treatment with hormone replacement therapy will relieve symptoms of oestrogen deprivation and initiate the resumption of menstrual periods.

2. *Exercise*

    Female athletes are commonly amenorrhoeic, and the mechanism is one of suppression of GnRH production. This condition is related to the much reduced body fat (although not necessarily body weight), stress and to exercise itself. Again, oestrogen replacement (with added cyclical gestogens) should be considered.

3. *Kallmann's syndrome*

    This is a rare condition of congenital hypogonadotrophic hypogonadism in association with anosmia. Secondary sexual characteristics are absent. Ovulation can be induced with gonadotrophins.

INVESTIGATION OF AMENORRHOEA

In most cases, the failure to menstruate is due to some abnormality in the control mechanism involving the hypothalamic-pituitary pathway. A careful history and physical examination is essential and may provide pointers to likely abnormalities.

The history should include:
> change in weight
> presence of galactorrhoea
> presence of hirsutes (excess body or facial hair)
> presence of stress
> questions about excessive exercise

A full physical examination should be performed. This should include:
> assessment of patient's BMI ([weight in kg^2/height in m)
> presence of galactorrhoea
> presence of hirsutes
> blood pressure
> urinalysis
> assessment of secondary sexual characteristics
> assessment of external genitalia
> pelvic examination to assess internal genitalia

In women who are virgo intacta, a pelvic examination should not be performed. If necessary, information about the presence of a uterus can be gained from ultrasound examination. However, inspection of external genitalia can still be performed and may reveal a condition such as cliteromegaly.

Investigation

The simplified scheme of investigation shown will identify which compartment is responsible for the amenorrhoea. In practice, estimation of serum prolactin and thyroid stimulating hormone (TSH) is performed concurrently with a progesterone challenge test.

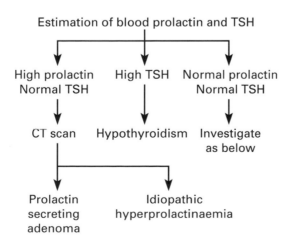

INVESTIGATION OF AMENORRHOEA

The progesterone challenge test involves giving a progesterone, e.g. medroxyprogesterone acetate 10 mg daily for 5 days. It is essential to exclude pregnancy first. If the woman bleeds after progesterone is withdrawn, this indicates firstly that a uterus is present, and secondly that there is some circulating oestrogen. If the progesterone challenge test is negative, it is appropriate to give oestrogen and progesterone, (e.g. 1.25 mg of conjugated oestrogens for 21 days, with the addition of a progesterone for the last 5 days). Failure to bleed in response to this treatment confirms a uterine problem.

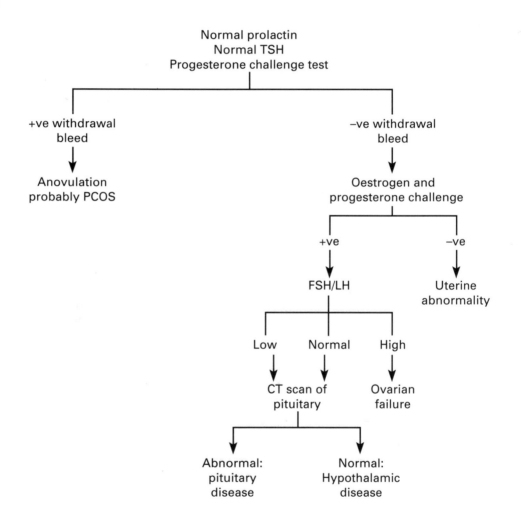

INVESTIGATION OF AMENORRHOEA

If the results of these tests are inconclusive it suggests that the cause lies between the pituitary and ovaries and further laboratory exploration must be undertaken, e.g.

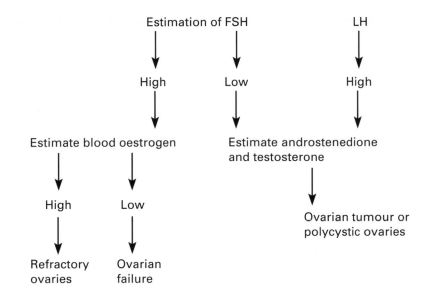

HIRSUTISM

HIRSUTISM in the female means an excessive production of hair with a tendency to male distribution. 'Excessive' is defined as beyond social acceptability or causing embarrassment to the patient.

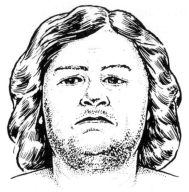

Normal pattern Hair is of two types-

- (i) fine downy, vellus hair which is non-pigmented.
- (ii) coarser pigmented terminal hair as in the axilla and pubis.

About one-third of women have some visible pigmented hair on the upper lip, and 5% have it on the chin and sides of the face.

Aetiology
1. Rise in secretion of free androgens.
2. Reduction in sex hormone binding globulin (SHBG).

SHBG level falls when testosterone production increases, and probably also in the case of drug-induced hirsutism.

Physiology of testosterone
The three principal androgens are dihydrotestosterone, testosterone, and androstenedione which is the least potent but is converted to dihydrotestosterone in the follicle cells.

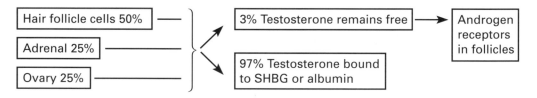

Causes:

1. Idiopathic hirsutism
By far the commonest, it has no apparent androgen increase, and is probably due to increased local testosterone production at the target organ.

2. Polycystic ovary disease
There is usually slight testosterone increase.

3. Androgen producing tumours
These may arise in the ovary or adrenal glands. They should be considered if serum testosterone is greater than 5 nmol/L or if the history is of sudden onset.

4. Congenital adrenal hyperplasia
This is an adrenal disease, caused by an enzyme defect (commonly 21-hydroxylase deficiency) resulting in elevated androgens. 17-hydroxyprogesterone is elevated.

5. Drugs such as:-
phenytoin (Epanutin) ⎫
diazoxide (Eudemine) ⎬ epilepsy
minoxidil (Loniten) ⎭ hypertension

androgen-containing compounds

HIRSUTISM

Investigation

serum testosterone
serum dehydroepiandrosterone sulphate (DHAS)
(elevated in adrenal disease)
17-hydroxyprogesterone (17-OHP)
(elevated in congenital adrenal hyperplasia)

24h urinary free cortisol if Cushing's syndrome is suspected

LOCAL TREATMENT

Ferriman Galwey charts
These charts provide a semi-objective scoring system for hirsutism. If they are completed at each patient visit, the change in symptoms may be assessed.

Shaving
This method has to be repeated frequently.

Electrolysis
Decomposition of the hair follicle by the passage of an electric current. Low galvanic current is used through a fine electrode. The hair is electrolysed after about 10 seconds and plucked out painlessly.

Diathermy
The follicle is coagulated instantly and the hair pulled out.

Electrical destruction of individual hairs is permanent but prolonged treatment is tedious and expensive and may cause scarring.

Depilatory creams
These are alkaline solutions which dissolve the hairs and allow them to be wiped away. They will injure the skin if left on too long.

Depilatory waxes
The wax is melted and spread on to the skin. When it sets it is pulled off, plucking the hairs with it. This is painful and leaves the skin tender and reddened.

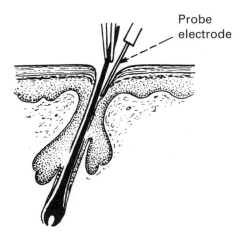

Probe electrode

HIRSUTISM

Drug treatment

1. *Low dose oral contraceptives*
   These drugs act firstly by suppressing LH production and thereby attenuating ovarian androgen synthesis. Secondly, the oestrogens stimulate SHBG production by the liver.

2. *Medroxyprogesterone acetate*
   Medroxyprogesterone acetate 30 mg daily acts by suppressing LH production and by increasing androgen clearance from the circulation.

3. *Cyproterone acetate*
   Cyproterone is a progesterone which inhibits LH production. It also binds to the androgen receptor and therefore acts as an antiandrogen. Two methods of administration of cyproterone acetate are used:
   (i) 50–100 mg cyproterone acetate daily from day 5–14, with 30–50 micrograms of ethinylestradiol on days 5–25 (the 'reverse sequential' regimen)
   (ii) 2 mg cyproterone acetate and 35 micrograms of ethinyloestradiol (the contraceptive pill 'Dianette')

   In practice, both regimens are probably equally efficacious in the treatment of hirsutism.

4. *Dexamethasone*
   Dexamethasone inhibits adrenal androgen production, and is useful in adrenal disease.

5. *GnRH analogues with addback HRT*
   This treatment is expensive, but has been shown to be effective in clinical trials.

   The following drugs may be effective in the treatment of hirsutism, but there is insufficient experience to recommend their use at present.

6. *Flutamide*
   Flutamide is a non-steroidal antiandrogen.

7. *Finasteride*
   Finasteride is 5α reductase inhibitor, and therefore inhibits the conversion of testosterone to dihydrotestosterone.

NB. With all of the above, it may be 3 months or more before an improvement in symptoms can be expected. The patient should be counselled about this.

VIRILISATION

Masculinisation and virilisation are terms for extreme androgen effects.

Clinical features

The symptoms and signs include:
> male pattern balding
> cliteromegaly
> deepening of the voice
> increased muscle mass
> male body habitus

- Alopecia
- Growth of moustache and beard
- Changes in larynx causing deepening of voice
- Flattened breasts
- Hirsutes of chest
- Hair on abdomen
- Enlargement of clitoris

Investigation

Investigation is as for the hirsute patient. An androgen secreting tumour of the ovary or adrenal gland is likely. Ultrasound, CT scanning and laparoscopy may be useful in making the diagnosis.

ABNORMAL MENSTRUAL BLEEDING

Abnormal menstrual bleeding is one of the commonest reasons why women in the Western world consult a gynaecologist.

Causes of abnormal bleeding patterns

Some of the causes of abnormal menstrual bleeding are illustrated below. Clearly, the age of the patient has a major influence on the likely cause of bleeding, e.g. endometrial carcinoma is uncommon in women under 35 years of age, and, similarly, endometriosis is uncommon in post-menopausal women.

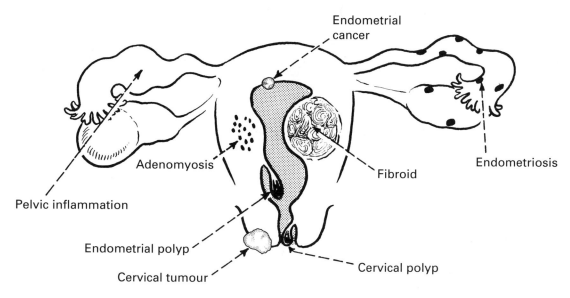

Other causes of abnormal bleeding include vaginitis, prolapse, cervicitis and cervical ectopy and urethral caruncle. In many cases of abnormal uterine bleeding no organic pathology will be found, and the condition is then called 'dysfunctional uterine bleeding'.

DYSFUNCTIONAL UTERINE BLEEDING

Dysfunctional uterine bleeding is one of the commonest causes of excessive menstrual bleeding in women of reproductive age.

Dysfunctional uterine bleeding is the term applied to cases of excessive bleeding where no organic lesion can be found. Presumably the cause lies in an abnormal function of the ovarian and endometrial control mechanisms associated with the menstrual cycle. The diagnosis of dysfunctional uterine bleeding should only be made after a thorough history is taken from the patient, and a careful examination, including pelvic examination, is made. If indicated, further investigations such as hysteroscopy or pelvic ultrasound should be performed to exclude organic disease.

Clinical features

The patient will complain of heavy and/or irregular bleeding.

Estimation of blood loss

1. *Subjective methods*
    The subjective estimation of menstrual blood loss is notoriously unreliable. What is normal to one woman may be regarded as abnormal by another. The simplest method of determining excessive menstrual loss is to ask the patient about the number of sanitary pads and/or tampons used daily. The use of pictures to indicate the amount of staining on each pad/tampon may improve accuracy. The passage of clots may also indicate excessive menstrual loss.

2. *Objective methods*
    Haemoglobin measurements will indicate if the patient is anaemic. An estimation of serum ferritin may show a depletion in iron stores. Whilst the detection of anaemia has important clinical implications, many women with a good diet are able to maintain normal haemoglobin levels despite excessive menstrual loss.

    The optimum method of assessing menstrual blood flow accurately is to ask the patient to collect her used pads and tampons over the course of one menstrual period. These can then be soaked in sodium hydroxide, and the optical density compared to a known standard. This technique is generally only available as a research tool, but reveals that many women who complain of menorrhagia have a menstrual loss within the normal range.

DYSFUNCTIONAL UTERINE BLEEDING

INVESTIGATION OF THE ENDOMETRIUM
If endometrial carcinoma is suspected, it can only be reliably excluded by one of the following methods.

Out-patient procedures

Hysteroscopy
Hysteroscopy is a technique used to visualise the endometrium under magnification. Abnormal areas of the endometrium can be seen, and a targeted biopsy taken. The procedure may be performed under local (cervical) anaesthesia as an outpatient if a sufficiently narrow hysteroscope and gaseous distension media are available.

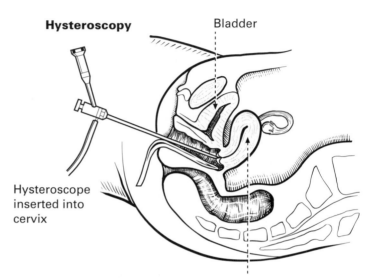

Hysteroscopy

Bladder

Hysteroscope inserted into cervix

Uterus

Pipelle de Cornier
The Pipelle is inserted into the uterine cavity and the plunger withdrawn to produce a vacuum. The endometrium is thereby sucked into the tube and subsequently expelled into fixative. This procedure is better tolerated than the Vabra curette but does not always produce sufficient tissue to evaluate histologically.

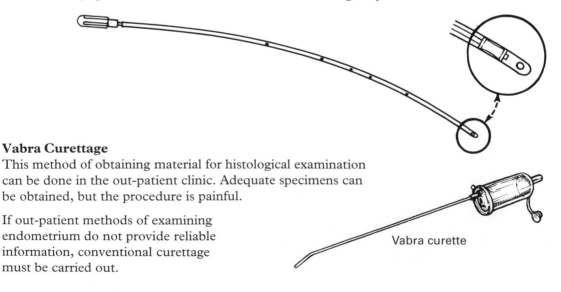

Vabra Curettage
This method of obtaining material for histological examination can be done in the out-patient clinic. Adequate specimens can be obtained, but the procedure is painful.

If out-patient methods of examining endometrium do not provide reliable information, conventional curettage must be carried out.

Vabra curette

DILATATION AND CURETTAGE

Prior to the introduction of hysteroscopy, D&C (dilatation and curettage) was the commonest method of obtaining endometrial tissue for examination and of excluding intra-uterine pathology. It is often necessary to dilate the cervical canal in order to pass the curette. This procedure is normally performed under general anaesthesia as an in-patient.

Technique
The dilator must be held firmly in one hand and pressed into the canal against traction in the opposite direction exerted by the other hand. Resistance must be overcome slowly, and the dilator must not be passed farther than the length of the uterine cavity measured by the sound.

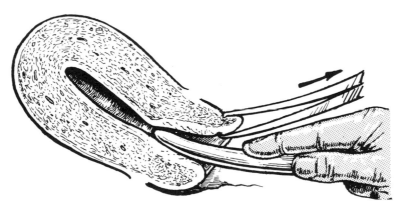

Curettage
Dilatation of the cervix is followed by curettage of the endometrium. The endometrium can then be examined histologically. Curettage is largely a diagnostic tool in the management of dysfunctional uterine bleeding, but in the uncommon situation in which pathology such as an endometrial polyp is present, it may be therapeutic.

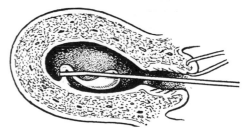

COMPLICATIONS OF DILATATION AND CURETTAGE

1. **Trauma to cervix**
   The volsellum forceps may tear the anterior lip of cervix if pulled on too forcibly.

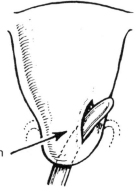

The cervix splits at about 8mm dilatation

The next dilatation enlarges the false passage

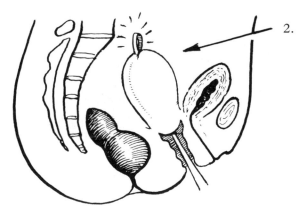

2. **Perforation of the uterus or cervix**
   This is not an uncommon occurrence and usually no ill-effects result. The usual site is the mid-line of the fundus and it becomes evident when the curette passes farther than the length of the cavity as shown by the uterine sound. Immediate laparoscopy and/or laparotomy is required if there is any suspicion of damage to extra-uterine viscera, or if the curettage has been carried out to complete an abortion, when bleeding is likely to be too heavy to ignore.

3. **Uterine synechiae**
   Over-vigorous curettage may remove all the endometrium from areas of anterior and posterior walls, permitting the myometrium to heal together forming adhesions - Asherman's syndrome.

MANAGEMENT OF DYSFUNCTIONAL UTERINE BLEEDING

SURGICAL MANAGEMENT

Hysterectomy

      abdominal   — total
                       — subtotal
      vaginal
      laparoscopically assisted vaginal hysterectomy

Endometrial ablation

TOTAL HYSTERECTOMY (Removal of uterus and cervix)

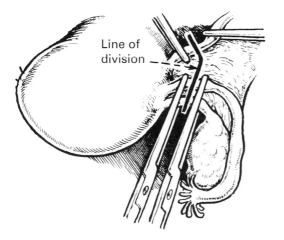

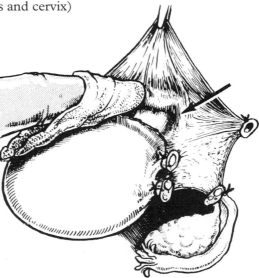

1.   Division of adnexa. The ovarian ligament, fallopian tube and round ligament are clamped and divided.

2.   Vesico-uterine peritoneum is opened up and bladder is being dissected off cervix. (The 'lateral vesico-uterine ligament' — marked by the arrow — conceals the ureter.)

MANAGEMENT OF DYSFUNCTIONAL UTERINE BLEEDING

Total hysterectomy *(cont.)*

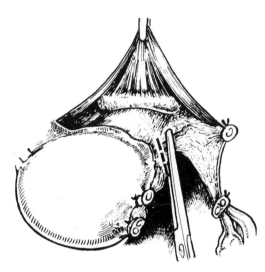

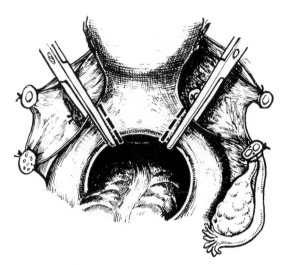

3.   Parametrium containing the uterine arteries is clamped and divided.

4.   The uterosacral ligaments are clamped and divided.

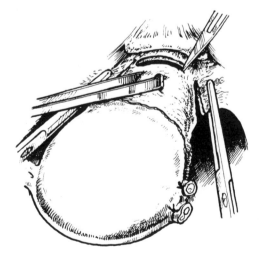

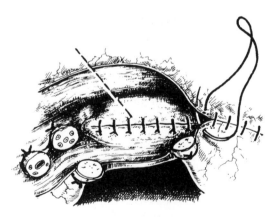

5.   The top of the vagina is now clear of bladder and ureters and can be opened to allow excision of uterus and cervix.

6.   After closing the vagina the raw area is reperitonised.

MANAGEMENT OF DYSFUNCTIONAL UTERINE BLEEDING

SUBTOTAL HYSTERECTOMY

Subtotal hysterectomy involves removal of the body of the uterus only. The cervix is conserved. The operation is easier and safer than total hysterectomy, particularly if there are adhesions around the cervix (e.g. from previous Caesarean section). The risk of ureteric damage is much less than with total hysterectomy. The major disadvantage of subtotal hysterectomy is the lack of protection from cervical carcinoma.

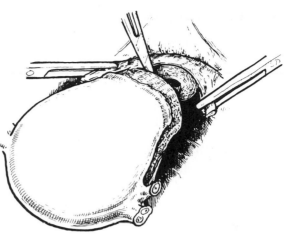

BILATERAL OOPHORECTOMY

Hysterectomy is often accompanied by bilateral oophorectomy. The pros and cons of this procedure are summarised below.

Advantages

reduces risk of ovarian cancer
effective treatment for PMS
may improve efficacy of treatment if pelvic pain is included in symptoms

Disadvantages

leads to premature menopause and effects of oestrogen withdrawal unless patient takes HRT

VAGINAL HYSTERECTOMY

In vaginal hysterectomy, the uterus and cervix are removed via a vaginal approach. This operation avoids the need for an abdominal scar, and recovery is often more rapid than from abdominal hysterectomy. The operation is technically difficult in women without some degree of uterine prolapse.

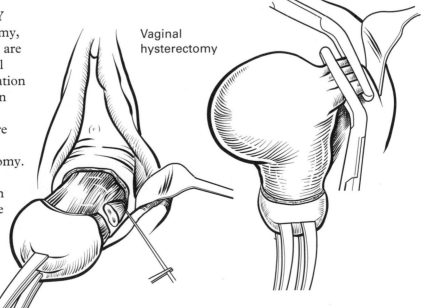

Vaginal hysterectomy

MANAGEMENT OF DYSFUNCTIONAL UTERINE BLEEDING

MINIMALLY INVASIVE SURGERY

Laparoscopically assisted vaginal hysterectomy (LAVH)

In laparoscopically assisted hysterectomy the broad ligaments, including the ovarian vessels, the round ligaments and the uterine arteries may be 'clamped and cut' by an endoscopic device which inserts multiple rows of stainless steel staples and divides the tissues. Alternatively, diathermy may be used to coagulate the tissues prior to division. The uterus is then removed vaginally and the vaginal vault closed per vaginam.

The putative advantage of LAVH over abdominal hysterectomy is a shorter in-patient stay.

Endometrial ablation techniques

1. Trans-cervical resection of endometrium (TCRE)
   Using an operating hysteroscope, the uterine cavity is distended with a glycine solution and either a wire loop diathermy instrument is used to cut strips of endometrium and underlying myometrium or a 'roller ball' electrode is used to coagulate the endometrium.

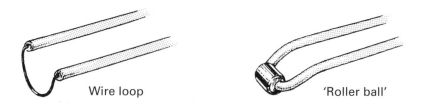

Wire loop   'Roller ball'

   Endometrial ablation rarely abolishes menstrual loss completely, but symptoms are improved in most women. Complications of the procedure include excessive fluid absorption and uterine perforation with damage to intra-abdominal organs. The major advantage of TCRE over abdominal hysterectomy is the shorter in-patient stay associated with this operation.

2. Hysteroscopic endometrial ablation by laser (HEAL) involves destruction of the endometrium using a fibre-optic transmitted YAG–Neodynium laser. This apparatus is more expensive, but is less likely to perforate the uterus than TCRE.

An endometrial biopsy to exclude endometrial carcinoma is essential prior to undertaking any of these procedures.

DYSFUNCTIONAL UTERINE BLEEDING

Pathology
Dysfunctional uterine bleeding may be associated with evidence of ovulation, or with anovulation. Endometrial sampling may be indicated to exclude endometrial carcinoma.

ANOVULATORY PATTERNS
e.g. Anovulatory with high oestrogen and high FSH
This produces a histological picture known as cystic glandular hyperplasia. The glandular epithelium shows mitotic activity. There is no inhibitory feedback to the pituitary and the anomalous position of high oestrogen, high FSH continues for months during which there is amenorrhoea. Ultimately the oestrogen level fluctuates and the fall produces excessive, prolonged bleeding. There is a risk of progression to carcinoma of the endometrium.

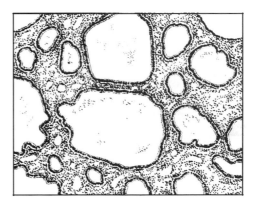

OVULATORY PATTERNS
e.g. Prolonged proliferative phase, short luteal phase
The illustration shows an endometrium in the early secretory phase although the specimen was taken on the 27th day. The prolonged oestrogenic phase has built up a thick endometrium. Progesterone is low. Excessive bleeding results when the oestrogen values decline and the endometrium is shed.

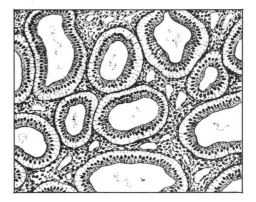

DYSFUNCTIONAL UTERINE BLEEDING

MEDICAL TREATMENT

Ovulatory bleeding

1. *Tranexamic acid*
   Administration: tranexamic acid 1–1.5 g qds during menstruation.
   Mode of action: inhibits clot breakdown within endometrial vasculature.
   Side effects include nausea, vomiting and diarrhoea.
   In women with true menorrhagia, a 40% reduction in menstrual loss can be achieved.

2. *Ethamsylate*
   Administration: ethamsylate 500 mg 4× daily during menses.
   Mode of action: reduces capillary fragility.
   Side effects include nausea, headache and rashes.
   In women with true menorrhagia, a 25% reduction in menstrual loss can be achieved.

3. *Prostaglandin synthetase inhibitors*
   Administration: e.g. mefenamic acid, 500 mg tid during menstruation.
   Mode of action: alters imbalance of vasodilator prostaglandin PGE2 and the vasoconstrictor prostaglandin PGF2a.
   Side effects include drowsiness, diarrhoea, rashes, thrombocytopenia and haemolytic anaemia.
   In women with true menorrhagia, a 25% reduction in menstrual loss can be achieved.

4. *Danazol*
   Administration: danazol 200 mg bd taken continuously throughout the menstrual cycle
   Mode of action: see, p.126
   A 70–80% reduction in menstrual loss can be achieved. Androgenic side effects may limit acceptability (see p.126).

5. *Combined contraceptive pill*
   Administration: usual contraceptive regimen.
   Mode of action: unknown.
   A reduction in menstrual loss can be seen in women both with and without menorrhagia.

6. *Levonorgestrel intrauterine system (LNG-IUS)*
   Administration: intrauterine system releasing 20 µg of levonorgestrel daily.
   Mode of action: inhibits endometrial proliferation.
   This device was originally designed as a contraceptive agent but is one of the most effective medical methods for reducing menstrual blood loss. One year after insertion, menstrual blood loss is reduced to 5% of the original amount. The main side effect of treatment is irregular bleeding in the first 3–6 months after insertion.

7. *Progesterone*
   Anovulatory bleeding.
   Cyclical gestogens.
   Administration: e.g. norethisterone 5 mg bd from days 5–26 of the menstrual cycle.
   Mode of action: thought to provide progestogenic support to the endometrium when endogenous progesterone is lacking.

ADENOMYOSIS

This is an infiltration of the myometrium by ectopic deposits of endometrium. It can normally only be diagnosed once the uterus is examined histologically following hysterectomy.

Pathology
The gross appearances are quite striking. The uterus is usually enlarged and this may be quite marked.

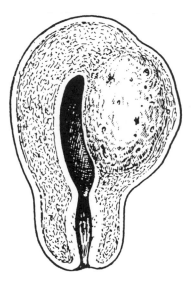

Microscopic appearances
The appearance of the endometrial deposits within the myometrium varies. In many cases they consist of typical glands and stroma although the stroma may be more prominent than the glands. Cyclical changes may be observed but this is not common. More often the endometrium is of immature type and if it does react it usually shows only proliferative changes. Clinical features are pain and menstrual upset.

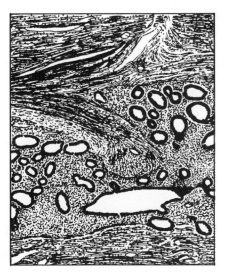

Endometrial deposits in the myometrium. Note the non-secretory gland epithelium. The surrounding myometrium undergoes moderate hyperplasia.

ENDOMETRIOSIS

Endometriosis involves deposits of endometrium outside the uterine cavity. Its manifestations are very variable and often bear no relation to the extent of the disease.

Pathology
The gross appearance shows ectopic deposits which can very in number from a few in one locality to large numbers distributed over the pelvic organs and peritoneum.

The commonest sites of these deposits are:
1. Ovary.
2. Peritoneum of the recto-vaginal cul-de-sac of the Pouch of Douglas.
3. Sigmoid colon.
4. Broad ligament.
5. Utero-sacral ligaments.

Less common are:
1. Cervix.
2. Round ligament.
3. Bladder.
4. Umbilicus.
5. Appendix.
6. Laparotomy scars.

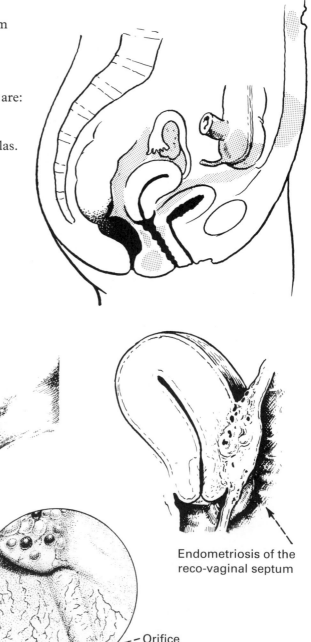

Endometriosis of a laparotomy scar

Endometriosis of the reco-vaginal septum

Endometriosis in the bladder

Orifice of ureter

ENDOMETRIOSIS

The commonest appearance of a typical lesion is that of a round protruding vesicle which shows a succession of colours from blue to black to brown. The variation in colour is due to haemorrhage with subsequent breakdown of the haemoglobin. Ultimately the area of haemorrhage heals by the formation of scar tissue. The result is a puckered area on the peritoneum. Commonly however the haemorrhage results in adhesion to surrounding structures. These adhesions are more apt to form between fixed structures such as the broad ligament, ovary, sigmoid colon or the posterior surfaces of the vagina and cervix.

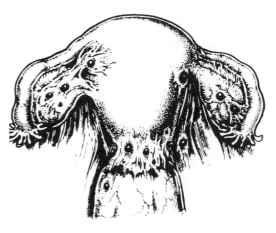

The ectopic deposits of endometrial tissue vary in size from pin-point to 5 mm or more. It is these larger deposits which tend to rupture leading to adhesions. These adhesions over the ovary can lead to the formation of quite large haemorrhagic cysts due to continued bleeding from deposits, the blood being unable to escape.

Investigation has shown that many lesions do not have a 'typical' appearance. The following is a list of other appearances which have been described.
1. White, slightly raised opacities due to retro-peritoneal deposits.
2. Red flame-like or vascular swellings, more common in the broad ligament or utero-sacral ligament.
3. Small excrescences like the surface of normal endometrium.
4. Adhesions under the ovary or between the ovary and the ovarian fossa peritoneum.
5. Café-au-lait patches often in the Pouch of Douglas, broad ligament or peritoneal surface of the bladder.
6. Peritoneal defects on utero-sacral ligament or broad ligament.
7. Areas of petechiae or hypervascularisation usually on the bladder and the broad ligament.

Secondary pathology
This is due to the adhesions between the endometriotic deposits and adjacent organs. In long-standing cases the pelvic cavity is obliterated by these adhesions. Retroversion of the uterus can be produced.

ENDOMETRIOSIS

Histology

While the deposits consist of endometrial elements rarely do they mirror the appearance of normal endometrium especially in their architecture. In place of the compact orderly arrangement of glands and stroma there are scattered patches of gland formations with some surrounding stroma. Sometimes gland formations predominate, occasionally only stromal cells can be seen.

Sometimes the deposits show evidence of cyclical activity but the activity does not always coincide with what is happening in the uterine endometrium.

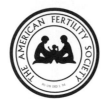

THE AMERICAN FERTILITY SOCIETY
REVISED CLASSIFICATION OF ENDOMETRIOSIS

Patient's name _____ Date _____

Stage I (Minimal)	– 1–5	Laparoscopy _____ Laparotomy _____ Photography _____
Stage II (Mild)	– 6–15	Recommended Treatment _____
Stage III (Moderate)	– 16–40	_____
Stage IV (Severe)	– >40	_____
Total _____		Prognosis _____

		ENDOMETRIOSIS	<1cm	1–3cm	>3cm
PERITONEUM		Superficial	1	2	?
		Deep	2	4	6
OVARY	R	Superficial	1	2	4
		Deep	4	16	20
	L	Superficial	1	2	4
		Deep	4	16	20
	POSTERIOR CUL DE SAC OBLITERATION		Partial		Complete
			4		40
	ADHESIONS		<1/3 Enclosure	1/3 – 2/3 Enclosure	>2/3 Enclosure
OVARY	R	Filmy	1	2	4
		Dense	4	8	16
	L	Filmy	1	2	4
		Dense	4	8	16
TUBE	R	Filmy	1	2	4
		Dense	4*	8*	16
	L	Filmy	1	2	4
		Dense	4*	8*	16

*If the fimbriated end of the fallopian tube is completely enclosed, change the point assessment to 16.

ENDOMETRIOSIS

Clinical findings

The incidence of endometriosis has been estimated at 3 to 7% of women but the true incidence is unknown. Quite often deposits are found incidentally in women who have no symptoms of endometriosis and are undergoing laparoscopy or laparotomy for some other condition. In addition, as indicated in the section on pathology, many peritoneal changes now known to be due to endometriosis were undiagnosed in the past.

The prevalence of endometriosis peaks between the ages of 30 and 45 years. Since ectopic endometrium is stimulated by the same ovarian steroid hormones as the endometrium lining the uterine cavity, endometriosis is almost never found outside the reproductive years.

Symptomatology

A. **Pain** affects more than 80% of women with endometriotic deposits. The pain tends to begin premenstrually reaching a peak during menstruation and subsiding slowly.

The character of pain may vary as does its apparent origin. It may be generalised throughout the abdomen and pelvis like the pain of severe dysmenorrhoea. Alternatively, pain may be localised to a particular site within the pelvis. Deep dyspareunia affects around 40% of women with endometriosis.

B. **Menstrual disturbance.** Menstrual disturbance affects around 20% of women with endometriosis. It may take the form of premenstrual 'spotting', menorrhagia or infrequent periods. Lesions in the wall of the bladder may result in 'menstrual haematuria'.

C. **Infertility.** Endometriosis is found more commonly in women undergoing investigation for infertility than in the 'normal' population. It is not clear which condition arises first. Approximately 30% of patients with endometriosis complain of infertility. When endometriosis is extensive, and both fallopian tubes are occluded, the mechanism by which endometriosis prevents conception is obvious. However, milder forms of endometriosis are also associated with subfertility, and here the pathophysiology is less clear. The most likely mechanism appears to be that immunological factors within the peritoneal cavity inhibit normal gamete function, thus reducing fertilisation rates.

Physical examination

Endometriosis cannot be diagnosed by physical examination alone. However, enlargement of the ovaries, fixed retroversion of the uterus and tender nodules within the pelvis may each raise the suspicion of the disease. Endometriosis should always be considered when patients have symptoms referable to the pelvic cavity.

Laparoscopy

Laparoscopic examination is the only way of making a positive diagnosis. The lesions can be seen and their number and location estimated. Endometriosis of long standing may be very difficult to diagnose due to obliteration of the pelvic cavity by adhesions. Histological confirmation must be obtained if feasible.

ENDOMETRIOSIS

Imaging techniques

Ultrasound, computerised tomography and magnetic resonance imaging may suggest the presence of endometriosis (e.g. by the demonstration of a particular type of ovarian cyst) but are by themselves insufficiently reliable to make the diagnosis.

Differential diagnosis

Due to the mixture of symptoms and the variation in appearance of the pelvic structures, conditions such as pelvic inflammatory disease and tumours of the ovary and bowel must be considered and eliminated.

Histogenesis

There are three theories.

1. Retrograde spill of menstrual debris through the tubes. Retrograde menstruation takes place in most women, but it is unclear why some women should develop endometriosis while others are unaffected.
2. Metaplasia of embryonic cells. These are derived from the primitive coelom and may remain in and around the pelvis and differentiate into Müllerian duct tissue.
3. Emboli of endometrial tissue may travel by lymphatics or blood vessels and become established in various sites.

The first of these theories is most favoured.

TREATMENT

Medical treatment

Any treatment must be aimed at treating symptoms. Since ovarian hormones are responsible for growth and activity in endometrium many medical therapies are designed to reduce ovarian steroid production or oppose their action.

1. *Progestogens*
    Progestogens in a relatively high dose (e.g. medroxyprogesterone acetate 10 mg tid) induce decidualisation, and sometimes resorption of ectopic endometrium. Side effects include weight gain, bloating and irregular vaginal bleeding.

2. *Combined contraceptive pill*
    The combined oral contraceptive pill also induces decidualisation of ectopic endometrium. It may be given continuously for up to 3 months.

3. *Danazol*
    Danazol is a steroid hormone closely related to testosterone, which inhibits pituitary gonadotrophins, is anti-oestrogenic, anti-progestational, slightly androgenic and anabolic. The dose of danazol given can be titrated to the patient's symptoms up to a maximum of 800 mg daily. If danazol can be tolerated, symptoms and objective signs of disease can be alleviated in the majority of patients. However, androgenic side effects including amenorrhoea, weight gain, acne, hirsutism and deepening of the voice may limit acceptability of the drug.

ENDOMETRIOSIS

Medical treament *(cont.)*

4. *Gestrinone*

    Gestrinone is a derivative of 19-nortestosterone. It has slight androgenic activity and is markedly anti-oestrogenic and anti-progestogenic. It interacts with the pituitary steroid receptors and decreases gonadotrophic secretion resulting in diminished follicular growth and anovulation. A bi-weekly oral dose of 2.5 to 5.0mg for 6 months induces amenorrhoea, disappearance of pain and regression of the endometrial deposits. Side effects include weight gain, acne, seborrhoea and mild hirsutism.

Gonadotrophic releasing hormone analogues (GnRH analogue)

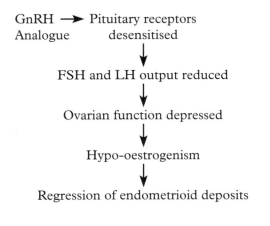

GnRH analogues are administered by depot injection or nasal spray. Their mode of action is shown above. Although these drugs are generally effective in treating symptoms, menopausal side effects, in particular bone loss, may preclude long term use. In the future, use of 'add back' regimens which include small supplementary doses of oestrogen may prove to be effective in treating the symptoms of endometriosis without the complications of total oestrogen deprivation.

Conclusion

As with medical therapies for other conditions, the optimum treatment is dictated by the side effect profile which is most acceptable to the patient. None of the drug treatments described will prevent recurrence of endometriosis once therapy has been stopped, although there may be a period of some months between stopping treatment and the re-emergence of symptoms. No medical treatment has been shown to improve subsequent fertility. Notwithstanding, none of the above, with the exception of the combined pill, is a proper contraceptive agent and patients should be advised to use barrier contraception to avoid the potential teratogenic effects of drugs such as danazol if they are at risk of becoming pregnant.

ENDOMETRIOSIS

Surgical treatment

Where infertility is not a problem radical surgery to remove both ovaries is said to be a lasting cure for endometriosis, since it removes the oestrogenic stimulus to endometrial growth.

In many cases the patient wishes relief from pain but also desires to retain the possibility of future pregnancy. In these circumstances only conservative surgery can be employed.

The intentions in conservative surgery are:

1. To ablate as many endometrial deposits in the pelvic cavity as possible.
2. To restructure the pelvic anatomy by destroying adhesions which interfere with ovarian and tubal function.
3. To destroy endometrial deposits in the ovaries.
4. To deal with sensory nerve pathways.

In view of the many vital structures such as the bladder, rectum, colon and ureters in close proximity to each other, conventional open surgery is not always feasible. Laser surgery under laparoscopy, with its almost microscopic accuracy, may be employed. Endometrial deposits and adhesions can be vaporised easily without damaging tissue outside a radius of a fraction of a millimetre from the target. Similarly the laser destruction of ovarian lesions can be carried out without destroying any of the functional tissue.

The question of dealing with sensory nerve pathways is difficult to answer. Severe pain is a feature of a number of gynaecological conditions, especially those related to malignancy. Elsewhere in this book operative techniques are described which involve interfering with sensory conductivity centrally, i.e. at the spinal cord level. Recently, a local operative procedure, paracervical uterine denervation, has been recommended. This consists of vaporising the utero-sacral ligaments by laser at their attachment to the posterior aspect of the cervix where the sensory fibres emerge from the uterus. Two difficulties are associated with this procedure. First, the ureters must be avoided and, secondly, veins lying lateral to the ligaments must not be injured. Unfortunately severe pain is often associated with severe endometriosis and adhesions may make the operation very difficult.

Reports in the literature record complete relief from pain in 50% of patients followed for more than a year and another 41% obtained moderate relief.

DYSMENORRHOEA

Dysmenorrhoea implies pain during menstruation, and most women experience some degree of pain at least on the first day of the period when the loss is heaviest.

Many women will also describe varying sorts of discomfort before the period starts, but this symptom should be regarded as a manifestation of the Premenstrual Tension Syndrome (see p.132).

The pain may be secondary to organic disease such as endometriosis or infection, but primary dysmenorrhoea, which is being discussed here, occurs in the presence of a normal genital tract.

Nature of the pain
It is usually described as having two components: a continuous lower abdominal pain attributed to vascular congestion, which radiates through to the back and sometimes down the thighs; and an intermittent cramping pain.

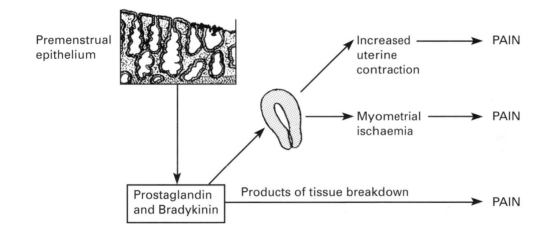

Aetiology
There is increased myometrial activity during the periods in women with dysmenorrhoea and uterine blood flow is reduced, especially during intense contractions. It is thought that this hyperactivity is the result of excessive quantities of prostaglandins synthesised during the breakdown of the premenstrual endometrium.

DYSMENORRHOEA

Clinical features of primary dysmenorrhoea

The patient is usually a nulliparous woman between 16 and 26 who is becoming increasingly disabled at the time of her periods, is incapable of work and often has to spend 1 or 2 days in bed.

Prostaglandin synthesis inhibitors have been shown experimentally to abolish uterine contraction and ischaemia and the pain which accompanies them.

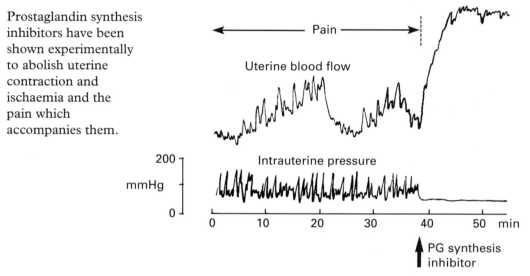

Management

In mild or moderate disease, treatment can be commenced after a full history and examination. In severe or unresponsive disease, organic disease must be excluded, usually by examination under anaesthesia and by laparoscopy. Thereafter the problem is to find a suitable drug which will alleviate the pain sufficiently to allow a normal existence during the period time.

If drug treatment is ineffective, which is very unlikely, some consideration may be given to the advisability of presacral neurectomy.

DYSMENORRHOEA

Drug treatment

1. **The contraceptive pill.** Dysmenorrhoea is very unlikely in the absence of ovulation, probably because of the pseudo-atrophy of the endometrium. The disadvantages of this efficacious treatment are the well-known side effects and perhaps the prevention of pregnancy.

2. **Prostaglandin synthetase inhibitors** such as mefenamic acid inhibit prostaglandin production, reduce uterine contractions and thereby alleviate dysmenorrhoea. In controlled studies, up to 90% of women report an improvement of symptoms with mefenamic acid. Other prostaglandin synthetase inhibitors, with the exception of aspirin, may also be worth trying.

3. **Progesterones**
    Prolonged treatment with progesterones may also reduce dysmenorrhoea. The mechanism of action is presumably myometrial relaxation induced by progesterone. A suggested regimen is dydrogesterone 10 mg bd taken from day 5 to day 25 of the menstrual cycle.

4. **Nifedipine**
    Nifedipine 20–40mg daily is effective in the treatment of dysmenorrhoea. Side effects include headache and flushing.

FUTURE PERSPECTIVES

Oxytocin antagonists
Oxytocin antagonists are being developed for the treatment of preterm labour. They are likely to be effective in the treatment of dysmenorrhoea.

PREMENSTRUAL SYNDROME

The premenstrual tension syndrome (PMS) includes a large group of symptoms which appear regularly and predictably in the week before the onset of menstruation. The symptom pattern will vary with the individual, but 95% of women will acknowledge at least one of the symptoms listed below. Symptoms resolve completely by the end of menstruation.

WATER RETENTION

Weight gain (up to 7lb)
Painful breasts
Abdominal distension
Feeling of bloatedness

PAIN

Headache
Backache
Tiredness
Muscle stiffness

AUTONOMIC REACTIONS

Dizziness/faintness
Cold sweats
Nausea/vomiting
Hot flushes

MOOD CHANGES

Tension
Irritability
Depression
Crying spells

LOSS OF CONCENTRATION

Forgetfulness
Clumsiness
Difficulty in
  making decisions
Poor sleeping

MISCELLANEOUS

Feelings of suffocation
Chest pains
Heart pounding
Numbness, tingling

Clinical features

Although the aetiology of premenstrual syndrome is unknown, it is clearly related to cyclical ovarian activity. Women who have no cyclical variation in sex steroids (e.g. post-menopausal women and women who have had bilateral oophorectomy) do not have PMS.

Investigations

There is no test which 'confirms' a diagnosis of PMS. It is helpful to ask the patient to complete a symptom diary (e.g. the Moos' Menstrual Distress Questionnaire) on a daily basis over the course of several cycles in order to demonstrate that symptoms are related to the premenstrual phase.

In a few women it may be helpful to institute treatment with a GnRH analogue for three months. This drug reliably suppresses ovarian activity. If symptoms are still present by the third month of treatment, they are unlikely to be related to the premenstrual syndrome.

PREMENSTRUAL SYNDROME

Treatment is empirical. Many regimes are used and none is universally effective.

1. **Pyridoxine (vitamin B6)**
   This is based on disordered tryptophan metabolism in sufferers from endogenous depression. Pyridoxine corrects the reduced brain 5-hydroxytryptamine. 20mg twice daily or more can give subjective relief.

2. **Oil of evening primrose**
   Oil of evening primrose is widely prescribed for the treatment of PMS. It is available 'over the counter' and has few adverse effects. Placebo-controlled studies have shown some limited benefits in the treatment of headache, bloatedness, clumsiness and depression.

3. **Progesterone**
   Progesterones are widely prescribed for the treatment of PMS. In the many placebo-controlled studies in which they have been evaluated, they have repeatedly been shown to be ineffective.

4. **Bromocriptine (Parlodel)**
   The dose of 2.5 mg twice daily orally needs to be achieved gradually to minimise nausea. Lassitude and dizziness may occur on bromocriptine and it is best reserved for subjects who complain principally of breast pain.

5. **Danazol**
   Danazol has been shown in double-blind crossover studies to relieve the symptoms of premenstrual syndrome in a significant number of women. 200 mg daily continuously for several months is as effective as higher doses and produces fewer side effects. Side effects such as weight gain, nausea and acne may occur. Benefit to PMS is not dependent on producing amenorrhoea.

6. **Selective serotonin uptake inhibitors (SSRIs)**
   SSRIs such as fluoxetine have been shown to be significantly better than placebo for the treatment of PMS in controlled trials. Since altered serotonergic function has been demonstrated in women with PMS, there is a clear rationale for their use.

7. **GnRH analogues**
   GnRH analogues are extremely effective in the treatment of PMS, and indeed may be useful in making the diagnosis (see above). Unfortunately, the menopausal side effects, associated bone loss and expense mean these drugs are unsuitable as long term treatments for the condition.

8. **Hysterectomy and bilateral salpingoophorectomy**
   Bilateral oophorectomy is extremely effective in the treatment of PMS. When combined with hysterectomy, oestrogen replacement can safely be given with no increase in symptoms. Clearly, hysterectomy and bilateral oophorectomy will rarely be indicated for the treatment of PMS alone. However, in women undergoing hysterectomy, the presence of significant PMS may be an indication for bilateral oophorectomy.

CHAPTER 7

GYNAECOLOGICAL INFECTIONS

INFLAMMATION IN THE LOWER GYNAECOLOGICAL TRACT

The vulva, vagina and ectocervix under normal conditions are the habitat of various types of infective agents, but they are only a threat if normal defence mechanisms are altered.

Defence mechanisms
1. Vaginal acidity.

Glycogen is produced by vaginal epithelium influenced by oestrogens and is converted to lactic acid by Doderlein's bacillus (a type of B.acidophilus). This maintains the vaginal pH between 3 and 4 which inhibits most other organisms.

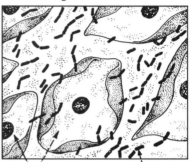

Normal vaginal flora

Desquamated cells   Organisms mostly lactobacilli

(Note absence of pus cells)

2. Thick layer of vaginal squamous epithelium.

This is a considerable physical barrier to infection. Continual desquamation of the superficial kerato-hyalin layer and glycogen production, both dependent upon ovarian oestrogen action, combat bacteria. In children and post-menopausal patients the epithelium lacks oestrogen stimulation and is thin and easily traumatised or infected.

3. Closure of the introitus.

In children and virgin adults the vaginal canal is only a potential space kept closed by the surrounding muscles and provides another physical barrier. This, however, alters and becomes of little importance following sexual activity and pregnancy.

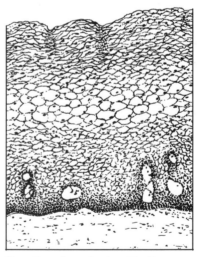

Functional vaginal epithelium: intermediate cells rich in glycogen

4. **Glandular secretions** from the cervix and Bartholin's glands maintain an outward fluid current helping to clear the canal of debris. In addition, cervical secretion contains immunoglobulins, especially IgA, and there are varying numbers of polymorphs, lymphocytes and macrophages.

VULVAL INFLAMMATION

Vulval inflammation is not uncommon but is usually an extension of infection from the vagina. A mild reaction may arise due to physical and anatomical conditions in the area, such as (a) moistness and (b) proximity of urethra and anus.

The area is not only naturally moist but also warm, particularly in obese patients. The folds of fat harbour moisture, and chafing occurs between them. The proliferation of bacteria is encouraged. Urinary incontinence and unsuspected glycosuria may add to this. It is important to test the urine for sugar in all patients.

Incidental factors may intensify any reaction resulting from these conditions e.g. the wearing of nylon underwear which is heat-retaining and non-absorptive. Associated with this may be chemical factors increasing the reaction such as washing underclothes with detergents, using toilet powders, perfumes and deodorants. The clinical result is irritation and itching leading to scratching. Continual itch-scratch-itch leads to maceration of the skin and may invite infection. Careful attention to personal hygiene is essential. Obese patients should be encouraged to lose weight and all of the incidental factors mentioned above should be avoided.

It must be remembered that itching may be a sign of a more serious disease such as impending liver failure or Hodgkin's disease.

Search for lice or scabies should be made where circumstances suggest the possibility.

One of the complications of vulvar inflammation is **obstruction of the duct of Bartholin's gland.** Cystic dilatation and abscess formation are apt to follow. The condition occurs during a woman's sexual life. Any organism, staphylococcal, coliform or gonococcal may be found.

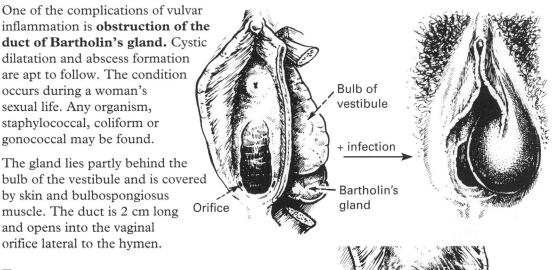

Bulb of vestibule

+ infection

Orifice

Bartholin's gland

The gland lies partly behind the bulb of the vestibule and is covered by skin and bulbospongiosus muscle. The duct is 2 cm long and opens into the vaginal orifice lateral to the hymen.

Treatment
Marsupialisation (Gk. marsipos, a bag)
The cyst or abscess is widely opened within the labium minus and drained and its walls sutured to the skin leaving a large orifice which it is hoped will form a new duct orifice and allow conservation of the gland. A ribbon-gauze pack is inserted for 48 hours by some operators.

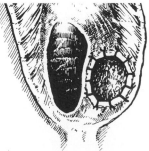

137

VAGINAL DISCHARGE AND INFECTION

A small amount of vaginal discharge is normal in adult life and may be excessive in the presence of ectropion or cervical tears.

Composition
Tissue fluid, cell debris, carbohydrate, lactobacilli, lactic acid. The pH is about 4.5, a degree of acidity which inhibits the growth of organisms other than the lactobacilli.

Source of Vaginal Discharge

Vulva: Greater vestibular glands, glands of vulval skin.

Vagina: Mainly desquamated epithelial cells which liberate glycogen. The lactobacilli metabolise the glycogen to lactic acid. Vaginal transudate (secretion from tissues and capillaries of the mature vagina) is often described: vaginal epithelium is certainly not water resistant (like transitional epithelium).
There are no mucosal glands.

Cervix: Alkaline mucous secretion which becomes copious and watery during ovulation.
Uterine glands also discharge into the vagina.

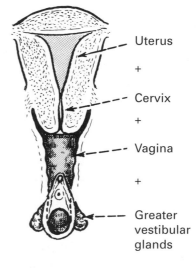

Uterus
+
Cervix
+
Vagina
+
Greater vestibular glands

Clinical Features

Volume: The need to wear a pad or tampon continuously suggests excessive discharge.

Onset: Sudden onset means infection. Onset can be associated with the end of a pregnancy, the contraceptive pill, a course of antibiotic, a sexual adventure.

Colour: Normal discharge is white but stains yellow or pale brown on clothing or pads. A greenish-yellow colour suggests pyogenic infection, commonly accompanied by an unpleasant odour. A red or dark brown suggests blood.

Irritation: Any discharge can in time excoriate the vulva but only candida and trichomonas cause itching.

COMPLAINTS OF VAGINAL DISCHARGE

Women will complain if:
   (a) there appears to be an excessive amount of staining on the clothing.
   (b) they detect an offensive smell.
   (c) they suffer local irritation.

There is often little correlation between symptoms and signs. Fastidious or neurotic women will complain of what is really normal; and gynaecologists regularly observe heavy and purulent discharge in women who deny any symptoms at all.

Examination

1. Vulva, perineum and thighs are inspected for signs of excoriation. The vestibular glands and urethral meatus are observed and palpated.

2. Vaginal walls and cervix are examined through a speculum. Normal vaginal epithelium is pink, the rugae are well marked and the epithelial surface of the cervix smooth and moist. Normal discharge is like curdled milk and is white and odourless.

3. A bimanual examination should always be made.

4. Specimens of discharge are taken for microscopy and culture, and a cervical smear for cytology. Chlamydia must be excluded. Cervical, rather than vaginal swabs should be taken and a separate swab and appropriate medium are essential for chlamydia. A urethral swab may give better detection of chlamydia.

LEUCORRHOEA

This means an excessive amount of normal discharge — a very subjective assessment. The patient will complain of constantly having to change her clothes but there will be no irritation and appearance will be normal. The smell will be the normal vulval odour (from the action of commensal bacteria on the secretions of the apocrine sex glands), microscopy will reveal normal appearances and culture will grow only lactobacilli.

The patient should be reassured and given an explanation of normal physiology. No local treatment is necessary.

Almost 20% of all patients attending gynaecological clinics complain of vaginal discharge, indicating some form of infection. The infective agents form three groups:

1. In 90% of cases the inflammation is usually relatively mild and is due to one of three agents:
   (a) Candida albicans
   (b) Gardnerella vaginalis
   (c) Trichomonas vaginalis.

2. The remaining 10% are more serious. They may cause painful sores, tumour-like lesions, spread into the pelvis or cause generalised infection.

3. Chlamydia trachomatis is a major cause of gynaecological morbidity (see p.146).

VAGINAL DISCHARGE

CANDIDA ALBICANS

This is yeast and exists in two forms — slender branching hyphae or as a small globular spore which multiplies by budding.

Source of infection

This organism may exist as a normal commensal in the rectum and small numbers may be found in the vagina, the acid medium suiting their survival without symptoms arising. The patient's fingernails may harbour the yeast. Sexual transmission is also possible. Symptomatic infection is most likely to arise when there are predisposing conditions e.g.

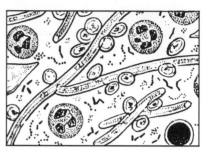

Mycelia and spores of C.albicans. Notethe presence of leucocytes.

1. **Pregnancy.** The vagina provides a tropical micro-climate and the high concentration of sex steroids in the blood maintains an increased glycogen formation in the vaginal epithelium and may alter the local pH.
2. **Immunosuppressive Therapy.** This includes cytotoxic drugs and corticosteroids. There is also thought to be a natural degree of immunosuppression during pregnancy.
3. **Glycosuria**. This may be due to undiscovered diabetes, but again a mild degree of glycosuria may exist in a normal pregnancy due to lowering of the renal threshold for sugar.
4. **Antibiotic Therapy.** Systemic antibiotics destroy the normal bacteria thus reducing the competition for nutrients leaving the field clear for C. albicans.
5. **Chronic Anaemia.** Normal iron stores are needed to maintain an adequate immune reaction. This also entails adequate folic acid intake. The angular stomatitis of chronic anaemia is due to Candida infection.
6. Rarely, deficient cell mediated immunity is a predisposing condition.

Clinical features

The patient is usually between 20 and 40, when oestrogen support of the epithelial glycogen content is at its highest. The complaint is of irritant discharge and dyspareunia. Examination reveals an inflamed and tender vagina and vulva with white plaques resembling curdled milk adhering to the vaginal wall and vulva. Removal of the plaque reveals a red inflamed area. Pre-pubertal or post-menopausal infection is uncommon, but if it does occur after the menopause the symptoms tend to be severe.

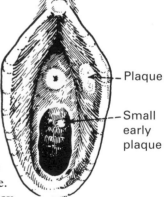

Plaque

Small early plaque

Treatment

A single 500 mg clotrimazole pessary, with external application of 1% clotrimazole cream offers convenient therapy. There is now doubt about the need to treat sexual partners, formerly advised. In persistent or recurrent infection, confirmation of the diagnosis by culture and determination of sensitivity to treatment are important. Oral fluconazole 150 mg or itraconazole 200 mg as a single dose, or monthly for 6 months may be effective. Nystatin 500,000 i.u. orally 4 × daily and Nystatin pessaries 2 × day for 3 or 4 months may be added. Boilable or disposable underwear should be worn.

VAGINAL DISCHARGE

GARDNERELLA VAGINALIS — BACTERIAL VAGINOSIS

For a long time a large number of cases of vaginitis were labelled non-specific because of disagreement regarding the infective agent. These cases were characterised by a non-irritating, foul smelling discharge. Ultimately, careful bacteriological studies have established the fact that although the discharge contains a mixture of bacteria, the one constant feature in 90% of cases is the presence of a tiny gram-negative cocco-bacillus which is a facultative anaerobe — Gardnerella vaginalis.

Clinical features

The patient complains of a foul-smelling discharge, and examination confirms both the discharge and the odour. In appearance the discharge is thin, greyish and sometimes shows bubbles. A vaginal smear reveals the presence of 'clue' cells. Gram staining is usually negative but can be variable.

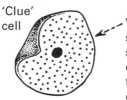

'Clue' cell

Vaginal squame showing stippling of cytoplasm due to adherent cocco-bacilli

Pus cells tend to be few in number. Doderlein's bacilli are also scanty but frequently many other bacteria are present. The pH of the fluid is raised. Although the main complaint is of malodorous discharge some patients will have pruritus, frequency, dysuria and dyspareunia.

Treatment

Oral Metronidazole 200 mg t.i.d. for 7 days or a single dose of 2 g appears to be effective. Clindamycin vaginal cream may also be employed. Male partners should also be treated.

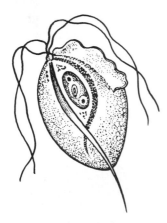

TRICHOMONAS VAGINALIS

Trichomonas vaginalis is a protozoan organism, which infests the vagina in the female and the urethra, prepuce and prostate in the male. It is a common cause of irritant vaginal discharge.

T.Vaginalis is a single-cell organism about 20μ x 10μ, with four flagellae and an undulating membrane which gives it a characteristic jerky movement. It is transmitted mainly during sexual intercourse but can be acquired from infected articles such as a contaminated speculum.

VAGINAL DISCHARGE

TRICHOMONAS VAGINALIS *(contd)*

Clinical features

In the acute phase the patient complains of severe vaginal tenderness and pain, and an irritant discharge. The vagina is seen to be inflamed, sometimes with a patchy strawberry vaginitis, and there is a copious offensive, frothy discharge. Frequently there is a burning sensation, pruritus, dysuria and dyspareunia. In the latent or dormant phases there are no symptoms although the presence of the organism can be demonstrated, often in a cervical smear.

Incidence

Perhaps 18% of the female population. T.vaginalis is commonly found in patients with gonorrhoea, and has an association with cervical dysplasia. No cause-and-effect relationship has been proved.

Diagnosis

Diagnosis is by observation of the motile organisms in a fresh smear diluted with saline and by laboratory culture.

Treatment

Always systemic and, if possible, including the patient's sexual partner. Metronidazole (Flagyl) 200 mg thrice daily for a week, or 2 g orally once, avoiding concurrent alcohol ingestion. Nimorazole (Naxogin) 2 gm as a single dose taken with food.

Short courses are useful with patients whose cooperation is uncertain, but are more likely to cause nausea and gastritis.

The post-treatment vaginal smear should be normal, but T. vaginalis can linger in the urethra, Skene's and Bartholin's glands, and reinfection of the vagina may call for further treatment.

The nitro-imidazoles are complex drugs and at least one of them, metronidazole, is active against anaerobic organisms and has also been used in alcoholism, Crohn's disease and rheumatoid arthritis. It is also effective as a potentiator of radiotherapy applied to hypoxic cancer cells, and a case of peripheral neuropathy has been reported after prolonged dosage. Care is necessary if the drug is being given to a pregnant woman, although no harmful effects on the fetus have been demonstrated.

Pathology

Passing from host to host during coitus T.vaginalis attaches itself to the vaginal epithelium and multiplies rapidly, taking glycogen away from Doderlein's bacilli which disappear. The vaginal pH rises to about 5.5, allowing the increase of bacterial pathogens which aggravate the infection and resulting discharge.

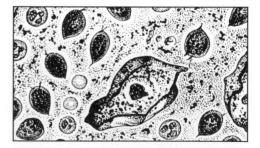

VAGINITIS

ATROPHIC or SENILE VAGINITIS

This sometimes arises at times when ovarian activity ceases with the onset of the menopause, after surgical removal of the ovaries or following ablation by radiotherapy or chemotherapy.

Clinical features

Symptoms may be mild, consisting of irritation with discharge. In other patients the changes may be severe. Pain can be the main feature and the discharge purulent. Examination of the vaginal mucosa reveals a rash of petechial haemorrhages and there may be ulceration. Smears show rounded epithelial cells, with no glycogen, many polymorphs and bacteria. In neglected cases intra-vaginal adhesions may develop. Fortunately the condition is becoming increasingly uncommon with hormone replacement therapy. Oestrogen quickly reverses the changes.

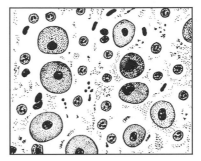

Vaginal smear of atrophic type, with numerous polymorphs, a mixed bacterial content and para-basal epithelial cells.

Oestriol vaginal cream or pessaries and very low dose oestradiol preparations such as 0.025 mg vaginal tablet (Vagifem) or silastic ring pessary (Estring) give local benefits without significant systemic oestrogen effects.

VULVO-VAGINITIS in CHILDREN

This is a rare condition and only arises in certain circumstances viz.

    (a) Sexual interference.

    (b) Insertion of foreign bodies by the child herself.

    (c) Threadworm infestation.

In (a) the changes will be those of physical damage to the tissues. Infection will depend to some extent on whether the person guilty of the offence is a carrier of a specific agent.

    (b) In this case infection may arise from bowel commensals.

    (c) The diagnosis may be made by applying Sellotape (Scotch tape) to the vulva then pressing the tape onto a microscope slide for microscopic examination.

Many of the examples of vulvo-vaginitis may arise from the irritation caused by threadworms. Scratching will lead to maceration of the skin which in turn will encourage bacterial contamination.

Vaginitis due to foreign bodies is sometimes seen in adults. Tampons, contraceptive devices and supportive pessaries used for prolapse may be left, forgotten, in situ. These give rise to an offensive purulent discharge. Bacteriological investigation will give an indication of the type of infection and the appropriate treatment following removal of the offending body.

A secondary vaginitis may arise due to contamination of the vagina through fistulous openings (vesico-vaginal or recto-vaginal) following injury, surgical operations or tumour growth. Repeated attacks of infection may occur. Treatment is obviously repair of the fistula where this is possible.

In all cases of vaginal discharge the possibility of malignant disease in the tract must be considered.

VAGINAL DISCHARGE AND INFECTIONS

The second group, the 10% of infections which cause serious disease or present difficulties in diagnosis, are almost all sexually transmitted. In addition to being a serious threat to the individual they present a public health problem. If their presence is suspected or diagnosed it is better that they be dealt with by a specialised department experienced in their treatment and possessing the laboratory facilities for continuing assessment.

VIRAL DISEASES

GENITAL HERPES
Herpes Simplex virus (HSV) types 1 and 2 may affect the lower genital tract or the mouth. It is highly infectious — 80% of women in contact with male carriers become infected. The initial attack may be severe. There may be, in 50% of victims, less severe recurring attacks every 3 or 4 weeks and they represent a potential for wide dissemination to others in the immediate environment. The incubation period is short — 3 to 7 days.

Clinical findings
The disease affects the vulvo-vaginal and peri-anal regions but may be transmitted to the mouth. The patient complains of burning, itching and hyperaesthesia of the area and the skin shows evidence of acute inflammation — oedema and erythema. There is usually a vaginal discharge. If the peri-urethral area is involved there may be dysuria and retention of urine.

The specific lesions start as small indurated tender papules which become vesicles and quickly break down to form shallow ulcers, 5 mm or more in diameter, with a yellowish grey slough in the base. These can be seen on the vulva and labia but in some cases they are confined to the vagina and cervix and there may be no external evidence of the disease. In these circumstances the ulcers may be large and could be mistaken for carcinoma of the cervix. The inguinal nodes are enlarged. The infection is accompanied by general symptoms of malaise, headache and even encephalitis. Sacral ganglion involvement causes neuralgia. There is no intense dyspareunia.

The acute phase lasts for 4–5 days. The lesions heal over 8–10 days and then a latent period ensues during which the virus remains in the sacral ganglia. Further attacks may follow. The disease may occur during pregnancy, and infection of the baby may prove fatal.

Diagnosis
Clinical suspicion is confirmed by tissue culture isolation of virus or detection of virus antigen by immuno-fluorescence or ELISA techniques. Some degree of immunity may be conferred during recurrent attacks and a search for antibodies will help to differentiate primary from second attacks.

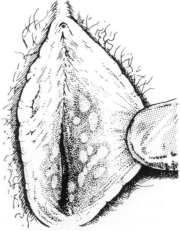

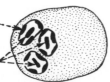

Chromatin at nuclear membrane

Eosinophilic inclusion bodies

VAGINAL DISCHARGE AND INFECTIONS

Herpes *(contd)*

Treatment

Ice packs, local analgesia (2% lignocaine), non-steroidal analgesic creams, saline bathing and systemic analgesics help relieve acute local symptoms. Acyclovir 3% ointment, applied repeatedly, is effective only if commenced at the onset of signs and symptoms. Oral Acyclovir, 200 mg 4 hourly for 5 days, may be commenced within 6 days of onset of a first episode. Antibiotics or povidone iodine control secondary infection. Acyclovir is less effective in recurrent episodes.

Acyclovir 800 mg daily, orally, has been used long-term when frequent recurrence is a problem. Famcyclovir and valciclovir have similar effect with less frequent administration.

CONDYLOMATA ACUMINATA

Commonly called genital warts, these are caused by human papilloma viruses (HPV) which are transmitted sexually, with more that 50% of contacts developing lesions. Numbers 6 and 11 are particularly associated with condylomata. Infectivity is greatest just after appearance of a wart. Incubation varies from a few weeks to 9 months or more.

Clinical findings

A single warty growth quickly spreads to form multiple growths showing a tendency to fuse. They are pinkish with dry surfaces unless macerated and are of softer consistency than the ordinary skin wart. The growths become luxuriant in moist areas and especially during pregnancy. They affect the labia, peri-anal area, perineum, the lower part of the vagina and may even spread on to the thighs. Secondary infection may give rise to purulent discharge.

Differential Diagnosis

1. **Syphilitic condylomata.** These are more widespread and not confined to the genital area. They are also flatter and more rounded. Treponemes can be found in the tissue fluid. Serological tests will of course confirm the diagnosis.
2. **Benign papilloma.** This is commonly single and similar to ordinary skin warts.
3. **Verrucous carcinoma.** This is a locally malignant lesion but vulval carcinoma is rare in pre-menopausal patients. Biopsy will differentiate the two conditions.
4. Sometimes condylomata affect the cervix and can resemble carcinoma.

Histology

The warts have a central core of connective tissue covered by a thick layer of prickle cells. Chronic inflammatory changes are present in the dermis.

Treatment

Podophyllin 20% in alcohol is often used, painted on the lesions. It may be ineffective and systemic absorption has proved fatal. It must not be used in pregnancy.

Podophyllotoxin, the active ingredient, is available as liquid and cream for self-treatment of both sexes.

Cryo-cautery, electro-cautery and laser ablation are employed. Lesions may recur.

VAGINAL DISCHARGE AND INFECTIONS

MOLLUSCUM CONTAGIOSUM

This is a highly infective pox virus, one of the largest known and can be seen under the microscope. It is commonly transmitted by sexual contact but towels and clothing can carry the infection. Whitish papules with dark umbilicated centres are produced. They are firm in consistency. Mostly they affect the genital region but can spread to other parts of the body. Spread is rapid. The disease is common in infants. Sometimes there is a cheesy discharge from the warts.

Histology

The epithelium undergoes hyperplasia extending deeply into the dermis.

The germinal layer of cells contains cytoplasmic inclusion bodies which push the nucleus aside. These cells desquamate when they reach the surface and spread the infection.

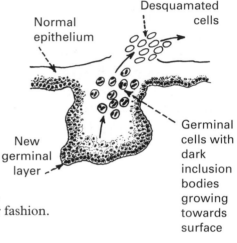

Treatment

This is a simple matter of killing the virus by local treatment to prevent spread of infection.
1. Phenol can be applied to the centre of a nodule.
2. Diathermy and cryosurgery are used in a similar fashion.

BACTERIAL INFECTIONS

CHLAMYDIA TRACHOMATIS This is a widespread gynaecological infection.

Clinical features

The initial symptoms in women are often mild. Discharge may be present, varying from watery to frankly purulent according to the severity of the reaction to the disease. In severe cases there is obvious cervicitis which looks like an infected erosion. Sometimes there is a punctate haemorrhagic inflammation with micro-abscesses. Occasionally there are few changes in the vagina and the first evidence of infection is the appearance of a salpingitis. It is an important cause of chronic pelvic inflammation. A gelatinous exudate is formed in the pouch of Douglas which proceeds to multiple adhesions and tubal occlusion. It is an important cause of infertility. Ophthalmia neonatorum is very common as there is over 50% chance of transmission during delivery.

Reiter's syndrome with urethritis, arthritis and conjunctivitis is more common in the infected male. There may be spread to cause perihepatitis with so-called violin string adhesions to the parietal peritoneum. This is accompanied by acute pain in the upper right quadrant. The condition may be mistaken for cholecystitis or pancreatitis. It has been suggested that chlamydia may be involved as an aetiological agent in carcinoma of the cervix.

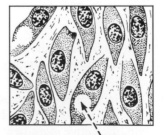

Chlamydia

VAGINAL DISCHARGE AND INFECTIONS

CHLAMYDIA TRACHOMATIS *(contd)*

Diagnosis

Endocervical cells, urethral cells or endosalpinx cells (salpingitis detected at laparotomy) must be obtained using a special cotton tipped swab and transferred *immediately* in special transport medium to an appropriate laboratory.

Nucleic acid amplification techniques are now commonly used to diagnose chlamydia from a vulval swab or a first-void urine sample, with 30% greater sensitivity than viral culture.

The organism can be seen under the microscope. It is intracellular. Staining by an immuno-fluorescence technique confirms the diagnosis. It multiplies like bacteria, but like viruses can only do so within cells. It contains both DNA and RNA.

Treatment: Tetracycline 500 mg at 6 hourly intervals for 2 weeks. If the patient is pregnant erythromycin is preferable since there is a danger of hepatic damage with tetracycline therapy.

LYMPHOGRANULOMA VENEREUM (LGV)

Previously thought to be viral, LGV is now attributed to a strain of chlamydia. Rare in the UK, it is mainly seen in the Far East, Africa and South America in seaports.

Clinical findings

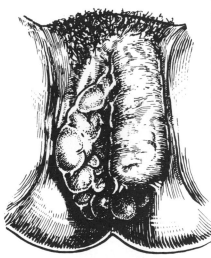

The primary lesion is a small painless ulcer with raised irregular borders which may involve the labia, clitoris or urethra. It appears 1 to 3 weeks after infection. Several weeks later the inguinal and iliac lymph nodes enlarge, become soft and fluctuant and this is followed by rupture creating discharging sinuses. The lesions eventually heal with the creation of large fibrous scars. In the process the urethra may be virtually destroyed and the rectum stenosed. Recto-vaginal fistulae may form and extensive surgical treatment may be required. The pelvic organs may be involved in the same way giving rise to intestinal obstruction and various fistulous communications.

Histologically the reaction is of granulomatous type. Lymph channels are often obstructed giving rise to elephantiasis of the vulva. The picture shows an advanced case of LGV.

Treatment: Tetracyclines or erythromycin are effective.

GRANULOMA INGUINALE

Another tropical ulcerative condition, caused by the intra-cellular Gram-negative Donovania granulomatis, this begins as a painless genital, inguinal or peri-anal nodule, which ulcerates. Local lymphatic glands enlarge, but do not ulcerate. In pregnancy, abortion often occurs or there is high fetal morbidity. Secondary infection is common.

Treatment: The condition responds to tetracycline given for 2 or 3 weeks. Both of these diseases may be followed by squamous carcinoma.

VAGINAL DISCHARGE AND INFECTIONS

CHANCROID

This lesion is due to infection by Haemophilus Ducreyii. After a short incubation period a red macule appears which quickly changes to a pustule and then an ulcer. The ulcers are numerous and vary in size from millimetres to several centimetres. They are well defined with projecting margins but shallow with a greenish slough in the base. These ulcers are soft and painful. This, together with the short incubation period helps to differentiate them from syphilitic lesions. The labia major, clitoris and peri-anal regions are affected. Two weeks later the local lymph nodes tend to enlarge and suppurate. There is usually secondary infection and the discharge is foul-smelling. Microscopically the lesions consist of granulation tissue infiltrated by lymphocytes and plasma cells. The bacillus can be demonstrated in scrapings from the ulcer stained by Giemsa.

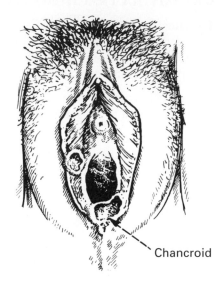

Chancroid

Treatment

Co-trimoxazole 960 mg twice a day by mouth is usually effective. Tetracycline may also be used. If the lymph nodes suppurate they should be aspirated through adjacent healthy skin, but do not incise.

GONORRHOEA

Gonorrhoea in the female carries a high risk of salpingitis and sterility, but early diagnosis is difficult to achieve. Symptoms are often mild or absent, and since the incubation period is about 2 weeks (longer than in the male) very few women consider the possibility of such an infection.

Clinical features

The classical history is of urethritis, vaginal discharge, menstrual upset of sudden onset, but any infection in the genital area however it presents, may be gonococcal. After the acute phase vaginal discharge will persist, followed in approximately 15% of cases by signs of pelvic inflammatory disease (PID).

'Metastatic' signs — conjunctivitis, dermatitis, arthritis — are very rare in gynecological practice.

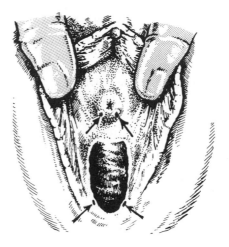

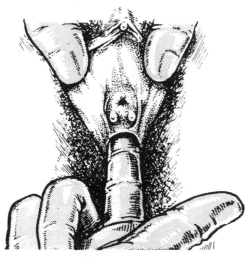

Examination

The labia are held apart, and the urethra, Skene's ducts and Bartholin's ducts examined for signs of infection. These ducts should be 'milked' for specimens of pus, if any, and swabs are taken from the cervix which is the main reservoir of infection.

Diagnosis is a laboratory procedure. Intracellular diplococci may be seen with Gram-staining, or the more time consuming immunofluorescent method, but the evidence of positive culture is essential as is antibiotic sensitivity determination. For trichomonas, candida, chlamydia, and syphilis.

Treatment

In the UK, 1.2 mega units of procaine penicillin with 2 g of probenecid, or Amoxycillin 3 g orally plus probenecid 1g orally are usually effective. In patient allergy or organism resistance, the latter very common outside of the UK, large oral doses of cephaloridine, tetracycline or doxycyline may be effective.

SYPHILIS

Syphilis is an uncommon disease in gynaecological practice, but any genital sore should come under suspicion. It is less uncommon in association with HIV.

PRIMARY SYPHILIS

The chancre (a corruption of 'cancer') has an incubation period of about a month and its appearance is often accompanied by pyrexia and malaise. The most common site is the vulva and then the cervix, but infection can occur anywhere. The chancre is the point at which the treponema enters the body.

The typical chancre is about 1cm in diameter and begins as a reddish papule which becomes ulcerated. It is painless and highly infective. The inguinal glands are markedly enlarged.

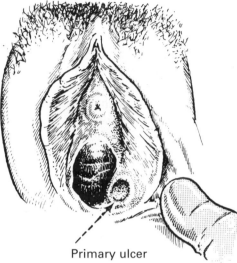

Primary ulcer

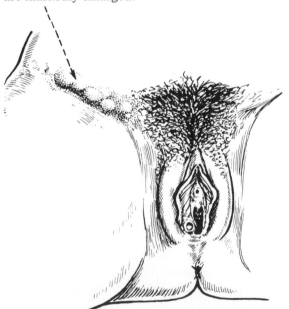

Diagnosis requires the identification of T. pallidum in the exudate of the chancre or in material aspirated from an enlarged gland. Treponemata are not easily recognisable in stained preparations and the dark-ground illumination of fresh specimens is used. Light is reflected off the edges of the organisms, making them easy to perceive and they are recognised by their shape and movement.
T. pallidum must be distinguished from other treponemata.

DIAGNOSIS OF SYPHILIS

Positive identification of T. pallidum is difficult for various reasons including the failure, so far, to grow the organism in vitro. The usual method of diagnosis is by serological tests which become positive 4–6 weeks after infection.

Reagin This is a non-specific antibody which appears in the tissues after infection with syphilis and many other bacteria and viruses. Its presence is detected by complement-fixation tests which are modifications of the original Wasserman reaction (WR) or by flocculation tests in which a reaction is observed under the microscope between infected serum and cardiolipin antigen.

False positives are usually weaker than a reaction due to syphilis, but if a positive result is obtained further tests are made. A false positive reaction may be obtained in the presence of latent yaws.

Reiter's Test is a complement-fixation test using a non-syphilitic treponeme as the antigen. A positive result means that the reagin is present because of a treponeme, and of course probably T. pallidum.

Treponemal Immobilisation Test (TPI).
This is a specific for syphilis but is expensive. Live T. pallida are used (from a rabbit chancre) and are seen to be immobilised if combined with syphilitic serum.

Fluorescent Treponemal Antibody Tests are becoming very widely used for verification of the 'positive WR'.

Principle of Fluorescent Tests (FTA)

1. Anti-human globulin is combined with fluorescein.

2. Dead treponeme is combined with test serum. If subject is infected, the treponeme acquires a coating of globulin antibody.

3. 1 and 2 are combined and the treponeme becomes fluorescent.

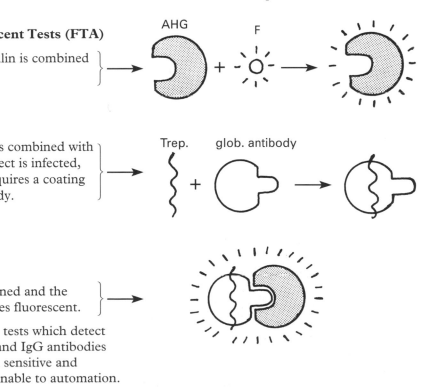

Enzyme immunoassay tests which detect anti-treponemal IgM and IgG antibodies are claimed to be both sensitive and specific. They are amenable to automation.

SYPHILIS

Signs and symptoms of the spread of T. pallidum throughout the whole body appear usually about 2 months after the primary stage, and the disease may present in this phase to the gynaecologist.

There is likely to be a mild pyrexia and malaise, but the dominating signs are a generalised lymphadenopathy and mucocutaneous lesions. 'Snail track' ulcers appear on mucosal surfaces, and the skin develops a very wide variety of macular and papular rashes. In warm moist areas such as the breast flexures and the vulva, the papules become hypertrophic and flattened and present as 'condylomata lata' which are highly infective.

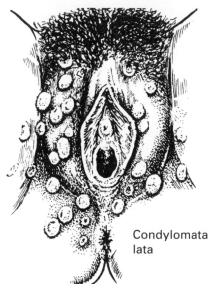

Condylomata lata

Diagnosis is by the demonstration of T. pallidum in the lesions and by serological tests.

Treatment of early contagious syphilis

T. pallidum is sensitive to many antibiotics, but reactions are common and care is required in treatment. Most patients receiving effective treatment for early syphilis with any antibiotic will display some degree of the Jarisch-Herxheimer reaction — rigors, sweating, headache, for about 24 hours. It can be modified by giving prednisolone 5 mg 6–hourly.

Penicillin

This is the drug of choice, but the large doses required may induce some hypersensitive reaction, vaso-vagal, or even anaphylactoid.

The requirement is a blood level of 3 μg per cent for about 2 weeks, and one mega-unit of procaine penicillin intramuscularly every day for 14 days is regarded as curative. The oral route is unreliable because of variable rates of absorption, and the uncertainty of patient cooperation.

Other Antibiotics

If the patient is sensitive to penicillin, many other drugs are available, including the tetracyclines, erythromycin, and doxycycline. These are given orally for 10–15 days, double the usual dosage, and Vitamin B and nystatin should be given concurrently because of the tendency to diarrhoea, pruritus ani, and candida infection.

If not treated in the early stages syphilis leads to a complex immune reaction with a chronic host–parasite relationship. The final stage involving cardiovascular and nervous lesions can appear months later.

TOXIC SHOCK SYNDROME

TOXIC SHOCK SYNDROME

This is an uncommon syndrome which can arise in women using tampons. It is caused by staphylococci which may be carried by the woman herself in various sites such as the vagina, cervix, perineum or nasopharynx. It is extremely dangerous and may prove fatal. The infection becomes established in the vagina, usually aided by the presence of a tampon.

Clinical signs

There is a rapid onset of fever often with vomiting, diarrhoea, muscular aches and skin erythema. The blood pressure drops to very low levels and the patient becomes confused and stuporose. Swabs should be taken from the various sites where the organism may be carried and tests of function should be made so far as possible in relation to the kidney, liver, muscle, central nervous system and blood platelets.

Treatment

Crystalloid solutions and plasma should be given rapidly to reverse the hypotension. Methicillin or oxacillin 1–2 g every 4 hours can be administered to subdue the infection. Check for a retained tampon.

Prophylaxis

Strict genital hygiene should be maintained with frequent baths. Tampons must be changed frequently — 3–4 times daily and an external pad worn at night — no internal tampon.

Following recovery, checks should be made to see if the patient is still carrying staphylococci.

Finally

In many cases of vaginal discharge the bacterial population is mixed and no specific cause for the symptoms can be discovered. Sometimes the complaint has begun as a specific infection e.g. trichomonas, but other contaminants have overgrown the initial organism. Good hygiene is necessary to clear up the general growth. Subsequent tests may reveal the offending organism.

INFLAMMATION OF THE UPPER GYNAECOLOGICAL TRACT

This is the result of:

1. Spread from the lower tract of infections such as chlamydia, gonococcus or trichomonas and it begins in the cervix. It may not spread farther but it remains a potential threat.

or 2. Diseases blood-borne from other parts of the body.

or 3. A few cases may be related to obstetrical trauma or abortion.

CERVICAL ECTOPY

An overgrowth of columnar epithelium replacing the squamous epithelium round the cervical os. It has a raw appearance and a velvety feel. It is an ectopy of columnar epithelium and in modern terminology is so described. This is physiological and no treatment is required.

Aetiology:

1. Parturition:
2. Contraceptive pill.
3. Persistence of a condition which is normal in infancy.

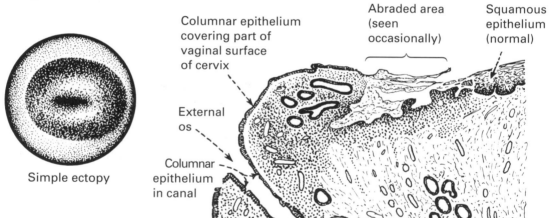

Simple ectopy

Columnar epithelium covering part of vaginal surface of cervix

External os

Columnar epithelium in canal

Abraded area (seen occasionally)

Squamous epithelium (normal)

CERVICITIS

An infection of the cervical epithelium and stroma, usually following ectopy.

Symptoms

There may be no symptoms with any of these conditions which are observed at examination, but usually there is a complaint of discharge, and they are potential causes of post-coital bleeding. Cervicitis has never been proved to have a special liability to malignant change.

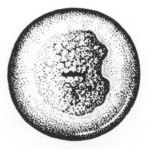

CERVICAL ECTOPY AND CERVICITIS

CRYOSURGERY This has been developed as an alternative to cautery and diathermy and is useful as an outpatient procedure.

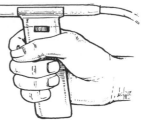

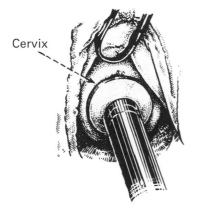

Cervix

The cryoprobe temperature is reduced to about -50°C over 2 minutes by the endothermic action of nitrous oxide, taking in its latent heat as it is decompressed after being forced at high pressure through a narrow orifice.

Treatment takes about 2 minutes and is almost painless. Extreme cold causes adherence between tissues and metal and 30 seconds must be allowed for thawing before the probe is removed. The patient will have a watery discharge for 2 weeks, and coitus should be avoided for a fortnight.

DIATHERMY

More extensive lesions must be treated by surgical excision or by diathermy.

In diathermy the infected tissue is destroyed by the great heat generated where the diathermy probe or point touches the cervix and sends high frequency current through the body to the indifferent electrode strapped to the leg.

The burnt tissue sloughs off over 2 weeks and the raw area is gradually re-epithelialised. This method requires general anaesthesia, and the discharge is more offensive than that following cryosurgery.

LASER

Laser therapy may be employed at a colposcopy clinic.

RARE CAUSES OF CERVICITIS

CHANCRE

Secondary infection is uncommon so the characteristic hard indurated base does not form. A chancre may be papular or ulcerative in which case it looks like an erosion. On palpation it may be mistaken for cancer.

A herpes simplex infection of the cervix may resemble a chancre.

TUBERCULOSIS

This is a very rare condition usually secondary to tubal and uterine infection and may be proliferative or ulcerative — in appearance not unlike ectopy.

It is usually found in association with chronic pelvic inflammation and infertility, and the diagnosis is histological.

If there is any doubt about the nature of a cervical lesion, a biopsy should always be taken before employing cryosurgery, diathermy or laser.

155

INFECTION OF THE UTERUS

ENDOMETRITIS

Acute inflammation may develop in response to infection following childbirth or abortion, or the insertion of a contraceptive device or as part of a gonorrhoeal infection. Actinomyces infection may be associated with neglected intra-uterine contraceptive devices and may be detected on a Papanicolaou smear.

Chronic Endometritis is a rare condition because of the frequency with which the endometrium is shed. The diagnosis is histological and there are no specific signs or symptoms, but the microscopic appearances are of infiltration mainly by plasma cells and lymphocytes. (For TB endometritis see p.159).

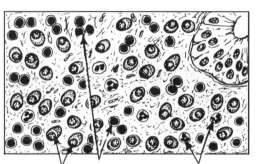

Plasma cells   Lymphocytes   Leucocytes

Senile Endometritis

Post-menopausal endometrium has little resistance to infection, and endometritis may arise from cervicitis or from tumour. If the cervix is stenosed by infection or tumour, the uterus becomes distended with pus and the condition is known as pyometra. Cervical dilatation will release the pus but curettage must be done to exclude malignancy and in such a situation it is very easy to perforate the uterus.

Metritis

Acute inflammation of the myometrium is a serious condition resulting from infection introduced during childbirth or abortion (see septic abortion p.342).

Treatment

If there is no organic cause, the menstrual irregularity may respond to sex steroid hormones. In the woman over 40 who wishes no more family, there is much to be said for simple hysterectomy. There may be a role here for progestogen releasing IUDs as these reduce the duration and amount of menstrual loss as well as giving excellent contraception.

PELVIC INFLAMMATORY DISEASE (PID)

Infection of the fallopian tubes usually involves the ovaries and peritoneum, and the combined infection is called pelvic inflammatory disease (PID). It results from ascending infection by microorganisms from the vagina or cervix. Its incidence is closely related to that of sexually transmitted diseases and it is predominantly a disease of young, sexually active, women.

ACUTE PID

The history is often of a prolonged period followed by the gradual onset of pelvic pain and irregular bleeding. The patient is pyrexial and on examination there is abdominal tenderness and guarding, and extreme tenderness of the vaginal fornices and cervical excitation.

Acute PID may follow operations, but it is usually a result of ascending infection, and may be associated with the intrauterine device. It must be treated actively to avoid the development of a chronic infection and minimise fallopian tube damage.

Bacteriology

It is unusual to be able to isolate pathogens from the infected area, but their demonstration in the cervix points to the probable cause.
N. gonorrhoea and Chlamydia trachomatis are said to be commonest, but anaerobic organisms are often found in pelvic abscesses. Bacterial vaginosis and mycoplasma have not been shown to cause acute PID.

Differential diagnosis

Appendicitis

Signs are mainly right sided, and the menstrual cycle is undisturbed.

Diverticulitis

This is a disease mainly of older women and signs are left sided.

Torsion of pedicle of a cyst

There may be a history of intermittent pain over several months. A cyst should be palpable.

Tubal pregnancy

The history may be helpful, but in young women in whom salpingitis and tubal pregnancy may co-cxist the distinction can be very difficult. A β-hCG pregnancy test aids diagnosis.

Management

A laparoscopy is advisable if there is any doubt, especially as this nearly always makes it possible to exclude tubal pregnancy. An intrauterine device, if in the uterus, should be removed. After swabs have been taken from the vagina and cervix a broad spectrum antibiotic such as doxycycline, azithromycin or ampicillin should be given. If acute signs and symptoms persist, a laparotomy should be carried out to search for abscess formation. No surgical procedure beyond drainage should be performed.

Referral to a genito-urinary medicine clinic is advisable. Without tracing and treatment of contacts, reinfection is likely. Acute PID may be relatively asymptomatic, but this does not preclude tubal damage, infertility and ectopic pregnancy. Ectopic pregnancy follows in almost 10% of subjects compared with a background rate of 1.5%.

PELVIC INFLAMMATORY DISEASE

CHRONIC PID

The patient complains of pelvic pain made worse during the periods which are irregular and heavy. Dyspareunia is common. There is a 10 fold increase in hysterectomy after PID.

Examination

Some swelling may be felt but often there is little to find except tenderness in the fornices. An exact diagnosis and estimate of the degree of PID cannot be made without laparoscopy.

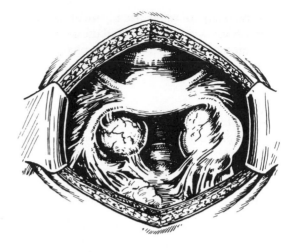

Pathology

All degrees of inflammation are met with from salpingitis alone to a widespread inflammatory reaction involving all the pelvic tissues. It is rare to recover any organism in chronic PID, other than in the case of tuberculosis. The ascending infection first attacks the tubes which are sealed off by oedema and adhesions. The tubes either swell up with watery exudate forming a hydrosalpinx or pyosalpinx; or they become very thickened and adherent to the ovary. The ovary may also be the seat of abscess formation, and the uterus and adnexa, normally mobile, become fixed by adhesions.

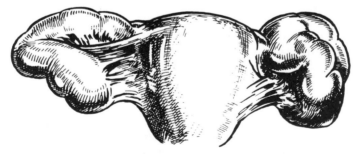

Blocked and distended tubes in PID

Treatment

The course of chronic PID is not predictable, and mild degrees may resolve spontaneously. In such cases the patient should be treated by rest, and although the infective organism may not be identified, a broad spectrum antibiotic is usually given. Hydrosalpinx and any abscess formation must be relieved by laparotomy and drainage, and dyspareunia may be relieved by correcting the uterine retroversion with a sling operation (p.237). In advanced cases however the only effective treatment is operation to remove the uterus and tubes and perhaps the ovaries as well.

GENITAL TUBERCULOSIS

Tuberculosis is a rare disease in gynaecology. It attacks the fallopian tubes and the endometrium, and lesions elsewhere in the genital tract are uncommon. It is possible that infection may be acquired from a sexual partner. The emergence of drug resistant strains of M.tuberculosis and the occurrence of tuberculosis in HIV-affected women and in developing countries may lead to a resurgence of genital tuberculosis.

Clinical Features

The patient is usually a young woman seeking treatment for primary infertility or complaining of irregular menstruation or perhaps abdominal pain.

Diagnosis

1. Histological evidence from curettings. This is the commonest method and it is assumed that the tubes are also infected.

2. Laboratory culture (formerly guinea-pig inoculation).

3. Biopsy from any suspicious ulcerated area in the vagina or vulva.

4. By laparoscopic inspection and biopsy.

Once evidence of genital infection is obtained, the respiratory and urinary tracts must also be investigated.

Pathology

This infection is blood borne, usually from a primary focus in the lung or kidney, and it infects the tubes, spreading thence to the endometrium.

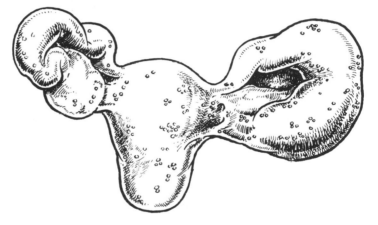

The tubes may appear normal (endosalpingitis) but usually display the distortion and swelling of chronic infection, and small pinhead tubercles appear on the serosa.

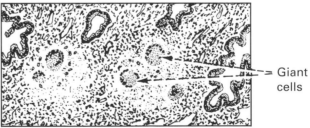

Giant cells

The endometrium also shows tuberculous follicles, best developed in the premenstrual phase. There may be debris in endometrial glands.

GENITAL TUBERCULOSIS

Treatment

Chemotherapy

A combination of rifampicin, isoniazid and ethambutol has been used effectively in recent years. Dosage is based on body weight and the first two drugs are given in combination for a year. The ethambutol is withdrawn after 90 days. Cure may be assumed if the endometrium shows no signs of tubercle, and the patient's menstrual cycle is normal.

Surgery

This means removal of uterus, tubes and ovaries, although conservation of one ovary would be permissible in a young woman. Surgery is indicated when chemotherapy has failed (about 5% of cases) or in combination with chemotherapy in the older woman. All infected tissue must be removed to avoid subsequent fistulous openings in bowel or bladder.

Tuberculosis and Infertility

Failure to conceive is probably the most important consequence of genital tuberculosis, and 90% of women presenting with the disease will never have a pregnancy. Pregnancy after successful treatment may be looked for in about 10% of patients, but there is a considerable chance of ectopic gestation.

ACQUIRED IMMUNE DEFICIENCY SYNDROME — AIDS

AIDS is now the most serious of all gynaecological infections. It was first recognised as a new entity in 1981. It has reached pandemic proportions affecting almost all countries and regions. In some parts of the world such as the sub-Sahara region of Africa and in some sections of the public in western countries, e.g. drug addicts in the USA, there are epidemics. The incidence is low in Arab countries. It is due to the human immune deficiency virus (HIV) or, in scientific terms, retrovirus oncornavirus.

Transmission
There are several modes of infection and risk factors.

A. **Sexual**
1.   Relationships with prostitutes. Multiplicity of sexual partners increases the risks. The same dangers exist with promiscuity.
2.   Male homosexual activities. Again there are likely to be multiple partners.
3.   Sexual contact with individuals of the same or opposite sex in southern parts of Africa.
4.   Abrasions around the genital or anal regions increase the risk of infection.

B. **Non-sexual**
1.   Addicts using needles in common for intravenous drug injections. Although some authorities provide a free supply of sterile needles the very nature of drug-taking induces carelessness.
2.   Injection of blood or blood products can be dangerous if proper precautions are not employed. For a time and in certain areas, Factor VIII treatment for haemophilia was associated with the occurrence of AIDS in a number of patients. This was due to using contaminated blood for Factor VIII preparations. The danger has been eliminated by heating all Factor VIII material to destroy the virus. The same potential danger exists in relation to blood or plasma for transfusion. Blood donors require rigorous testing for evidence of viral infection. Production of fractions by re-combinant DNA techniques avoids the risk of HIV contamination.
3.   Surgical injuries or needle-stick injuries in the course of treating infected subjects. Hepatitis is actually more infectious than HIV.

It is difficult to provide an adequate description of this disease. The symptomatology is such that almost every organ may appear to be affected at one time or another. There is a mixture of:
1.   Constitutional disease with fever, sweating, etc.
2.   Neurological symptoms and lesions.
3.   Malignant tumours.
4.   Liver or renal failure.
5.   Secondary infections.

The course of the disease is erratic, associated with progressive loss of immune resistance. Death is almost inevitable but may be delayed for years. To understand the main features of the disease it is necessary to recall some of the mechanisms involved in the normal immune process.

NORMAL IMMUNE MECHANISM

This depends upon the activities of lymphocytes, of which there are two basic types, B and T.

B lymphocytes
These are so called because they were first discovered in the bursa of Fabricius in the bowel of chickens.

When the body is invaded by a foreign antigen, such as in an infection, B lymphocytes are transformed and become plasma cells capable of secreting specific antibodies into the tissues and blood causing destruction of the antigen. This reaction is very rapid, almost immediate, and results in humoral immunity.

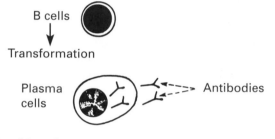

These B cells form 25% of the blood lymphocytes.

T lymphocytes are named thus because they are processed in the Thymus. They form 70% of blood lymphocytes.

T cells are also stimulated by foreign antigens and undergo transformation into several specific types whose function is to control and aid the B cells. There are 3 main types:

1. T cells which control the production of B cell antibodies.

2. T cells which control the over-all production of lymphocytes.

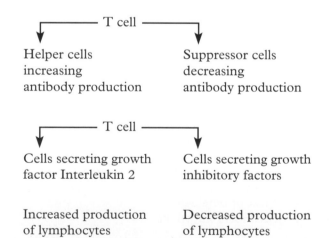

These changes in T cells follow the B cell phase and are therefore delayed. They produce cell mediated immunity. The various activities of the T cells make certain, in normal circumstances, that the immune reaction is tailored to the needs of the body at any particular phase of infection.

162

3. Killer cells. These kill other cells by direct contact if the latter have been infected.

HIV INFECTION AND THE IMMUNE SYSTEM

The Human Immunodeficiency Virus (HIV) and the B lymphocytes

The reaction is very slow and up to 6 months may elapse before antibodies appear in the blood. Usually, however, their appearance coincides with the eruption of symptoms. They seem to have little or no influence on the course of the disease and in the later stages they may disappear from the blood.

HIV and the T cells

Although B cells react and produce antibodies, initially it is the effect of HIV on the T cells which ultimately destroys the whole immune apparatus. The virus attacks T cells, especially those of the helper variety commonly called T4 lymphocytes which stimulate production of antibodies and increase the number of lymphocytes.

Curiously one of the antigens of these lymphocytes, the differentiation antigen CD4, has an affinity for the virus and acts as a receptor. On the other hand, although brain tissue and muscle may be infected by the virus, there is no CD4 antigen to act as a receptor in these regions.

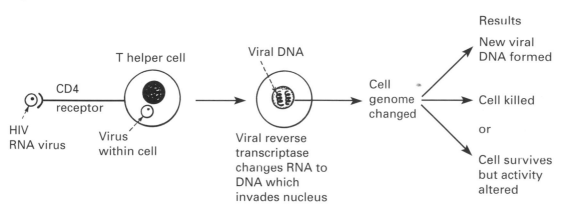

Ultimately there is a progressive lymphopenia affecting both B and T cells.

T cells also influence polymorphs and macrophages in much the same way as lymphocytes. Normally, in infection they increase chemotaxis and phagocytosis. With HIV infection these activities will diminish and this explains the ease with which secondary infections by organisms of very low pathogenicity can establish themselves, spread rapidly and cause septicaemia.

ACQUIRED IMMUNE DEFICIENCY SYNDROME — AIDS

The progress of the disease can be roughly divided into 4 phases, but these phases are ill-defined, variable in time of onset and duration.

Phase 1
Following infection there may be no symptoms but in a considerable proportion of infected individuals an acute illness resembling infectious mononucleosis appears with fever, night sweats, enlarged lymph nodes, diarrhoea and a blood lymphocytosis. Antibody formation occurs. In other individuals this feverish episode is delayed for varying periods.

Phase 2
A symptomless period usually ensues which may last for 7 years or more. Despite the lack of symptoms the virus goes on replicating within the body. During this period there is frequently enlargement of lymph nodes in various parts of the body. As a result the name 'Persistent generalised lymphadenopathy' is often applied to indicate a particular phase.

Phase 3
This is the turning point in the disease when the virus has replicated and is beginning to reduce the ability of the patient to mount an effective immune response to ordinary infections. Symptoms of the type observed in the initial phase may reappear. Further development means a change from mere infection by HIV to full-blown AIDS syndrome. Fifty per cent of infected individuals progress to phase 4 within 10 years. The phrase 'AIDS related complex' is used to indicate a particular stage in the disease but this phrase is not particularly useful because of the erratic behaviour of the infection.

Phase 4
The final phase is characterised by repeated attacks of intercurrent infection due to progressive immuno-deficiency. The core antigen increases. T4 helper lymphocytes progressively diminish. The viral DNA is integrated into the genome of infected cells producing more HIV.

Pneumonia due to pneumocystis carinii is one of the commonest complications but the list of secondary infections is very large and includes parasites, viruses, bacteria, fungi etc. They are almost entirely of the type which cause minor, localised lesions in normally immune individuals, but in AIDS patients they spread rapidly and can be fatal.

Three conditions are particularly characteristic of the immuno-deficiency state:
1. Kaposi sarcoma, usually an indolent growth in the skin, becomes aggressive.
2. Hairy leukoplakia of the tongue.
3. Lymphomas are common in AIDS patients and lymphoma of the brain is almost diagnostic.

ACQUIRED IMMUNE DEFICIENCY SYNDROME — AIDS

Intercurrent infections frequently found in AIDS patients

Minor infections and infestations which remain localised in normally immune persons and produce mild symptoms if any, spread rapidly and cause life-threatening clinical conditions in the AIDS patient whose immunity is seriously compromised.

Infective Agents	Clinical Results
Parasites	
Pneumocystis carinii	Pneumonia
Cryptosporidium	Severe diarrhoea
Strongyloides stercoralis	Severe diarrhoea
Toxoplasma gondii	Chorio-retinitis
Viruses	
Herpes	Pneumonia
J.C. virus	Leuco-encephalopathy
Bacteria	
Species usually causing .... minor lesions e.g. skin spots	Septicaemia
Fungi	
Cryptococcus neoformans	Pneumonia Meningitis

The final condition of the patient is pathetic due to these infections, wasting and possibly dementia.

Paediatric AIDS

Infection of the fetus or newborn from the mother can occur in utero, intrapartum or, through breast feeding, post-partum. Zidovudine has been shown to reduce vertical transmission of HIV-1.

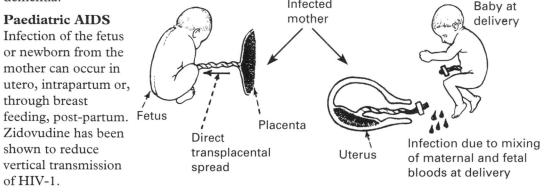

Infected mother

Baby at delivery

Fetus

Direct transplacental spread

Placenta

Uterus

Infection due to mixing of maternal and fetal bloods at delivery

Spread to the offspring occurs in one third of all AIDS patients. Symptoms are similar to those occurring in the adult but, in addition, lymphoid interstitial pneumonia and parotid gland enlargement occur in the infant.

Initial tests for antibody may be positive in the infant but if they become negative the child is not infected. If infection has occurred further tests at 15 months will be positive. In most cases of infection however, the child dies within 1 year.

Haemophilic children who were infected by contaminated Factor VIII show a slow progress of the syndrome with prolonged asymptomatic periods.

165

ACQUIRED IMMUNE DEFICIENCY SYNDROME — AIDS

Management

With the rapid spread of HIV infection it is inevitable that general practitioners will be drawn into the treatment and management of cases. The practitioner should take all precautionary measures in the way of protective clothing including disposable gloves, and should arrange for some method of dealing with blood which may be spilled. In regard to the patient the following routine should be established.

1. Regular follow up every 3 months to determine progress.
2. Check weight.
3. Full blood count.
4. Erythrocyte sedimentation rate.
5. Examine especially for tumour growth e.g. Kaposi sarcoma, lymphoma.
6. Watch for opportunistic infection and treat immediately.
7. Arrange for expert psychological handling when necessary.
8. If possible leave HIV positive cases who require surgery to the end of a list so that special precautions can be observed.

Prevention of spread

1. Educate patients regarding risks of multiple sexual partners.
2. Indicate the use of barrier contraception.
3. Blood for transfusion must always be tested for HIV antibodies. If circumstances make this impossible, withdraw blood from the patient and store for future use.
4. In cases of infertility where donor semen is to be used for in vitro fertilisation, store it in cryo-preservation conditions for 3 months until certain that the donor is free of infection.
5. There are a large number of factors which can only be controlled by education and legislation. Some of these are:
   (a) Drug production, pushing and dealing.
   (b) Drug consumption.
   (c) All new drugs or other substances which may be habit forming.
   (d) Prostitution, both male and female.
   (e) The current fashion of casual sex. Television, newspapers and magazines must bear a great deal of blame for this.

Ethical considerations

Guidelines have been laid down by the General Medical Council and the British Medical Association. The main features are:

1. Confidentiality must be maintained at all times. The only exception to this rule is when the practitioner establishes that the health of another person is threatened. This must be explained to the parties concerned.
2. Tests must not be carried out without the consent of the patient.
3. Care must be exercised in dealing with the family and sexual partner of the patient. It is essential to establish a frank and open relationship with the patient so that both practitioner and patient can trust each other and all matters can be discussed freely.
4. Doctors who are themselves HIV positive must make every effort to protect patients, limiting their practice including treatment methods such as minor surgical procedures which carry a risk of transmitting the infection.

ACQUIRED IMMUNE DEFICIENCY SYNDROME — AIDS

Treatment

Specialised knowledge and experience are essential. Earlier forms of treatment were aimed at preventing and treating secondary infection in the final phases of the disease. They were directed especially at pneumonia due to pneumocystis carinii which is common in these patients and, if untreated, causes death within 1 year.

Drugs have been used in a prophylactic manner to prevent secondary infection occurring. There are several preparations but some, such as nebulised pentamidine, while being effective against pneumocystis, are too specific and have no influence on other common infections such as toxoplasmosis. Oral drugs e.g. co-trimoxazole, sulpha-methoxazole-pyrimethamine, dapsone and dapsone-pyrimethamine, have a more general action.

Four methods of treating or preventing the viral infection itself are in various stages of development:

1. Anti-viral drugs

These show some promise but whether they can produce a cure or merely modify the course of the disease is not yet clear. Zidovudine, lamivudine, indinavir, didanosine, nevirapine and didoxyinosine are such. The last has a disadvantage in that diabetes mellitus and Raynaud's syndrome have occurred during therapy. Combination therapies are more effective than single agents.

2. Gene therapy

An altered virus, a so-called mirror image of the AIDS virus has been constructed. The apparent idea is that the individual will be 'infected' with the artificial virus which will then occupy the viral receptors on T lymphocytes thus preventing entry of the AIDS virus and protecting the immune system.

3. Vaccination

It is obviously impossible to use whole AIDS antigen for vaccination for fear of actually infecting the individual. Sub-units of the antigen have been used and there are indications of some success but, unfortunately, while treatment may protect against systemic infection there is no protection against the mucosal invasion during sexual activity. There is also evidence that the antigenic sub-units can vary and so also does the degree of immunity.

4. A new drug treatment with **benzodiazepine derivatives** is being tried.

These drugs are known to interfere with reverse transcriptase reaction and would therefore stop the replication process.

A new viral disease similar to AIDS and named HIV2 has appeared in West Africa. It produces a milder symptomatic form of the disease but can end in the fully developed AIDS. Already it has spread to France, Portugal and West African communities in Britain, especially London. It is believed to have originated in West African Mangabey monkey species, whereas HIV-1 and HIV-0 came from chimpanzee hosts.

CHAPTER 8

DISEASES OF THE VULVA

VULVAL DERMATOSES

The skin of the vulva appears to react differently from skin elsewhere. It is more easily irritated by friction and by local application of antiseptic, anaesthetic and antihistamine creams, and it has long been recognised that the treatment of vulval carcinoma by radiotherapy produces a much more intense inflammatory reaction in vulval skin than in other parts of the epidermis. Transepidermal water loss is higher in the vulva, and it more readily becomes dry and irritable.

Vulval dermatoses is the term applied to non-infective non-neoplastic diseases of the vulval skin. Their management is moving more and more into the province of the dermatologist, but the symptoms of itching, soreness and dyspareunia will usually take the patient in the first place to the gynaecologist.

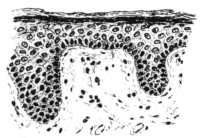

Normal vulva

Classification

The following classification is recommended by the International Society for the Study of Vulvar Disease (1989)

A.   Non-neoplastic disorders of the vulva
    lichen sclerosus
    squamous cell hyperplasia
    other dermatoses

B.   Vulval intraepithelial neoplasia (VIN)
    Squamous VIN
        VIN 1 — mild dysplasia
        VIN 2 — moderate dysplasia
        VIN 3 — severe dysplasia/carcinoma in situ
    Paget's disease

VULVAL DERMATOSES

LICHEN SCLEROSUS

Lichen sclerosus is the commonest condition found in elderly women complaining of vulval itch. The aetiology is unknown, but it appears to be associated with autoimmune disorders.

Although the disease can affect both sexes at all ages in any area of skin, it is most commonly seen in the vulvo-perineal skin of middle-aged women.

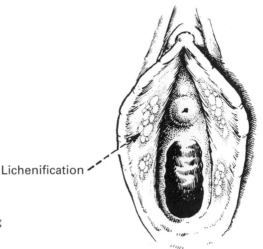

Lichenification

Appearance

The disease starts as a flat pinkish-white macula. The vulval contours disappear, and adhesions may form between the labia. Scratching may induce lichenification (thickening).

Histology

There is atrophic thinning of the epidermis with some hyalinisation of the dermis. The keratinised layer is thickened, giving a whitened appearance ('leukoplakia').

Some hyperkeratosis   Thin atrophic epithelium

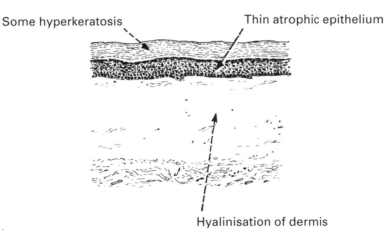

Hyalinisation of dermis

Management

1. Asymptomatic: no treatment
2. Itching may be relieved by one of the following:
    aqueous cream
    1% hydrocortisone tds
    more potent steroid (eg. clobetasol proprionate) for a short period
    2% testosterone ointment bd for six weeks

There is no place for vulvectomy in the management of this condition.

Malignant associations

There is uncertainty about the risk of malignant transformation in women with lichen sclerosus. A recent estimate suggests that 4% of women with lichen sclerosus will develop invasive cancer.

171

BENIGN TUMOURS OF THE VULVA

The complaint is usually of a 'lump' or 'swelling' at the vaginal introitus. (In many cases the patient may mistake prolapse of various types or hernia for tumour growth.)

NON-NEOPLASTIC SWELLINGS

These are the result of blockage of ducts of glands, congenital malformations or due to trauma.

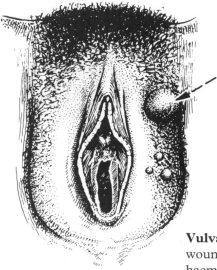

Cyst of Bartholin's gland This is the commonest simple tumour of the vulva. Caused by obstruction of the duct, the cyst almost always becomes infected and requires surgical treatment (see p.137).

Sebaceous cyst of the vulva occurs in the hairy region of the labium majus. The cyst may become infected and cause pain. On examination, multiple cysts are usually found, mostly small. If painful they can be removed. The cyst contains whitish, cheesy sebaceous material.

Vulval varicosities may produce tumour-like swellings. Treatment is by excision or injection of sclerosing agents.

Vulval haematoma is a result of direct violence or wounding (it is most commonly found with childbirth). The haematoma spreads widely because of the loose tissue structure. Treatment is by incision, evacuation and drainage.

Endometriosis is uncommon in the labia majora or other parts of the vulva. It may enlarge and become tender during menstruation. Treatment is by excision.

Ectopic breast tissue may enlarge during pregnancy.

NEOPLASTIC SWELLINGS

Lipoma is found rarely. It arises from the subcutaneous tissues of the vulva and usually becomes pedunculated and dependent with growth. Treatment is by excision.

Fibroma is also uncommon but presents as a pedunculated tumour like a lipoma but is firmer. It arises from the fibrous tissue of the round ligament and the vulvar connective tissue. Treatment is by excision. Very rarely it is found to be a myoma. These tumours on occasion become sarcomatous.

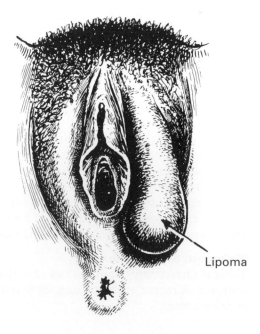

Lipoma

VIN

VULVAR INTRA-EPITHELIAL NEOPLASIA (VIN)

In all cases of marked 'dermatosis' the possibility of early malignant change should be considered. It is helpful to apply acetic acid to the area. Areas of hyperplasia show up as white spots. These can then be biopsied and studied microscopically.

VIN is a multifocal disease with histological features and terminology similar to that of CIN. The malignant potential of VIN is thought to be less than that of CIN.

VIN may present with vulval pruritus. Alternatively, VIN may be found when the vulva is biopsied after treatment for preinvasive cervical carcinoma.

Treatment of VIN

There is uncertainty about the best treatment for VIN. The following are treatment options:

1. careful observation only
2. topical steroids
3. excision biopsy
4. CO_2 laser vaporisation.

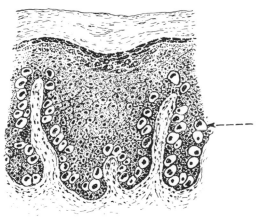

PAGET's DISEASE of the VULVA (Adenocarcinoma in situ)

This malignant disease starts as an erythematous, irritant plaque which becomes eczematous (oedema and exudate) and spreads. Histology shows the characteristic Paget's cells — large round, clear-staining cells with large nuclei, often mitotic. Adenocarcinoma of the apocrine glands is found in one third of patients. In a proportion of the remainder, there is cancer of the vulva, cervix, bladder, ovary or other organs. Total vulvectomy is the treatment of choice.

CARCINOMA OF THE VULVA

Incidence: 3 per 100 000 per year (UK)

Aetiology
The aetiology of vulval cancer is unknown.
Some vulval cancers contain viral antigens
(e.g. HSV 2), but the importance of these in
the aetiology of the disease is uncertain.

Histology
Squamous carcinoma: 85%
Melanoma: 5%

Clinical features
The majority of patients with vulval cancer are
over 60. The presenting features include vulval
irritation and pruritus (70%), a vulval mass (60%)
and bleeding (30%).

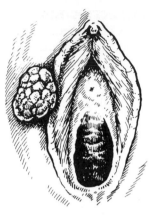

Squamous carcinoma

The diagnosis is often delayed, partly due to the patient's reluctance to seek medical help,
and partly due to delay in performing a clinical examination once the patient presents.

Any lump on the vulva must be examined and biopsied.

The inguinal lymph nodes may be enlarged, but absence of enlargement does not guarantee
absence of lymphatic spread.

The FIGO staging of vulvar cancer (1995)

Stage	Definition
Stage Ia	Confined to vulva and/or perineum, 2 cm or less maximum diameter. Groin nodes not palpable. Stromal invasion no greater than 1 mm
Stage Ib	As for Ia but stromal invasion greater than 1 mm
Stage II	Confined to vulva and/or perineum, more than 2 cm maximum diameter. Groin nodes not palpable
Stage III	Extends beyond the vulva, vagina, lower urethra or anus; or unilateral regional lymph node metastasis
Stage IVa	Involves the mucosa of rectum or bladder; upper urethra; or pelvic bone; and/or bilateral regional lymph node metastases
Stage IVb	Any distant metastasis, including pelvic lymph node

CARCINOMA OF THE VULVA

LYMPHATIC SPREAD

1. To the superficial inguinal glands which lie along the inguinal ligament and the saphenous vein (vertical group). These nodes lie between the layers of the superficial fascia in relation to numerous superficial vessels.

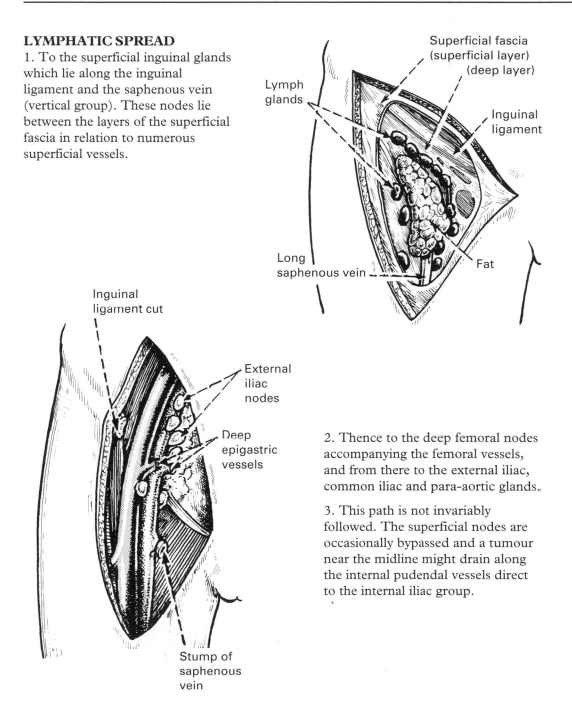

2. Thence to the deep femoral nodes accompanying the femoral vessels, and from there to the external iliac, common iliac and para-aortic glands.

3. This path is not invariably followed. The superficial nodes are occasionally bypassed and a tumour near the midline might drain along the internal pudendal vessels direct to the internal iliac group.

175

CARCINOMA OF THE VULVA

Surgical treatment
Surgery is the optimum treatment for vulval cancer. The conventional operation is radical vulvectomy with dissection of the superficial and deep inguinal glands and the external iliac glands. Such surgery has increased the five year survival for the disease which is now 75%.

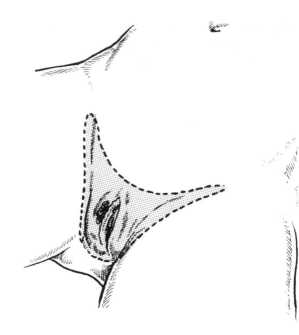

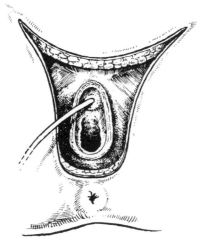

The whole vulva, skin and subcutaneous tissue are excised down to the periosteum.

The wound should be closed completely if possible, undercutting and mobilising skin if necessary. In this picture closure is incomplete, but the small raw area should heal in a few weeks. Drains are shown which remain in place for the first few days.

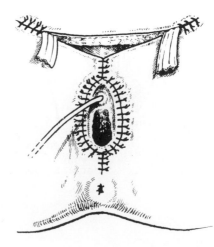

CARCINOMA OF THE VULVA

Radical vulvectomy with en bloc dissection and removal of the inguinal and iliac lymph glands is associated with significant morbidity. The following variations in technique have been introduced to reduce morbidity.

1. Separate groin incisions
In vuval cancer, lymphatic metastases develop initially by embolisation. In early disease there is no need to remove the lymphatic channels between the tumour and the groin nodes. Therefore, three separate incisions can be used to remove the tumour and the nodes on each side. Such an approach is associated with lower morbidity than conventional surgery.

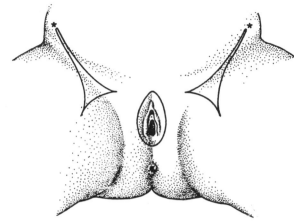

2. Modified radical vulvectomy
If the primary tumour is small, and confined to one area, a more limited operation may be as effective as radical vulvectomy. In modified radical vulvectomy, the lesion and surrounding area is removed, leaving the reminder of the perineum intact. A 2–3 cm margin of healthy tissue should be removed along with the tumour.

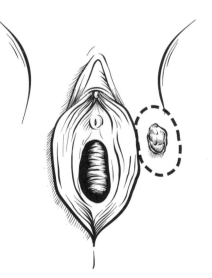

3. Ipsilateral lymphadenectomy
If the tumour is confined to one side of the vulva only and the groin nodes appear clinically tumour free, ipsilateral lymphadenectomy may be sufficient to detect lymph node disease. However, if tumour is found in the ipsilateral lymph nodes, the opposite groin should also be explored.

177

CARCINOMA OF THE VULVA

Complications
1. Wound breakdown and infection.
   The incidence of this complication is reduced by the use of the three incision technique.
2. Thromboembolic disease.
   This may be minimised by the use of subcutaneous heparin.
3. Secondary haemorrhage.
4. Chronic leg oedema.
5. Paraesthesia over the upper legs.
6. Impaired sexual function.

Prognosis of vulval carcinoma
The prognosis depends on the staging, the more advanced the disease, the worse the prognosis. In a recent British series, the overall five year survival was 75%.

Radiotherapy
Radiotherapy is useful for treatment of groin node disease after inguinofemoral lymphadenectomy. Pre-operative radiotherapy has been used for advanced tumours. In the situation (rare nowadays) where the patient is unfit for surgery, radiotherapy is preferable to no treatment.

DISEASES OF THE URETHRA

PROLAPSE of the URETHRAL MUCOSA

This forms a swelling round the meatus. Symptomatic urethral mucosal prolapse may be treated by cautery.

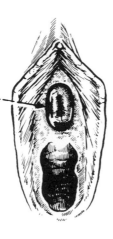

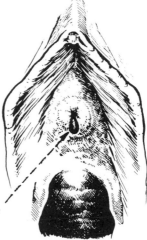

CARUNCLE

A small tumour arising from the lower end of the urethra. It is composed of a very vascular stroma, almost a haemangioma, usually infected and covered with squamous or transitional epithelium.

Clinical Features

Caruncles are red in colour because of their vascularity, and extremely sensitive. The patient is usually an elderly woman complaining of dysuria and bleeding.

Treatment

Caruncles should be excised and sent for histological examination although malignant change is rare. The base of the tumour on the urethral mucosa should be cauterised.

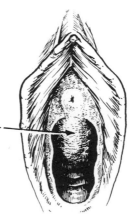

URETHROCELE

This is a descent of the urethra from its position under the pubic arch. It is sometimes a cause of stress incontinence and may exist by itself or in company with a cystocele.

Treatment is described in the section on prolapse.

OPERATIONS ON THE PERINEUM: POSTERIOR REPAIR

Posterior colpoperineorrhaphy

The indications for this operation are the treatment of rectocele (enterocele repair is covered in chapter 12). Women should only be treated if they are symptomatic, since over enthusiastic surgery will lead to coital difficulties.

The operation may be difficult if there is scarring from a previous episiotomy or tear. Care should be taken not to damage the rectum, which is close to the overlying vaginal skin and levator muscle.

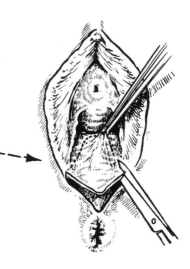

1. The vaginal wall has been dissected off the perineum and rectum. Excess tissue is being excised.

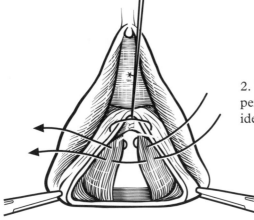

2. The levator and other perineal muscles are identified and opposed.

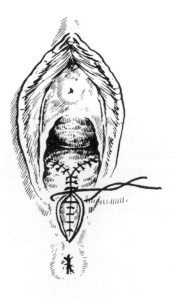

3. The skin is closed in the usual manner.

OPERATION FOR ENLARGING THE VAGINAL OUTLET

PERINEOPLASTY

The principle is to divide all the fibres of the perineal body except the anal sphincter.

1. Making the longitudinal incision through skin and muscle. The finger in the rectum allows the surgeon to know how near his knife is to the rectal wall.

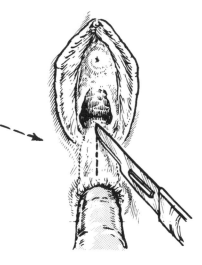

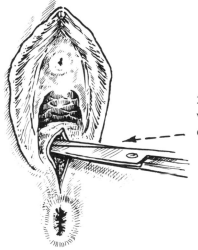

2. The cut muscles retract laterally, and the vaginal wall is further mobilised to allow closure without tension.

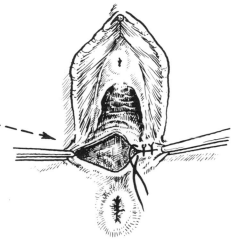

3. The longitudinal wound is then closed transversely with interrupted sutures.

Vaginal dilators are used once the sutures are removed and continued with for several weeks until all tenderness is gone and coitus can be resumed.

CHAPTER 9

DISEASES OF THE VAGINA

CYSTS OF THE VAGINA

Vaginal cysts are relatively common but rarely large. They are found in the anterior or lateral walls of the lower third of the vagina and in the posterior wall of the upper third, seldom larger than a walnut, sometimes multiple, and may be mistaken for a cystocele. These cysts are occasionally a cause of dyspareunia but usually cause no symptoms at all.

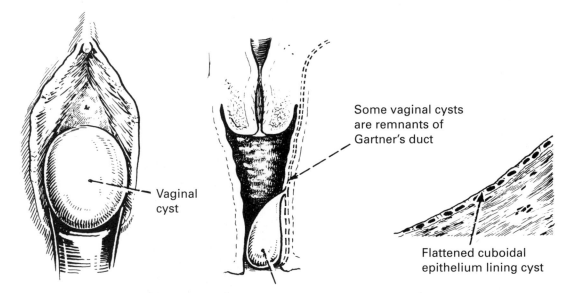

Vaginal cyst

Some vaginal cysts are remnants of Gartner's duct

Flattened cuboidal epithelium lining cyst

Treatment is by excision or marsupialisation.

TRAUMATIC EPITHELIAL CYSTS (inclusion cysts) are found usually in the lower vagina, and are caused by infolding of epithelium at repair operations. If they cause symptoms they should be excised or marsupialised.

VAGINAL INFECTIONS See pages 135–167.

VAGINAL INTRAEPITHELIAL NEOPLASIA (VAIN)
This is similar to CIN I to III but remains superficial until an invasive tumour develops as the vaginal epithelium lacks the crypts of cervical epithelium. VAIN may be buried at vault closure after hysterectomy. Rarely, it is seen after radiotherapy to the cervix.

Diagnosis is by colposcopy (technically difficult access) or by histology after hysterectomy.

Treatment may be by CO_2 laser, but after hysterectomy surgical excision is essential because VAIN may be buried above the vault closure. Radiotherapy may be employed in older patients in whom access for surgery may be difficult.

CARCINOMA OF THE VAGINA

Primary growths of the vagina are rare and the average gynaecologist will see only one such tumour for 30 of the cervix. Pre-invasive lesions (VAIN) are now more frequently diagnosed. They may proceed to cancer. There is little evidence for radiotherapy as a cause and intra-uterine exposure to di-ethyl stilboestrol (DES) in fact carried a very low risk of causing vaginal cancer as opposed to vaginal adenosis. Secondary growths are more common, especially extension from cervical cancer, and metastatic deposits may appear from disease elsewhere in the body.

Clinical Features

The patient is usually menopausal and most commonly complains of bleeding (60%). Discharge (15%) and pelvic pain (10% or less) may be present. If the bladder is involved, she will experience pain and dysuria.

The tumour is not at first painful and unless it appears in a woman who is still sexually active, it is not likely to present until it has penetrated the vaginal wall and caused bleeding. Old women often believe or affect to believe that all bleeding is from haemorrhoids.

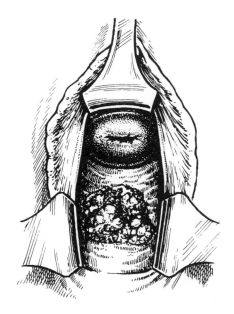

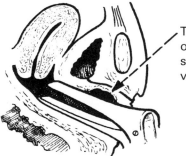

Tumour obscured by speculum in vagina

An early tumour can easily be missed if it is obscured by the blade of a metal speculum. The whole vagina should always be inspected, and cytological smears taken from any lesion at all unusual.

Colposcopy, cystoscopy and proctosigmoidoscopy are indicated to detect spread.

Histology

Eighty-five per cent are squamous carcinomas, occurring in women over 60. The remainder include melanoma, sarcoma, adenocarcinoma and clear cell carcinoma, all of which tend to be associated with middle-aged or even young women.

185

CARCINOMA OF THE VAGINA

Site and Spread

Tumours of the lower third (25–30% of cases) have a much poorer prognosis than those of the upper and middle thirds, partly because spread to the inguinal nodes is quicker and because of the danger to the bladder.

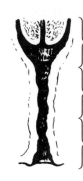

Upper third: approximately same drainage as cervix.

Middle third: any pelvic lymphatic channel may be involved.

Lower third: approximately same drainage as vulva.

Clinical staging		Five Year Survival Rates
Stage 0	Intraepithelial carcinoma.	Should be curable. Beware buried VAIN
Stage I	Invasive. Confined to the vaginal mucosa.	75-90%
Stage II	Invading subvaginal tissues, but not to pelvic wall.	45%
Stage III	Extension to the pelvic wall.	30-40%
Stage IVa	Extension to mucosa of bladder or rectum.	$\not> 20\%$
Stage IVb	Extension beyond the pelvis.	$\not< 20\%$

Prognosis depends on the stage, which depends on when the patient goes to her doctor, and on the position in the vagina. The lower third with its much quicker lymphatic spread is the least favourable.

Treatment

In stage 0 growths, good results have been obtained with local application of 5-fluorouracil cream, but for stage I onwards, radiotherapy is the usual treatment.
1. It can be applied at any stage.
2. It is more readily available than skilled radical surgery.
3. The patients are often elderly and poor surgical risks.

Radical surgery (radical hysterectomy, vaginectomy, lymphadenectomy) is claimed to give good results in experienced hands, and a cure rate of over 80% has been achieved for stage I. In stage IV where radiotherapy is only palliative, surgery which includes some form of exenteration is the better treatment if the patient is fit and the gynaecologist has the necessary experience.

Vaginal melanoma is almost always fatal, with poor results from radiotherapy and no appropriate chemotherapy available.

Sarcoma botrioides is a rare tumour of young children, presenting as grape-like masses with bleeding. Chemotherapy with vincristine, actinomycin D and cyclophosphamide gives good results.

PLASTIC SURGERY OF THE VAGINA

This is required when the patient is prevented from coitus by congenital absence of the vagina or by distortion and contractures due to injury. Such a situation is rare; but various operations have been devised. Small bowel has been used successfully in male to female sex change procedures.

The McIndoe-Bannister Operation — using a free skin graft from the thigh.

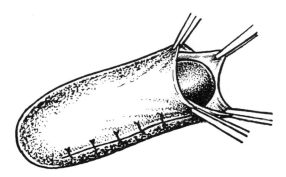

1. A plastic mould is covered with skin from the thigh. (This is done by a plastic surgeon.)

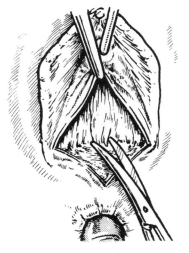

2. The space between urethra/bladder and rectum is opened up. The finger in the anus helps the surgeon to avoid damaging the rectum.

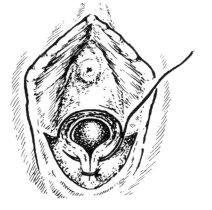

3. Mould and graft are inserted and kept in place by suturing the split ends of the labia minora. (The vaginal orifice may need enlarging later on.)

The mould must be kept in situ for several months and once it is removed the patient should have regular and frequent coitus to prevent contraction of the new vagina.

The main complications to be avoided are graft failure due to venous oozing or sepsis; and pressure necrosis of bladder or rectal wall from too large a mould.

187

PLASTIC SURGERY OF THE VAGINA

Williams' Operation
The formation of a cul-de-sac by suturing the labia majora in two layers. This means that the anterior wall of the new 'vagina' is the vulva. It is a simple operation which seems to provide a satisfying coitus for both parties.

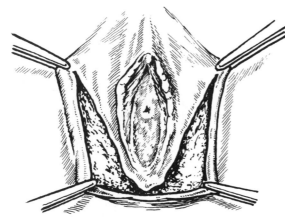

1. The labia majora are split down to the perineal muscles. Bleeding is copious.

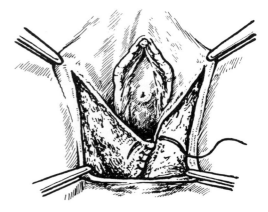

2. The inner margins of the labia are sutured together.

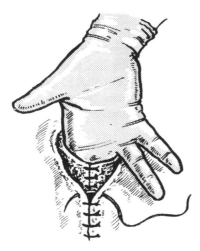

3. The outer margins are sutured. The resulting cavity should accommodate two fingers.

Other methods include the use of pedicle grafts from the labia, and encouraging natural epithelialisation of the dissected cavity without any grafting. There is sometimes a rudimentary vaginal depression already developed which can be enlarged to a functional size by using a pessary to maintain prolonged upward pressure.

CHAPTER 10

DISEASES OF THE CERVIX

NORMAL CERVICAL EPITHELIUM

ANATOMY OF THE CERVIX

The cervix constitutes the lower third of the uterus.

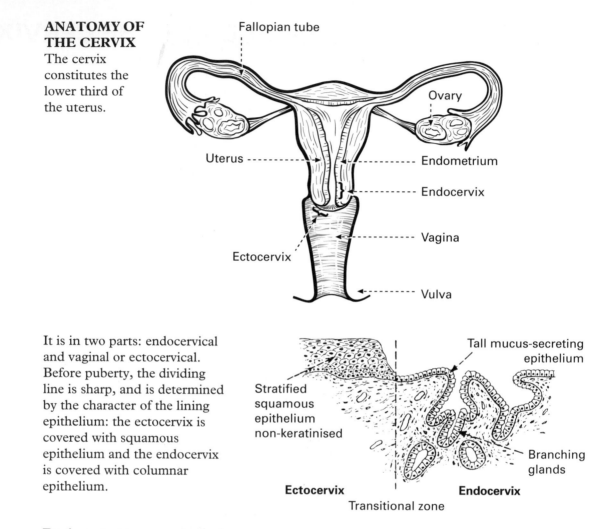

It is in two parts: endocervical and vaginal or ectocervical. Before puberty, the dividing line is sharp, and is determined by the character of the lining epithelium: the ectocervix is covered with squamous epithelium and the endocervix is covered with columnar epithelium.

Benign squamous metaplasia

Stratification well defined with:

Squames at surface

Oval polygonal cells form several layers

Basal cells usually a single layer at right angles to the surface

Under the influence of oestrogen (e.g. at puberty, during pregnancy or when the combined pill is taken), the cervix enlarges, so that the columnar epithelium of the endocervix can be seen on the ectocervix. This region, formerly endocervix which is now anatomically ectocervix, is known as the 'transformation zone'. The transformation zone undergoes squamous metaplasia, which is a benign condition. Occasionally, the transformation zone gives rise to dysplastic change, and ultimately, cervical cancer.

CERVICAL DYSPLASIA

DYSPLASIA

Dysplasia is when the squamous epithelium shows a degree of proliferative activity with some cellular atypia. It is regarded as the first of a series of changes which may lead to **cervical intra-epithelial neoplasia (CIN)** and subsequently to invasive carcinoma. The pathological features of mild, moderate and severe dysplasia are shown. In practice there is significant inter- and intra-observer variation between these categories.

CIN 1 ≡ mild dysplasia

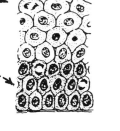

Upper two thirds stratified squames i.e. normal

Cells of basal third have high nucleocytoplasmic ratio; pleomorphic nuclei in layers at this level.

CIN 2 ≡ moderate dysplasia

Upper half of epithelium shows stratification and maturation

Abnormal basal cells occupy lower half →

CIN 3 ≡ severe dysplasia

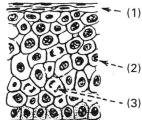

(1) There may be one or two layers of stratified epithelium on surface.

(2) Remainder is immature with large nuclei.

(3) Mitoses are common.

Risk of progression of cervical dysplasia

The risk of progression of CIN I to CIN III has been estimated at 25% over a two year period.

The risk of progression of CIN to invasive cancer is difficult to quantify. However, in women with CIN III who received treatment which was unsuccessful, 30–40% developed invasive cancer within 20 years.

CARCINOMA OF THE CERVIX

SCREENING FOR CERVICAL CANCER

Premalignant cervical conditions can be detected by performing cervical smears in all women, and colposcopy in women who have an abnormal smear. Treatment of CIN significantly reduces the risk of developing cervical cancer. For these reasons, many countries, including the UK, have set up a national screening programme to reduce the mortality of cervical cancer.

METHODS OF SCREENING

1. **The cervical smear.**

   A cervical smear can be taken as an outpatient procedure. Minimal discomfort is experienced by the patient. The cervix is visualised using a speculum. An Ayre's spatula is placed in the cervical canal and rotated through 360°. The superficial layer of cells overlying the squamocolumnar junction is removed and smeared on a slide. The slide is fixed, stained using Papanicolou's method, and examined under a microscope. Abnormal cells can be identified, and the patients referred for colposcopy.

The following system of cervical screening is in place in the UK (1990)

— All women between 20 and 60 years should be screened 3–5 yearly
— Routine screening can stop aged 60 provided the woman has had at least two normal smears and no abnormal smears over the previous 10 years
— Routine screening is not required in women who have had a hysterectomy for benign disease
— Immunocompromised / immunosuppressed women should be screened annually

An abnormal smear is usually an indication for colposcopy (see p.194)

2. **Colposcopy**

Colposcopy is an integral part of the screening programme. It should be performed in all women with abnormal smears, prior to treatment (see p.194).

CERVICAL SMEARS

INTERPRETATION OF CERVICAL SMEARS

Smears are reported in six main categories:

1. Normal   No signs of CIN

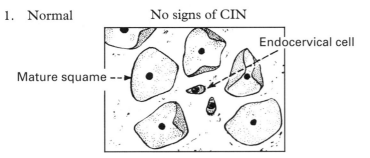

II. Inflammatory *or* borderline nuclear changes

III. Mild dyskaryosis
       Moderate dyskaryosis

The smear shows a mixture of
normal cells and dyskaryotic
(abnormal nuclei) cells

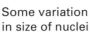

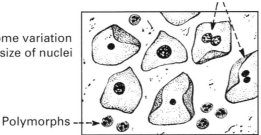
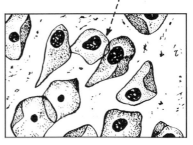

IV. Severe dyskaryosis   The cells area almost all abnormal
                                  and show larger
                                  nuclei with coarse
                                  chromatin.

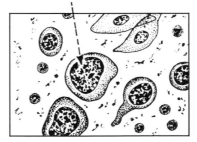

V. Invasion suspected

Abnormal glandular cells

In general, the more severe the dyskaryosis, the more likely the patient is to have CIN II
or CIN III. However, even in women with a mildly dyskaryotic smear, the incidence of
CIN II–III is 50%.

Most programmes recommend immediate referral for colposcopy for all women with mild
dyskaryosis and more severe lesions. A repeat smear is justified in women with inflammatory
or borderline nuclear changes. However, if these abnormalities persist, colposcopy is
indicated.

COLPOSCOPY

Colposcopy means binocular inspection of the cervix with a magnification of up to 20 times.

The colposcopist recognises two kinds of epithelium, the 'native' which may be squamous or columnar; and the metaplastic squamous epithelium which arises in the physiological transformation zone.

The transformation zone lies between the cervical canal and the squamo-columnar junction.

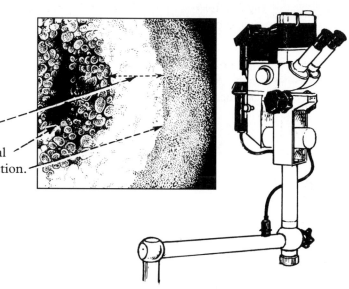

Atypical epithelium

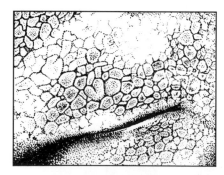

Mosaic appearance

Prior to examination with the colposcope the cervix is swabbed with acetic acid. Any focus of increased cellularity becomes white in colour indicating the areas requiring close attention.

Atypical epithelium may have a mosaic or tiled appearance because of the arrangement of the epithelial capillaries.

An experienced colposcopist can detect suspicious areas with great accuracy and take multiple punch biopsies without trauma. Biopsies are examined histologically and the degree of CIN determined.

TREATMENT OF CIN

1. ABLATIVE TECHNIQUES

All these techniques destroy abnormal cervical tissue. In contrast to excisional methods, there is no tissue for analysis after treatment. Hence it is essential to exclude invasive disease by colposcopically directed biopsy prior to treatment.

CRYOSURGERY

This allows destruction of affected tissue to a depth of 3 mm. It is quick and sufficiently painless to be used in the conscious patient.

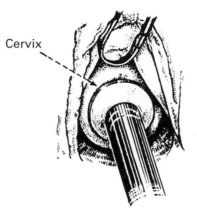

Cervix

DIATHERMY

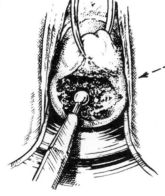

Diathermy under general anaestheia will destroy tissue to a depth of 7–8 mm

CO$_2$ LASER

This instrument emits very powerful electromagnetic radiations which vaporise tissue to a depth of 7–9 mm. It can be used with great precision and causes very little trauma. The diameter of the laser beam at its focal point is 1.8 mm.

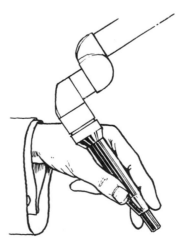

TREATMENT OF CIN

2. EXCISIONAL TECHNIQUES

Excisional techniques have the major advantage over ablative methods that tissue is obtained and can be examined histologically. The original diagnosis can be confirmed. Ideally, the biopsy will show disease free margins around the lesion.

Many operators prefer to perform excisional techniques on all patients. Others may reserve these techniques for women with the following indications:

1. suspected invasive disease
2. suspected glandular abnormality
3. inability to see the squamocolumnar junction
4. previous cervical surgery

The following techniques are in current use:

1. Large loop electrodiathermy of the transformation zone (LLETZ)

This method has become one of the most popular for treating premaligant cervical disease. A thin wire loop is used to excise the transformation zone using a blended diathermy current.

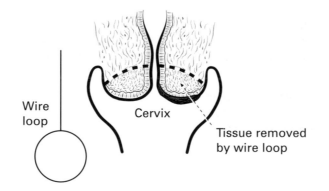

TREATMENT OF CIN

Excisional techniques *(contd)*

2. Knife cone biopsy

Prior to the introduction of LLETZ, this technique was extremely popular. However, it requires a general anaesthetic and is now rarely used. Complications include bleeding, infection, and cervical stenosis or incompetence in a subsequent pregnancy.

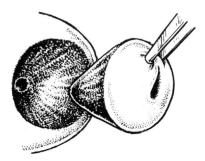

3. Laser cone biopsy

In laser cone biopsy, a cone of tissue is removed as above. However, the procedure may be done under local anaesthesia. The costs of the equipment reduce its potential popularity. Laser does have the advantage that co-existing VAIN may be treated at the same time.

Follow up
Despite the efficacy of the above techniques in treating cervical intraepithelial neoplasia, recurrence is common. All women who have had CIN should be followed up with annual smears for a minimum of ten years.

MICRO-INVASIVE CARCINOMA

Stage 1a

This is the stage between CIN III and clinical invasive carcinoma. It is characterised by the spread of malignant cells in two directions: a depth of no more than 5 mm from the nearest basement membrane and a total width of not more than 7 mm.

Treatment

If the lesion is completely excised by biopsy, no further treatment may be necessary. Many gynaecologists would treat this lesion by total abdominal hysterectomy, particularly in women who wish to have no more children.

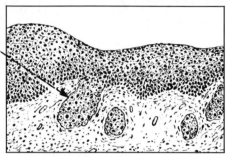

Histological assessment requires a good deal of experience. The diagnosis is entirely histological but colposcopists claim to be able to identify likely areas of micro-invasiveness with considerable accuracy.

CIN DURING PREGNANCY

When persistently abnormal smears are obtained during pregnancy further investigation is hindered by the danger of severe haemorrhage associated with cervical biopsy during pregnancy. The bleeding is such that hysterectomy has, on occasion, been necessary, and there is a considerable risk of abortion.

Colposcopy is now regarded as a reliable method of screening. Difficulty arises when micro-invasion is suspected, and in such cases a wedge biopsy may be required.

CIN III is not affected by the pregnancy and further investigation and treatment may be delayed.

CARCINOMA OF THE UTERINE CERVIX

Carcinoma of the cervix is the commonest malignant tumour of the female genital tract. The incidence varies from country to country and appears to be significantly reduced where there is a vigorous campaign for early diagnosis and eradication of carcinoma in situ.

The growth is a squamous cell carcinoma in 90% of cases, the remaining 10% being almost always adenocarcinomas.

Clinical finding

The cervix becomes very indurated; necrosis and ulceration commonly follow quickly.

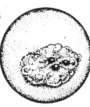

Later, a large fungating mass is produced. Sloughing may leave an excavated crater.

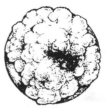

The tumour may form a proliferating growth which protrudes into the vagina — a 'cauliflower', 'exophytic', 'everting' growth. This type bleeds easily and soon becomes ulcerated.

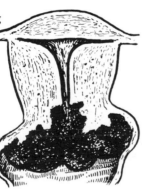

Sometimes the spread is in the substance of the cervix — 'excavating', 'endophytic', 'inverting' growth. The cervix becomes stony hard and enlarged — the 'barrel-shaped' cervix.

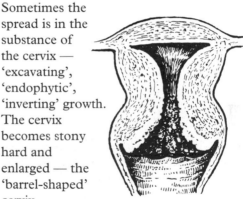

Histology of Squamous cell carcinoma

The appearances are typical, but cell nests are absent and keratinisation is rarely seen.

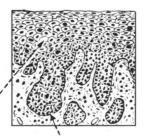

Central cells ovoid and obviously of squamous type

Peripheral cells cuboidal

199

CARCINOMA OF THE CERVIX

ADENOCARCINOMA

This less common form of cervical malignancy usually arises from the columnar epithelium of the endocervix. The histological type of lesion does not appear to alter the behaviour or spread of the tumour.

The appearances in this form are typical of adenocarcinoma in other organs.

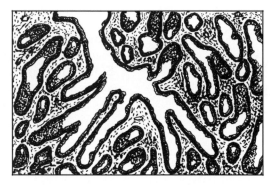

Low power. Tubular processes spread out from the lumina of the glands. The characteristic pattern is an aggressive adenomatous formation with very little fibrous stroma.

Many indeterminate patterns are seen on microscopic examination. Sometimes both glandular and squamous malignant cells appear together — adenocanthoma — and squamous metaplasia is common.

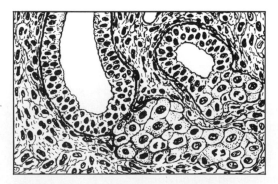

High power appearance of squamous epithelium which appears to originate by metaplasia from columnar epithelium.

AETIOLOGY OF CARCINOMA OF THE CERVIX

AETIOLOGY

1. Number of sexual partners
Cervical cancer is more common in women who have had many sexual partners. Young age at first intercourse is a weak risk factor.

2. Smoking
Several epidemiological studies have shown that smoking is an independent risk factor for cervical cancer.

3. Contraception
The use of barrier contraception appears to reduce the risk of cervical cancer.

4. Viral agents
Viral agents are now thought to be of minor importance only in the aetiology of cervical cancer.

a. Human papilloma virus (HPV)
    Many studies have examined the association between HPV, particularly types 16 and 18, and cervical cancer. These viruses can transform cells into malignant cells in vitro. However, it is becoming increasingly clear that infection with HPV is common in normal healthy women, and it seems unlikely therefore that HPV alone causes cervical cancer

b. Herpes simplex virus-2 (HSV-2)
    HSV-2 was formerly a candidate virus for malignant transformation in cervical carcinoma. However, it is now clear that HSV has little role to play in this disease.

CARCINOMA OF THE CERVIX

Spread

Direct spread into adjacent tissues usually occurs first. Involvement of the corpus uteri may cause pyometra. Further spread to the parametrium induces the same signs and symptoms as chronic pelvic inflammation.

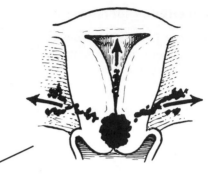

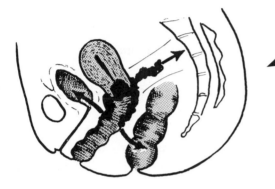

Spread downwards into the vaginal wall inevitably involves bladder or rectum causing fistulae. Backwards spread along the uterosacral ligaments leads to involvement of the sacral plexus causing intractable sciatic pain.

Lymphatic spread usually follows but may precede direct spread.

From the cervical lymphatics the spread is usually along the paracervical lymph tract to the external iliac nodes. Occasionally the extension is backwards to the internal iliac group.

Blood borne spread is exceptional.

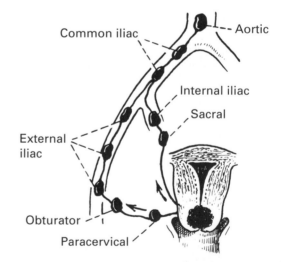

Symptoms

1. Irregular bleeding is one of the first complaints, either post-menopausal or post-coital. It is not often due to carcinoma but the possibility must be kept in mind.

2. Infection. The growth is soon infected from the vagina and a foul discharge is common.

3. Pain. This is due to spread of the growth to the pelvic cavity and is a late sign.

4. Cachexia occurs in advanced cases due to prolonged infection. There is mild but persistent fever, weight loss and anaemia.

DIFFERENTIAL DIAGNOSIS OF CERVICAL CARCINOMA

Biopsy is necessary for histological confirmation, but in very few cases is there any doubt. If the growth is early, some normal tissue should be removed as well, and a diagram provided to show the pathologist where the biopsy was taken. It should be no bigger than necessary and cone biopsy is not done in the presence of naked eye evidence of malignant growth. Curettage should also be done if the external os is accessible.

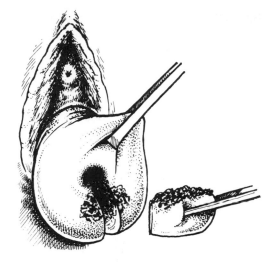

Very occasionally what appears to be a definitely malignant lesion turns out to be benign.

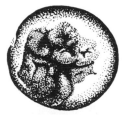

Cervicitis with ectopy is the commonest cervical lesion and if florid can be most misleading.

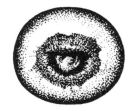

Mucous cervical polyps when infected can present a very suspicious appearance. (But all polyps require examination.)

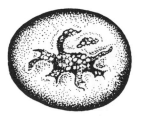

Tuberculosis is rare in the cervix. There is nearly always a history of genital tuberculosis.

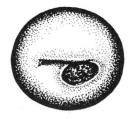

A primary chancre (syphilis) can appear in the cervix: ulcerated hard and indurated. In the United Kingdom it is rare.

CLINICAL STAGING OF CERVICAL CARCINOMA

Each growth is allocated to a stage according to the extent of spread (FIGO 1995).

Stage O CIN III
(Carcinoma-in-situ)

Stage Ia
Micro-invasive carcinoma not extending more than 5 mm beyond
the basement membrane and of a width less than 7 mm.

Stage Ib The growth is
confined to the cervix.

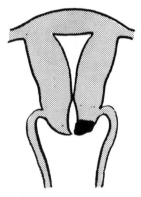

Stage IIa Extension to the vagina
not beyond the upper two thirds.

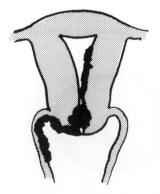

Stage IIb Extension into the parametrium
but not as far as the pelvic walls.

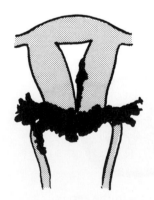

CLINICAL STAGING OF CERVICAL CARCINOMA

Stage III Extension to lower third of vagina or to pelvic wall.

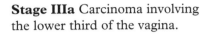

Stage IIIa Carcinoma involving the lower third of the vagina.

Stage IIIb Carcinoma extending to the pelvic side wall and/or hydronephrosis due to tumour.

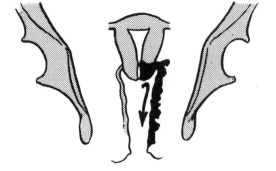

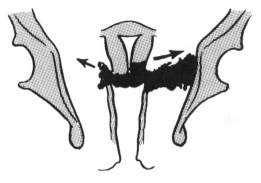

Stage IV Extension through vagina into bladder or outside pelvis.

Stage IVa Carcinoma involving bladder, rectum or outside the pelvis.

Stage IVb Carcinoma extending to distant organs.

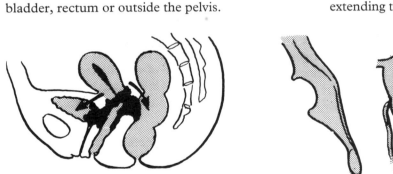

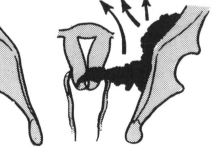

Classification (which is a clinical staging) is made after vaginal and rectal examination followed by cystoscopy and sigmoidoscopy when indicated, and doubtful cases are placed in the less advanced stage.

RADIOTHERAPY

Radiotherapy is the treatment of choice for some stage 1b tumours, and all tumours of a more advanced stage. A combination of external and intracavity therapy are employed.

Intracavity therapy

Hollow carriers are placed in the uterus and vaginal fornices under general anaesthesia. Radioactive sources can then be loaded into these tubes for treatment at a later date. Intracavity therapy allows high doses of radioactivity to be targeted to the cervix. Since the activity falls with increasing distance from the source, the tissues around the cervix (bladder, bowel etc.) receive a relatively low dose of radioactivity. This treatment may be used alone in early stage disease.

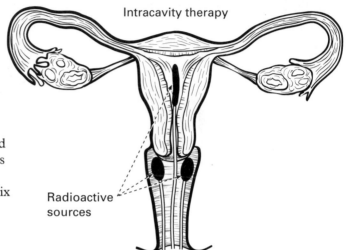

Intracavity therapy

Radioactive sources

Dose of treatment

The dose of intracavity radiotherapy is described by the radiation applied at two representative points: A and B. Point A is defined as 2 cm lateral to the central uterine canal and 2 cm above the external cervical os. Point B is 5 cm lateral to the central uterine canal and 2 cm above the cervical os. A total dose of 6000–8000 cGy is normally applied, in divided doses.

External beam therapy

External beam therapy is applied to the pelvis to control spread outwith the cervix. A total dose of up to 5000 cGy is used.

Results

Five year survival rates are dependent on disease staging. Mean five year survival is 55%, but this ranges from 80% in stage I disease to 14% in stage IV disease.

Complications

Short term (up to 100% of patients)
  Diarrhoea
  Acute urinary symptoms

Long term (5–10% of patients)
  Subacute bowel obstruction
  Diarrhoea
  Haematuria
  Vesicovaginal fistulae.

SURGERY FOR CERVICAL CARCINOMA

Wertheim's hysterectomy

This consists of removal of the uterus and adnexa, most of the vagina and the fatty-fibrous tissue which 'pads' the pelvis and contains the lymph glands.

The broad ligament is opened up and the ureter dissected off uterus and cervix. This is usually made difficult by the presence of inflammation.

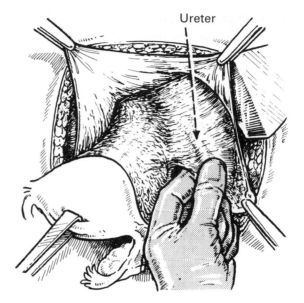

The ureter is being identified by palpation.

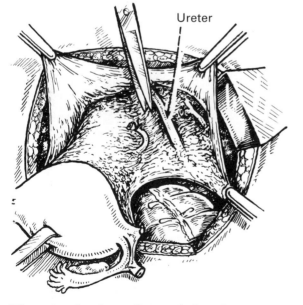

The ureter has been dissected clear down to the bladder and the uterine vessels divided.

The ureter can always be identified in the false pelvis and followed downwards, but dissection in the parametrium is difficult especially if the growth has infiltrated (stage II growth). The ureter has to be mobilised to protect it, but the more thorough the surgeon is, the greater the possibility of damage to the ureter's blood supply and development of fistula due to avascular necrosis.

207

SURGERY FOR CERVICAL CARCINOMA

RADICAL HYSTERECTOMY

After removal of the uterus the vaginal stump is usually closed, but sometimes a drain is required because of oozing.

In this description the hysterectomy is shown first, to be followed by the lymphadenectomy; but many surgeons carry out a 'block dissection' removing pelvic nodes and fat and then the uterus and vagina all in one piece. The essential end-result is to clear the pelvis down to the muscle fascia, leaving only vessels, nerves and the rectum and bladder.

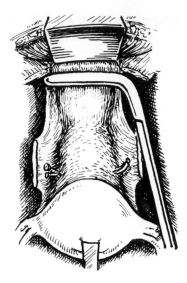

The vagina is severed below the special Wertheim clamp.

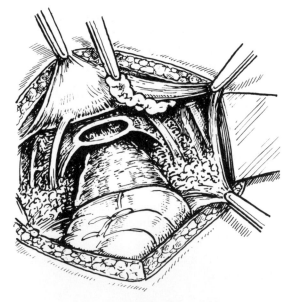

Dissecting out the fatty tissue and glands from the obturator fossa.

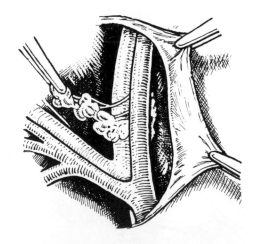

Dissecting out the external iliac glands. (Other accessible groups of nodes are also removed.)

SURGERY FOR CERVICAL CARCINOMA

RADICAL VAGINAL HYSTERECTOMY FOR CERVICAL CANCER

Modifications in technique

Some surgeons have described hysterectomy with extended lymph node dissection performed as a laparoscopic procedure. The risks and benefits of such an operation have not been fully evaluated, and an 'open' Wertheim's hysterectomy should be considered as the standard technique, outwith well conducted clinical trials.

Complications of surgical treatment for cervical cancer

Early
   Haemorrhage
   Damage to ureters or bladder
   Damage to intestinal tract
   Pulmonary embolism

Late
   Atonic bladder
   Ureteric/bladder fistulae (1–2%)

TREATMENT OF CERVICAL CARCINOMA: SURGERY OR RADIOTHERAPY?

Early stage cervical cancer is normally treated by surgery (up to and including stage 1a), later stage cervical cancer (stage IIa onwards) is treated by radiotherapy. There is debate about the optimum treatment for stage 1b disease. Small lesions in young fit women are probably best treated surgically, larger lesions in older women who may not tolerate surgery are best treated by radiotherapy.

The pros and cons of the two treatment types are shown below.

Advantages of surgery
   ovarian function retained
   normal vaginal function retained
   avoidance of effect of radiotherapy on bladder and bowel.

Advantages of radiotherapy
   suitable in women who are unfit for surgery.

Chemotherapy

Chemotherapy may be used as palliative treatment for cervical cancer. Agents which appear to be of benefit include cisplatin, bleomycin and methotrexate.

Palliative care

In women with advanced cancer, it may be unrealistic to seek to cure the disease with surgery, radiotherapy or chemotherapy. In some women, these procedures may be performed palliatively, to reduce symptoms.

The care of patients with advanced or terminal disease is now a specialty in itself, and help should be sought from palliative care specialists at an early stage. Such specialists are invaluable in minimising symptoms, including pain, whilst maximising quality of life.

CHAPTER 11

DISEASES OF THE UTERUS

UTERINE POLYPS

ENDOMETRIAL ADENOMATOUS or MUCOUS POLYP

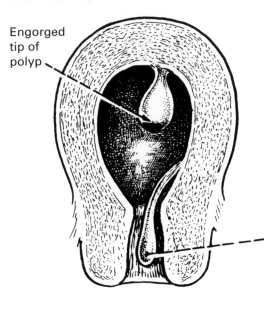

Engorged
tip of
polyp

Symptoms

Heavier but regular periods.
Post-menopausal bleeding.
Irregular bleeding on HRT.

Cramping pain — usually mild —
as uterus tries to expel polyp.

Intermenstrual staining — usually due to
congestion or necrosis, but malignant change
must always be considered.

The polyp may be visible in the external
os and there may be more than one.
Endometrial polyps may be visualised by
hysteroscopy. Vaginal ultrasound is less
reliable.

PLACENTAL POLYP

This is due to the survival of chorionic tissue from
a recent pregnancy. The tissue remains adherent
to the uterine wall and enlarges with the accretion
of fibrin and fibrous tissue.

Symptoms

Menorrhagia and intermenstrual bleeding which
may present some time after the pregnancy has
terminated or aborted. Examination will reveal an
enlarged uterus.

Treatment

All polyps must be removed, either by curettage,
avulsion or laser hysteroscopy and submitted to
pathology.

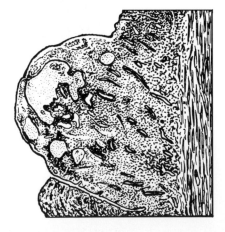

FIBROIDS

FIBROIDS (FIBROMYOMATA)

Fibroid is the gynaecological term for a leiomyoma of the uterus or, occasionally, of the cervix.

It is a circumscribed tumour of non-striped muscle with supporting fibrous tissue. ⟶

Fibroids develop in the myometrium and are not encapsulated, but they develop a false capsule of compressed myometrial tissue.

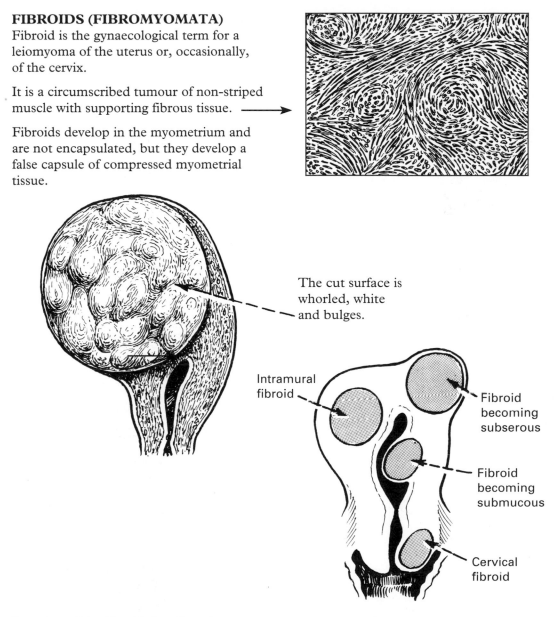

The cut surface is whorled, white and bulges.

Intramural fibroid

Fibroid becoming subserous

Fibroid becoming submucous

Cervical fibroid

Location of the fibroid describes the type.

They are sometimes conglomerate and multiple and vary in size from tiny (millet seed) to many centimetres in diameter.

Some fibroids develop a long pedicle and present as polyps.

Not uncommonly, hard faecal masses in gut are mistaken for uterine fibroids on bimanual examination.

213

FIBROIDS

The fibroid is the commonest tumour found in women (present in 15 to 20%) especially after 35 years of age.

They may make the uterus bulky and irregular and may enlarge the cavity so that there is a greater area of endometrium to be shed at menstruation. Menstruation tends to be heavy but the cycle is usually regular. Fibroids are associated with infertility and nulliparity.

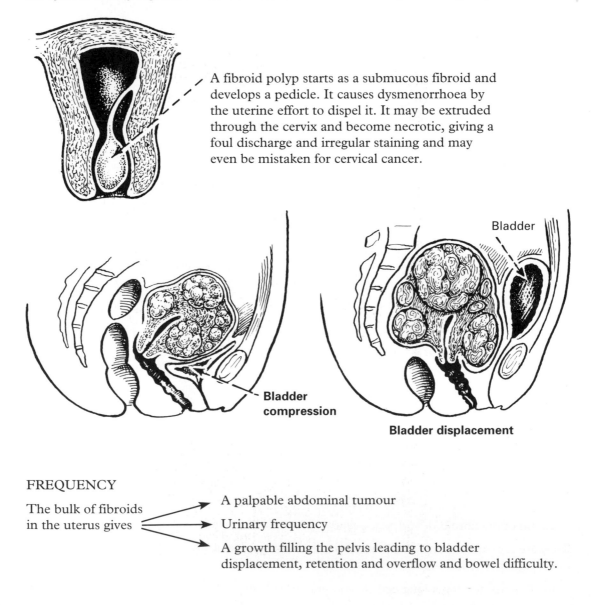

A fibroid polyp starts as a submucous fibroid and develops a pedicle. It causes dysmenorrhoea by the uterine effort to dispel it. It may be extruded through the cervix and become necrotic, giving a foul discharge and irregular staining and may even be mistaken for cervical cancer.

Bladder

Bladder compression

Bladder displacement

FREQUENCY

The bulk of fibroids in the uterus gives

→ A palpable abdominal tumour

→ Urinary frequency

→ A growth filling the pelvis leading to bladder displacement, retention and overflow and bowel difficulty.

FIBROIDS

DIAGNOSIS

1. This is suggested by a history of increasing menstrual blood loss in a woman commonly in her forties.

2. Large fibroids are palpable per abdomen. On bimanual examination, an irregularly shaped uterus suggests fibroids.

3. **Examination** under anaesthesia and curettage will allow a more accurate assessment and the exclusion of endometrial carcinoma.

4. If a doubt as to the nature of the mass remains, ultrasound scanning will make a distinction between fibroids and an ovarian cyst but not necessarily a solid ovarian mass.

5. The **diagnosis** may be made at laparoscopy.

COMPLICATIONS

1. **Sarcomatous change.** This is rare but occurs, and even asymptomatic fibroids must be kept under observation.

2. **Degeneration.** Fibroids tend to outgrow their blood supply and are subject to various forms of degeneration. **Necrobiosis** ('red degeneration') occurs in pregnancy and is a cause of pain. Usually this remits and no treatment is needed. **Hyaline, mucoid, cystic degeneration.** These changes may produce soft or hard fibroids, confusing the diagnosis.

3. **Torsion of the pedicle.** This can arise in the case of a polypoid subserous fibroid and gives rise to acute abdominal symptoms. If the torsion is subacute and the blood supply gradually reduced, the fibroid may develop a new vascularity through adhesions (parasitic tumour).

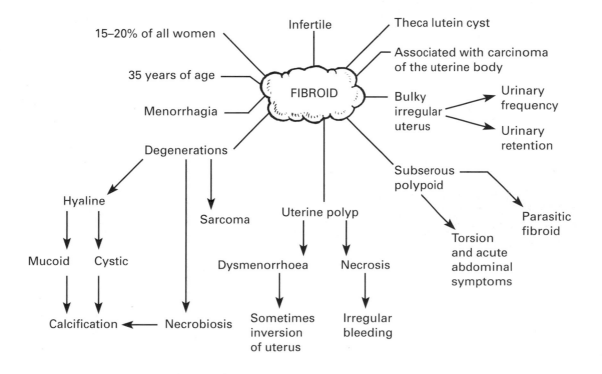

215

FIBROIDS

Treatment
Small, asymptomatic fibroids need not be treated.

1. Medical treatment with GnRH analogues, perhaps adding cyclical norethisterone to minimise bone loss and menopausal symptoms, may give 50% reduction in 6 months, but rapid return to former size follows cessation of this expensive therapy.

2. Surgical removal with conservation of uterus (myomectomy) <u>may</u> preserve fertility.

3. Removal of uterus with fibroids usually abdominally (hysterectomy).

MYOMECTOMY
The approach to the tumour is made through the uterine wall, and the fibroid is shelled out by scissors and finger dissection. The false capsule may make the plane of dissection difficult to identify.

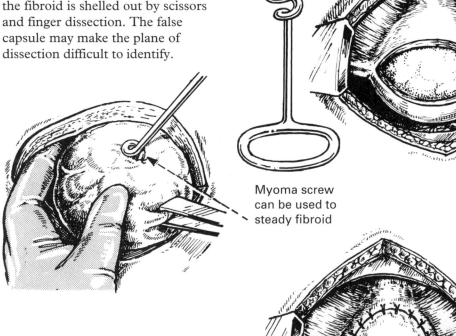

Myoma screw can be used to steady fibroid

The resultant cavity is obliterated by buried sutures and the uterine wall flapped over to bring the suture line as low on the uterine wall as possible to reduce the risk of adhesions to bowel.

The disadvantages of myomectomy are possible haematoma formation and recurrence of fibroids. Hysterectomy is the treatment of choice unless the patient wishes to become pregnant.

HYPERPLASTIC CONDITIONS OF THE ENDOMETRIUM

Being less accessible than lesions of vulvar, vaginal or cervical epithelium, endometrial pre-malignant conditions are less easily diagnosed and followed up. Any hyperplastic condition raises the question of development of cancer and assessment of risk is important. Hyperplasia and carcinoma may coexist.

Endometrial hyperplasia may be classified as simple (cystic), complex (adenomatous) or atypical.

Clinical Findings

Most patients are in the 3rd and 4th decades of life, but hyperplasia is not confined to these age groups. It is often found in association with anovulation in teenage women and post-menopausal women. Haemorrhage is the presenting symptom but the severity or frequency is not related to the degree of pathological change. Young women with simple, cystic hyperplasia may suffer bleeding suggestive of abortion.

Simple Hyperplasia

This is the most common type. Previously known as metropathia haemorrhagica, the endometrium has a characteristic appearance, often termed 'Swiss cheese' or cystic glandular hyperplasia.

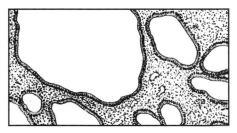

At low power magnification the pattern is a mixture of glands of varying sizes, a significant proportion of them being cystic. There is no crowding of the glands which are lined by cubical or columnar epithelium. Mitotic figures are present in small numbers. A similar gross picture may be seen in atrophic endometria but mitotic activity is absent. Other associated pathology is rare.

Complex Hyperplasia

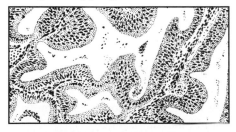

In this grade of hyperplasia the most striking feature is the evidence of quite obvious hyperplasia — crowding of glands so that they are back-to-back, the epithelium is stratified and mitoses are relatively frequent. There is, however, no epithelial atypia.

Atypical Hyperplasia

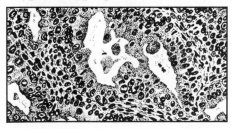

At this stage nuclear atypia is present. Intra-glandular polypoid formations and abnormal mitotic figures are seen. Severe cases may be indistinguishable from carcinoma and adjacent areas of endometrial carcinoma may occur.

217

HYPERPLASTIC CONDITIONS OF THE ENDOMETRIUM

These grades of epithelial change seem to form a graded series. Evidence of proof of this is difficult to find however. Some of the conclusions drawn from studies must be viewed with caution from an intellectual point of view, but in practice it must be accepted that any hyperplastic condition must be regarded with suspicion and treatment should be anticipatory.

Many cases have a history of profuse menstruation and some present clinical features which are said to be stigmata of the type of patient apt to develop endometrial carcinoma such as obesity, abnormal glucose tolerance curve and hypertension.

In some cases of localised adenocarcinoma of the endometrium, the surrounding endometrium shows evidence of hyperplasia, giving credence to the view that one condition develops out of the other. In addition, there are cases where it is microscopically difficult to state that the endometrial changes are hyperplastic but not malignant.

Claims are made for the likelihood of adenocarcinoma developing according to the grade of hyperplasia. Mild — 1%, moderate — 5%, severe — 30%, and the time taken for malignancy to appear, milder — 10 years, severe — 4 years.

Aetiology
Commonly, no cause is apparent. Unopposed oestrogen, as in anovulation, inappropriate hormone replacement therapy, oestrogen secreting ovarian tumours and tamoxifen therapy can cause hyperplasia of endometrium.

TREATMENT
This depends principally on the types of hyperplasia though the age of the patient and a desire to retain fertility are factors to consider. Endometrial and ovarian malignancy should be excluded by EUA, hysteroscopy, curettage, ultrasound and Ca125 assay and endogenous or exogenous sources of oestrogen sought.

Simple hyperplasia, with 1% risk of progression to carcinoma requires no routine follow-up. Recurrent abnormal bleeding would, of course, merit investigation.

Adenomatous hyperplasia is not thought to merit hysterectomy, and progestin therapy, such as levonorgestrel releasing IUCD is probably of greater value as a contraceptive and for reassurance of the gynaecologist than as a prophylactic against the risk of endometrial carcinoma. Subsequent care after diagnosis can reasonably be dictated by subsequent symptoms.

Atypical hyperplasia, with estimated risks of co-existence of, or progression to, endometrial carcinoma of between 20 and 80+% merits hysterectomy and bilateral salpingo-oophorectomy in most cases. Women who wish to remain potentially fertile may be treated with progestogens, oral, injectable or by IUCD but long-term data is scanty. Recurrence on cessation of therapy is reported and long-term surveillance with repeated curettage is mandatory.

CARCINOMA OF THE ENDOMETRIUM

One of the commonest gynaecological cancers, especially in white Americans, it occurs most often in postmenopausal women (up to 80% of cases) with less than 5% diagnosed under 40 years of age. Association with obesity, diabetes and polycystic ovarian syndrome is common. Postmenopausal American women may run a 1 in 1000 risk of endometrial carcinoma each year. There is no effective screening programme, but occasionally cervical smears contain endometrial cancer cells or double thickness endometrial ultrasonic thickness of 4 mm or more indicates a need for endometrial sampling.

Symptomatology

The usual presenting symptom of endometrial carcinoma is *postmenopausal bleeding* which carries a 10% risk of associated malignancy in the absence of hormone replacement therapy. Curettage, or endometrial sampling is *mandatory*. *Postmenopausal discharge* from pyometra carries a 50% risk of associated malignancy. *Pain* may occur with pyometra or metastatic spread.

Diagnosis

Hysteroscopy with endometrial curettage or endometrial sampling, curettage alone, or outpatient endometrial sampling alone, are essential. Curettage is not infallible. On the other hand, if a Pipelle has been correctly introduced (record how many cm) and the pathology is benign, or no tissue is obtained, it is most unlikely that malignancy exists.

Hysteroscopy, cervical smear (> 1% risk of concurrent cervical malignancy) and vaginal or abdominal ultrasound for ovarian pathology are advised, when endometrial malignancy is found.

Hysteroscopy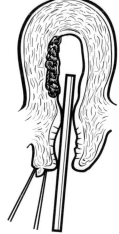

Curettage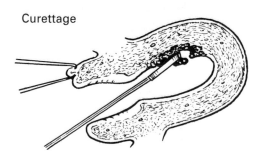

CARCINOMA OF THE ENDOMETRIUM

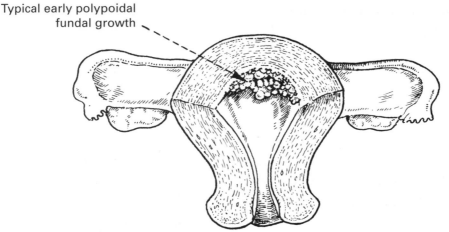

Typical early polypoidal
fundal growth

Histology

The majority of tumours (60%) are pure adenocarcinomata. They can be divided into
3 groups according to the degree of glandular differentiation.

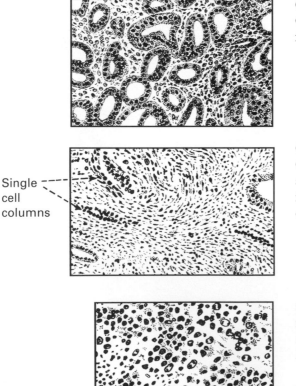

Grade 1 — well differentiated.
Gland forms are conspicuous. Mitotic
figures are moderately numerous.

Single
cell
columns

Grade 2 — patchy differentiation.
Gland forms are much less prominent
and many deposits consist of
infiltrating single cell columns
or solid masses.

Grade 3. This type consists of solid
masses of malignant cells of varying
sizes and shapes with little or no stroma.
Mitoses are numerous.

CARCINOMA OF THE ENDOMETRIUM

Further groups have been described.

Adeno-squamoid group
This has been divided into two groups:

1. If the squamous cells are well differentiated the tumour is termed adeno-acanthoma (Histological Grade 1).

2. Poorly differentiated squamous cells merit the name adeno-squamous carcinoma (Grade 2).

Adeno-acanthoma

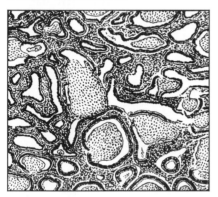

Adeno-squamous carcinoma

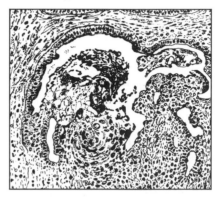

One other histological type is recognised and is apparently of prognostic significance.

Clear celled carcinoma

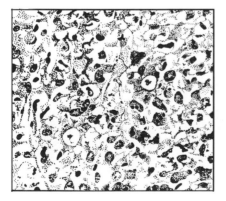

This tumour has a poor prognosis and is included with the Grade 3 adenocarcinomata. It occurs mainly in the elderly.

STAGING OF ENDOMETRIAL CARCINOMA

The classification given below is that of the Federation of Gynaecology and Obstetrics (FIGO).

Stage I Growth
confined to
(a) Endometrium
(b) <1/2 myometrium
(c) >1/2 myometrium

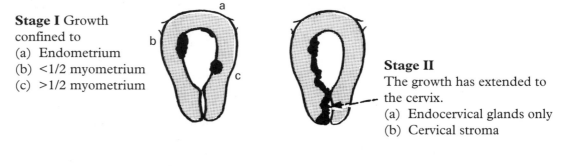

Stage II
The growth has extended to the cervix.
(a) Endocervical glands only
(b) Cervical stroma

Stage III
The growth has extended to
(a) Serosa and/or adnexa and/or +ve peritoneal washings cytology
(b) Vagina
(c) Pelvic or para-aortic lymph nodes

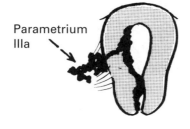

Parametrium
IIIa

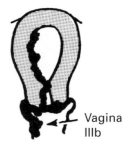

Vagina
IIIb

Stage IV
The growth has invaded
(a) the rectum or bladder or
(b) structures beyond the pelvis.

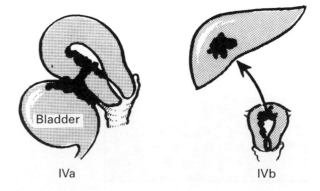

Bladder

IVa

IVb

Histological grading, G1, G2 or G3 is applied to Stages I, II and III only.

SPREAD OF ENDOMETRIAL CARCINOMA

In general this cancer is slow to spread from the uterine cavity, probably because the endometrium lacks lymphatics. A chest X-ray helps detect lung metastases. Magnetic resonance imaging is preferable to ultrasound for detection of myometrial invasion and pelvic spread.

Local Spread
Slow invasion of the myometrium is the commonest spread. It may produce considerable uterine enlargement; or spread may involve the vaginal vault.

Venous Spread
This pathway might account for the occasional appearance of a low vaginal metastasis; but venous spread is not a common feature of uterine cancer.

Lymphatic Spread
The incidence of this (it is much debated) seems to be somewhere between 10 and 30%. All pelvic nodes, including the internal iliacs, the parametrium, the ovaries, and the vagina may be involved, probably with equal frequency. Lymphatic spread is more likely to occur when the tumour is anaplastic and the uterine wall is deeply invaded.

Tubal Spread
Malignant cells can pass along the tube in the same way that peritoneal spill may occur during menstruation. This may account for isolated ovarian metastases.

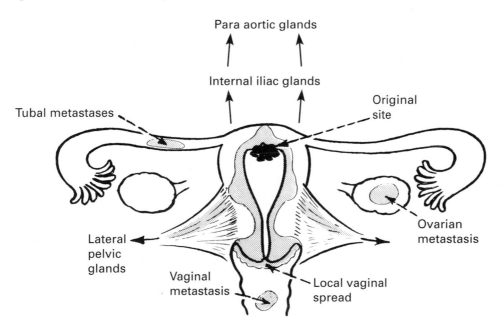

Most metastases occur in adjacent structures and peritoneum. In advanced cases distant metastases do occur, most commonly in lung, but occasionally in liver, vertebrae or other bones and in supraclavicular lymph nodes.

AETIOLOGICAL FACTORS IN ENDOMETRIAL CARCINOMA

The actual cause of this cancer is unknown. Argument has centred around the undoubted association between this tumour and oestrogen. Increased incidences have been reported in women given oestrogen alone as postmenopausal hormone replacement therapy and in obese and in diabetic women. They commonly have a high plasma oestradiol even postmenopausally related to increased peripheral conversion of adrenal androstenedione to oestrone in the body fat and decreased sex hormone binding globulin allowing a higher percentage of free oestrogen in the plasma. Oestrogen secreting tumours of the ovary are associated with an increased incidence of endometrial carcinoma.

The central position of oestrogen in the aetiology of endometrial cancer is strengthened by the fact that the addition of progestogen to the oestrogen in hormone replacement therapy appears to abolish the increased incidence of endometrial cancer. There can be no doubt that oestrogen can alter the behaviour of this tumour but there is still a question about oestrogen as a primary causal agent. Every normal woman is subject to the influence of unopposed oestrogen for 2 weeks out of every 4 for a matter of 30 years or more. Approximately 75% of cases of endometrial cancer occur in the postmenopausal period when oestrogen values are low and progesterone is absent. Nulliparity and PCO syndrome (with defective progesterone synthesis) carry an increased risk. Only a proportion of obese, diabetic and hypertensive women develop endometrial cancer and similarly only a proportion of women with endometrial cancer are obese, diabetic or hypertensive. The question remains whether oestrogen is a causal agent, or is acting in its normal capacity as a growth factor and is really to be regarded as a co-carcinogen. It may be that the lack of progestational activity alters the reaction to oestrogen.

In the Lynch II family syndrome, related to a chromosomal abnormality, endometrial carcinoma occurs more frequently, together with breast and colon cancer.

Oral contraception, especially after long term use, reduces the incidence of both endometrial and ovarian carcinomas.

The endometrial hyperplasia induced by Tamoxifen produces endometrial polyps. A report in the Lancet in 1999 suggested a four-fold increase in endometrial carcinoma. The selective oestrogen receptor modulator raloxifene (Evista) does not stimulate the endometrium.

PROGNOSIS OF ENDOMETRIAL CARCINOMA

With the exception of stage 1 tumours of histological grades I and II, the prognosis is less favourable than many gynaecologists believe, with an overall 5 year survival of 70% approximately. Fortunately over 80% of cases are diagnosed at stage 1.

Staging at diagnosis, extent of myometrial invasion and *histological grading* (differentiation) are the most important prognostic factors apart from competence of treatment.

Various figures are quoted but the following are an example of the 5-year survival rates according to clinical staging.

Stage	5-year survival
I	85%
II	68%
III	42%
IV	22%

Assessing 5-year survival rates according to Federation International Gynaecology Obstetrics (FIGO) histological grading is reported as follows:

Grading	Appearance	Percentage survival
G1	Highly differentiated	100
G2	Differentiated, part solid	66
G3	Mainly solid	57

Using both methods on similar cases we find that the 5-year survival rates for Stage I are the only ones altered significantly:

Stage and histology	5-year survival
I, G1 and 2	80%
I, G3	60%

Prognosis is also altered by individual findings. For instance, if the tumour has penetrated more than half-way through the myometrial thickness the prognosis is bad. In addition, the recurrence rate, up to 15%, is directly proportional to the histological grade. Early recurrence carries a poor prognosis.

TREATMENT OF ENDOMETRIAL CARCINOMA

This is essentialy *surgical*, with postoperative *radiotherapy* added when unfavourable prognostic features are found at surgery. Pre-operative clinical staging is inaccurate. *Progestogen therapy* is probably only of value in recurrent disease.

Few women are unfit for surgery, and caesium insertion radioactive therapy may be employed for these, but radiation alone is less effective than combined surgical and radiation treatment.

Stage I
Total abdominal hysterectomy and bilateral salpingo-oophorectomy without partial removal of vagina. Peritoneal saline washings are taken for cytology on opening the abdomen and the abdominal contents carefully examined. Vaginal hysterectomy with removal of ovaries, sometimes laparoscopy-assisted, has equal 5 year survival and lower operative mortality, in appropriate hands.

Radiotherapy is employed postoperatively for the 30% of cases in whom unfavourable prognostic features are found at surgery or pathology.

Post operative *vault* radiotherapy is a reasonable procedure in all cases, reducing vault recurrence.

Convincing evidence is lacking for adjuvant progestogen therapy in stage I, or for lymphadenectomy.

Stage II
Stage IIa carries a similar prognosis to stage I and may be treated as stage I.

Stage IIb, with clinical invasion of the cervix, has a poorer prognosis than stage I and radical hysterectomy, pelvic lymphadenectomy and para-aortic lymph node sampling are indicated, with a combination of local and external radiotherapy as an alternative treatment.

Stage III
Following the staging laparotomy, radical hysterectomy, lymphadenectomy, para-aortic node sampling and removal of as much malignant tissue as possible, omentectomy is carried out. Stage III diseases limited to the pelvis may be treated by radiotherapy.

Stage IV
Treatment of this stage is designed to control tumour growth and alleviate symptoms. Surgery, radiation therapy, cytotoxic therapy and adjuvant progestogen therapy all have a place.

The overall results are better than for carcinoma of the cervix, not because it is a less malignant tumour, but because treatment is usually given earlier. Post-menopausal bleeding is much more difficult to ignore than the irregular bleeding of the younger woman.

RECURRENCE OF ENDOMETRIAL CARCINOMA

The incidence of recurrence within 5 years is in the region of 30% and is accepted along with the 5-year survival rate as a measure of the effectiveness of the various systems of treatment. The majority of recurrences appear within 3 years of treatment. Early recurrence has a poor prognosis.

Sites
Local recurrence is the commonest especially in the pelvic walls and vaginal vault; but endometrial carcinoma also recurs outside the pelvis in the para-aortic glands, the lungs, the skeleton and the lower vagina. Vault recurrence is less common after vault irradiation.

Prophylaxis
Pre-operative vaginal irradiation will very much reduce the chance of vaginal recurrence, and some radiotherapists advise pelvic megavoltage treatment as well. The basis of radical surgery is an attempt to clear the pelvis of lymphatic tissue which is not possible; and there is no agreement on whether lymphadenectomy, if technically feasible, is worth doing except on principle.

Treatment
Modern radiotherapy permits an attempt at cure, especially if the recurrence is restricted to the accessible vagina, when up to 60% of recurrences may be cured. It also offers symptom relief in skeletal and lymph node metastatic disease. Surgery is rarely justified.

PROGESTOGENS
Many endometrial carcinomata are hormone dependent and progestogens have been used as part of a combined primary treatment as well as for recurrent or metastatic growths.

Between 15% and 50% of recurrences will respond. Medroxyprogesterone acetate, 400 mg to 600 mg daily, is most commonly employed and the addition of tamoxifen may improve the response.

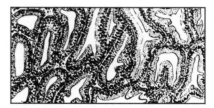
After progesterone

Chemotherapy
Cytotoxic chemotherapy has a limited place in advanced recurrence. Single agent therapy with adriamycin, cisplatinum, cyclophosphamide and hexamethylmelamine gives response rates between 20% and 40%.

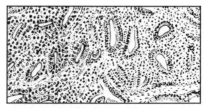
Before progesterone

MALIGNANT TUMOURS OF ENDOMETRIUM OF MIXED EPITHELIAL-STROMAL HISTOLOGY

These are rare tumours and show varying degrees of malignancy of either the glandular or stromal elements or both.

1. **Endometrial stromatosis.**
   (also called endolymphatic stromal myosis or endometrial stromal nodule).

   This forms a nodular growth of stromal cells extending in an expansile fashion rather than by infiltration. It may however appear to invade the local lymphatics, but does not form metastases and is essentially non-malignant.

2. **Endometrial stromal sarcomas.**

   These are tumours of endometrial stromal cells. They vary in degree of malignancy and form 2 groups:

   (a) **Low grade malignancy.**
   Cure may follow local removal but they sometimes recur years later in the pelvis. Occasionally they may form pulmonary metastases. The patient has a prolonged survival and may be cured after radiation therapy.

   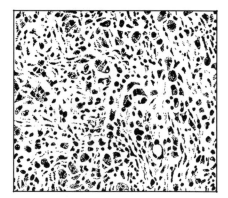

   (b) **High grade malignancy.**
   This type of stromal tumour shows numerous mitoses and is infiltrative from the start. There is early recurrence and widespread metastases occur even if there has been little local invasion of the myometrium. The prognosis is poor.

3. **Adeno-sarcoma.**
   This forms a polypoid mass in the uterine cavity consisting of a mixture of gland and stromal elements. The glandular tissue appears to be benign but the stroma shows the usual signs of malignancy — cellular atypia and mitotic activity. In 25% heterologous elements are found such as striated muscle and cartilage. Recurrences are confined to the pelvis. Distant metastases are rare.

4. **Carcino-sarcoma.**
   In this variant both epithelial and stromal elements are malignant. It forms a soft polypoid mass, usually haemorrhagic. Microscopically most of the growth is sarcomatous but there are foci of carcinoma — adeno, squamoid, undifferentiated or various mixtures of these. The sarcomatous parts show marked cellular atypia such as giant cells and other bizarre forms. The prognosis is poor. Treatment is surgical plus radiotherapy for recurrences and metastatic deposits.

MALIGNANT TUMOURS OF ENDOMETRIUM OF MIXED EPITHELIAL-STROMAL HISTOLOGY

5. **Mixed mesodermal tumours.**

These are often confused with carcino-sarcoma. They may be found in the vagina or cervix in children, but the uterine variety occurs in postmenopausal women. Treatment is as for endometrial carcinoma. These tumours are often well advanced at diagnosis. Cisplatin and adriamycin have a place in the management of advanced or recurrent tumours. The growth in children has a grape-like appearance — botryoid sarcoma.

Surgery gives poor results but chemotherapy, using vincristine, actinomycin D and cyclophosphamide has been reported as curative in 80% of children treated.

Bulky mixed mesodermal tumour showing haemorrhagic appearance

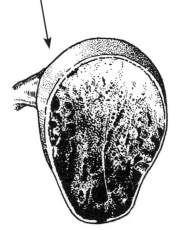

Microscopic appearance of mixed mesodermal tumour

Striated muscle

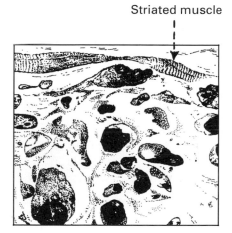

In the uterus it presents as a large white polypoid mass, semi-necrotic with areas of haemorrhage. Microscopically the tumour is pleomorphic with areas of myxomatous, cartilagenous and bony tissue. Growth is very rapid and it invades adjacent organs quickly. The prognosis is extremely poor, the 5-year survival rate being 20% at most. Blood borne metastases are common.

SARCOMA OF THE UTERUS

Histological Appearances

The tissues of origin are the connective tissue and muscle of the myometrium or leiomyoma or the endometrial stroma. These are composed of undifferentiated round- or spindle-celled masses. A special group of sarcomatous growths, the mixed mesodermal tumours, sometimes occur. In children, striated muscle is often a feature and a characteristic polypoidal growth occurs — sarcoma botryoides. Later in life carcinoma, sarcoma and various mesodermal tissues such as cartilage may be found.

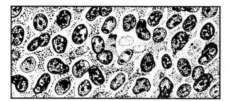

High power appearance
of round cell sarcoma

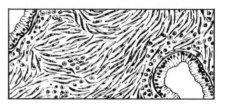

Low power view of
spindle-cell sarcoma

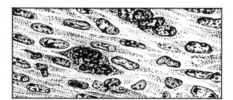

High power view of
smooth muscle sarcoma

Treatment

Sarcoma spreads by the blood stream and surgery should be limited to removal of the uterus and ovaries. The value of adjuvant radio- or chemotherapy has not been proven in early disease but vincristine, actinomycin and cyclophosphamide combination therapy, or cisplatinum, are of value in advanced disease or recurrence.

Prognosis

This depends on the degree of spread and the histological differentiation and is generally poor. Circumscribed and pedunculated growths have a better prognosis than infiltrating ones, and the most hopeful outlook is in the case of a chance histological finding in a fibromyoma thought at operation to be benign.

SARCOMA OF THE UTERUS

A malignant tumour arising from the connective tissue or muscle of the uterus. This is a rare disease in contrast to the common benign tumour of connective tissue and muscle, the leiomyoma or fibroid. Sarcomatous change may occur in between 0.1% and 1% of fibroids.

Clinical Features

The patient is usually over 50 and presents with a complaint of fairly heavy bleeding of recent origin, accompanied by pain. Pelvic examination reveals a large intra-uterine mass with friable tissue palpable through the os. The tumour may originate from the vagina in the younger woman and from the cervix in the child; but these are very rare conditions indeed.

Pathology

Tumour tissue may infiltrate the whole myometrium and fill the uterine cavity (diffuse, infiltrating) or arise from a pedicle (circumscribed type). This type often presents as a cervical or vaginal polyp. If the malignant change originates in a fibromyoma (which is very rare) the sarcomatous area has a yellowish fleshy appearance with areas of necrosis.

Differential Diagnosis

The growth is obviously malignant as a rule, but biopsy is required to distinguish sarcoma from the more common adenocarcinoma.

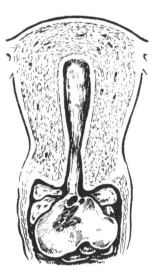

Pelvic examination on this case would suggest a cervical origin.

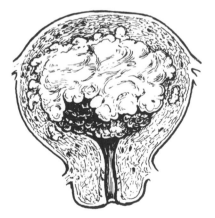

A diffuse infiltrating sarcoma.

CHAPTER 12

DISPLACEMENTS OF THE UTERUS

BACKWARD DISPLACEMENTS OF THE UTERUS

An alteration from the usual anteverted position of the uterus often with a change in the curve of the uterine axis. Most of the so-called displacements are merely variations of the normal and are of little clinical significance.

Anteverted Uterus
The uterus is approximately at right angles to the vagina and has a slight forward curve.

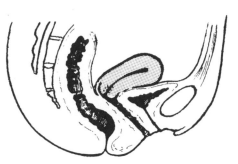

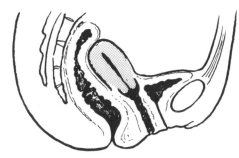

Retroversion
The long axis of the uterus is directed backwards.

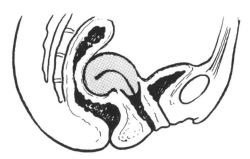

Retroflexion
The uterus is curved backwards. The cervix may remain in the normal position but is usually positioned as in retroversion.

Retroposition
The uterus is displaced backwards but the direction of its axis remains the same.

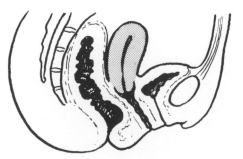

BACKWARD DISPLACEMENTS OF THE UTERUS

Causes of Displacement

Displacement may be due to the presence of some other condition such as a cyst or fibroid or endometriosis. However there may be no contributing cause; the uterus in some women appears to take up retro-displacement spontaneously.

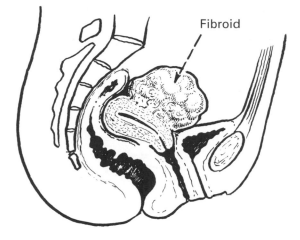

Fibroid

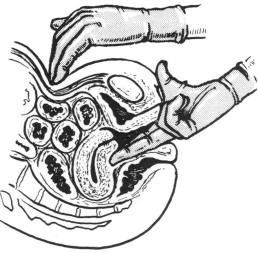

Diagnosis is by bimanual palpation. The vaginal hand palpates a mass in the Pouch of Douglas, the abdominal hand detects the absence of a uterine corpus in the expected place. The possibility of tumours and inflammatory masses must be considered. Ultrasound may be used to confirm the clinical findings.

SYMPTOMS AND TREATMENT OF DISPLACEMENT

Consequences of Uncomplicated Displacement

Usually none. However if the uterus is not mobile, coitus may be unbearable if the penis thrusts against the retroflexed uterus lying with prolapsed ovaries in the Pouch of Douglas. If such pain occurs it can easily be reproduced by pressing with the examining fingers. It is quite possible for the patient to present with a complaint of dyspareunia and to have a retroverted uterus which has nothing to do with her complaint.

Treatment

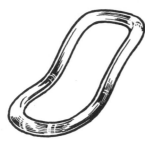

Insertion of Hodge Pessary:
This is a rigid plastic pessary, oblong in shape, which was designed for insertion into the vagina in such a way as to maintain a uterus in the anteverted position once the retroversion had been manually corrected. It is now becoming obsolete but is still occasionally used in the 'pessary test'.

Pessary Test:
This is applied to patients in whom a chronic retroversion is suspected of causing dyspareunia. The pessary is placed as shown and will certainly maintain the anteversion. If properly fitted it does not interfere in any way with coitus, and if it abolishes the dyspareunia it is removed. The retroversion and its symptoms may not recur but, if they do, a sling operation should be considered.

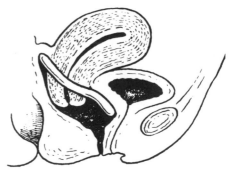

SLING OPERATION ON UTERUS

This is seldom required and indicated only after at least one positive pessary test. The operation makes use of the round ligaments to hold the uterus forward. These ligaments have a considerable capacity for stretching and a permanent correction can never be guaranteed.

Gilliam's Ventrosuspension Operation

The sutures are attached as shown and the loops of round ligament are pulled up through peritoneum and rectus muscle fibres, to be sutured to each other across the recti. This operation can also be performed under laparoscopic visualisation. The round ligaments are picked up with forceps and sutured to the rectus sheath through two small incisions, and there is no need for formal laparotomy. Synthetic absorbable sutures may be preferable as silk can cause abscess formation.

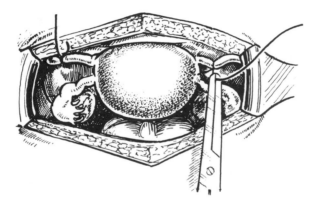

UTEROVAGINAL PROLAPSE

Herniation of the genital tract through the pelvic diaphragm.

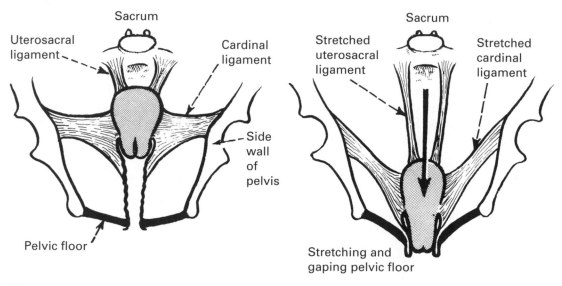

The uterus and vagina are held in the pelvis by the cardinal and utero-sacral ligaments and by the pelvic floor musculature, mainly the levatores ani.

When these ligaments and muscles become ineffective, the uterus and vagina descend (prolapse) through the gap between the muscles.

The Causes of Prolapse are:

1. The stretching of muscle and fibrous tissue which occurs with repeated childbirth and damage to the innervation of the pelvic floor.

2. Increased intra-abdominal pressure (as in fat women with chronic coughs) and in women who undertake heavy manual work.

3. A constitutional predisposition to stretching of the ligaments as a response presumably to years in the erect position. (Thus nulliparous women can develop prolapse: cf. the constitutional factor in the development of varicose veins.)

The incidence of this condition in the United Kingdom is greatly reduced with improvement in obstetric techniques. The more liberal use of caesarean section and the elimination of long labours are probably the two most important factors.

UTEROVAGINAL PROLAPSE

The uterus gradually descends in the axis of the vagina taking the vaginal wall with it. It may present clinically at any level, but is usually classified as one of three degrees.

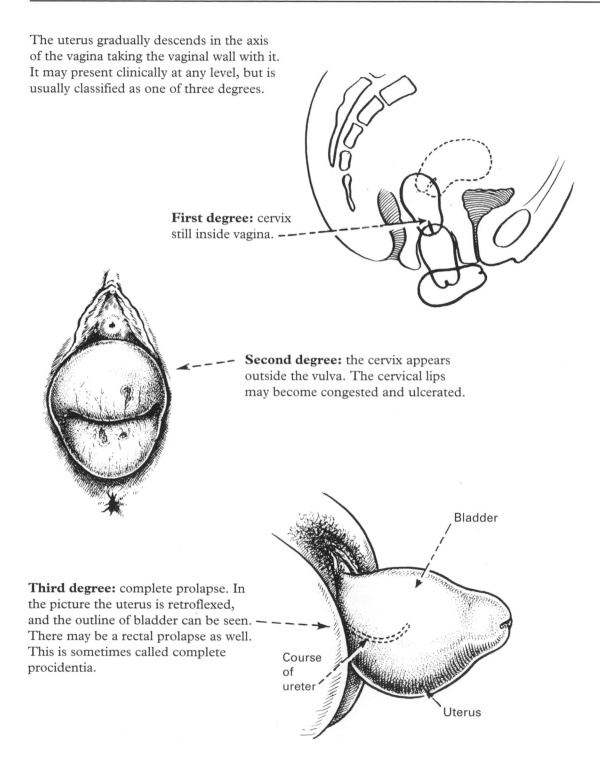

First degree: cervix still inside vagina.

Second degree: the cervix appears outside the vulva. The cervical lips may become congested and ulcerated.

Third degree: complete prolapse. In the picture the uterus is retroflexed, and the outline of bladder can be seen. There may be a rectal prolapse as well. This is sometimes called complete procidentia.

Bladder

Course of ureter

Uterus

VAGINAL PROLAPSE

The prolapse is confined to the vaginal walls and the related viscera. The cervix may come down as well because of elongation of the supravaginal cervix but the uterus stays in the pelvis.

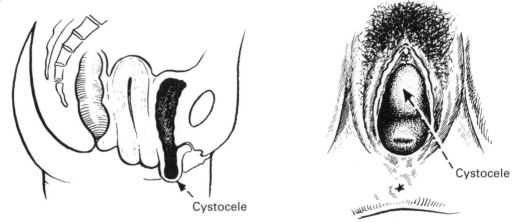

Anterior Prolapse
When the upper part of the anterior wall prolapses, there is an underlying failure of the investing fascia, and the bladder base also descends. This is called a cystocele.

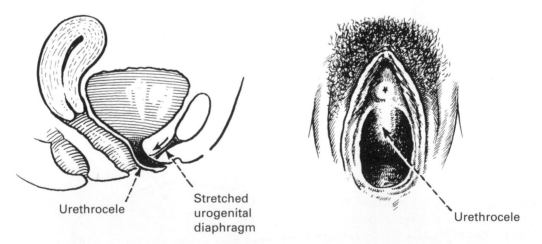

Sometimes the lower part of the vaginal wall prolapses and the urethra also descends. This is called a urethrocele and indicates stretching of the urogenital diaphragm which holds the urethra to the pubic bone.

PROLAPSE OF THE POSTERIOR WALL

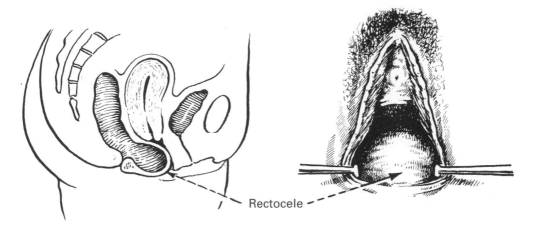

Rectocele

If the prolapse is at the level of the middle third of the vagina, the recto-vaginal septum is often involved and rectum prolapses with vaginal wall. This is called a rectocele. If the lowest part of the vagina prolapses, the perineal body is involved rather than the rectum.

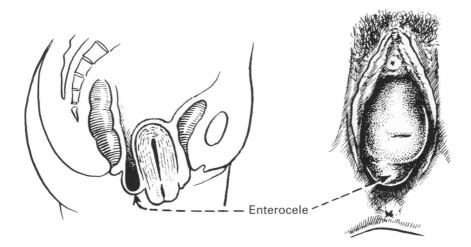

Enterocele

If the upper part of the posterior vaginal wall prolapses, the Pouch of Douglas is elongated and small bowel or omentum may descend. This is called an enterocele. Enterocele is usually associated with uterine prolapse, as in the picture, and is sometimes called 'vault prolapse' or 'hernia of the Pouch of Douglas'. The vaginal vault may prolapse after hysterectomy. This is a difficult condition to treat. One technique suspends the vault from the sacro-iliac ligaments using non-absorbable sutures.

CLINICAL FEATURES OF PROLAPSE

The common complaints are:

1. **'Something coming down'** when the patient is on her feet. The sensation is not there when she lies down.

2. **Backache.** This is often due simply to the patient being overweight.

3. **Increased frequency of micturition.**
   This is at first due to incomplete emptying, but sooner or later is aggravated by cystitis.

4. **A 'bearing down' sensation,** analogous to the parturient woman's desire to push. This is probably caused by pelvic venous congestion, and pressure from the abdominal contents on an inadequate pelvic floor.

5. **Stress Incontinence.**
   This is by no means always present. Sometimes it is found that reduction of the prolapse causes stress incontinence.

6. **Coital problems.** The patient may admit to difficulties with intercourse only on direct questioning.

7. **Difficulty in voiding urine and defaecating.** The patient may find that it is impossible to initiate micturition except by pushing up the cystocele with her finger. In the same way the rectocele must be pushed back to allow emptying of the rectum.

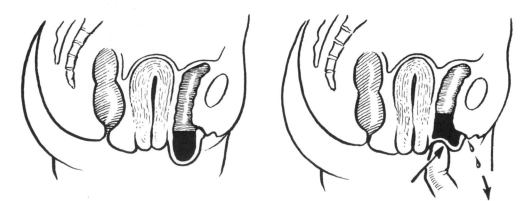

The onset may be gradual or quite sudden and is commoner after the menopause when the genital tract tissues begin to atrophy.

DIFFERENTIAL DIAGNOSIS OF PROLAPSE

Prolapse should be confirmed by vaginal examination. The following
conditions resemble prolapse on superficial examination.

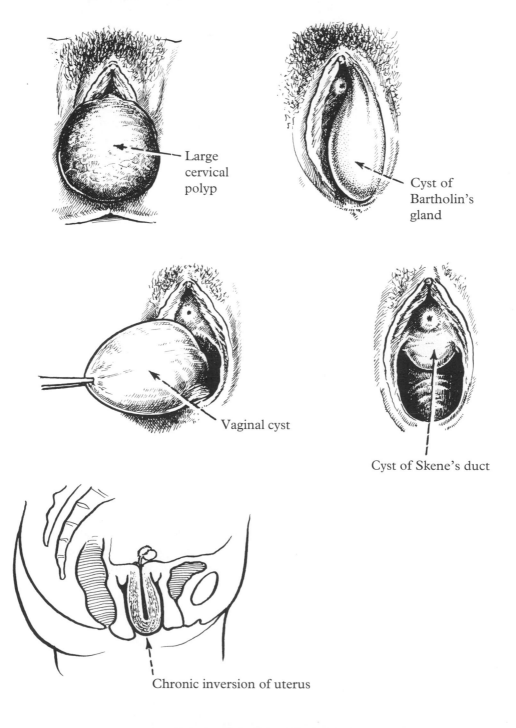

Large
cervical
polyp

Cyst of
Bartholin's
gland

Vaginal cyst

Cyst of Skene's duct

Chronic inversion of uterus

243

PESSARY TREATMENT

A ring pessary, usually of semi-rigid plastic, is inserted into the vagina and so stretches the vaginal walls that they cannot prolapse through the introitus.

The pessary is compressed into a long ovoid shape, lubricated and gently pushed into the vagina, where it resumes its circular shape and takes up a position in the coronal plane. It must not be too tight; and correct fitting is learnt by experience.

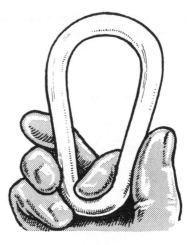

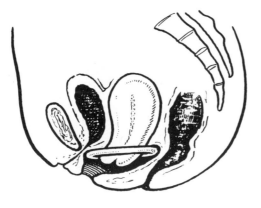

Indications for Pessary Treatment

1. The patient prefers a pessary. Pelvic surgery with its unavoidable risks should only be applied to a willing patient.

2. The prolapse is amenable to pessary support. If the perineal muscles are very deficient they will not hold a pessary. If too big a ring is required, the vaginal wall or cervix will prolapse through it.

3. The patient is not fit for surgery.

4. The patient wishes to delay operation temporarily (for example another pregnancy is anticipated).

Plastic rings should be changed once or twice a year, and if it has been properly fitted the patient will be unaware of its presence in her vagina even during coitus. An ill-fitting pessary is ineffective and may cause dyspareunia and discomfort. If it is too tight or left too long, ulceration of the vaginal wall will occur, and malignant change has been reported. Vaginal oestriol cream or vaginal oestradiol tablets (0.025 mg) help prevent atrophic vaginitis.

ANTERIOR COLPORRHAPHY (AND REPAIR OF CYSTOCELE)

Surgical restoration of the normal anatomy is the best treatment. Reconstitution of the fibrous 'scaffolding' of the pelvic organs allows the musculature to function efficiently, provided it is not itself too fibrotic from prolonged stretching.

Cystocele, rectocele and vaginal wall prolapse are dealt with by anterior and posterior colporrhaphy. Uterine prolapse calls for shortening of the cardinal and uterosacral ligaments. Each 'repair' must be adapted to the extent of the prolapse, and perineal repair is often required as well.

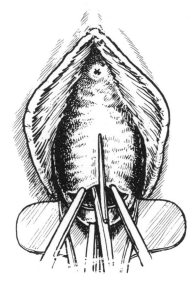

ANTERIOR REPAIR

1. Opening up the anterior vaginal wall.

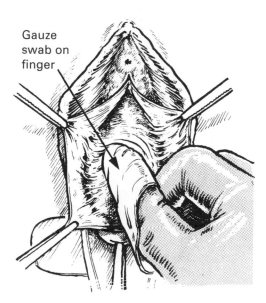

Gauze swab on finger

2. Mobilising cystocele from vaginal walls.

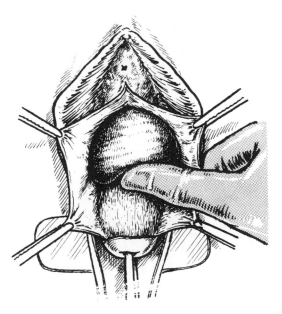

3. Mobilising cystocele from cervix.

ANTERIOR COLPORRHAPHY (AND REPAIR OF CYSTOCELE)

Anterior repair *(contd)*

The next step is obliteration of the cystocele protrusion by tightening the fascial layer between it and the vaginal wall, a layer which is often very difficult to identify. It has various names — pubovesical fascia, pubocervical ligaments (equating them with an anterior continuation of the transverse cervical ligaments), even fascia of Denonvillier. In practice, the bladder has a fascial envelope which can be used for the purpose.

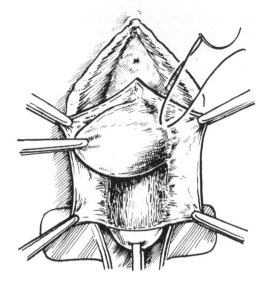

4. Placing the tightening sutures as far laterally as possible.

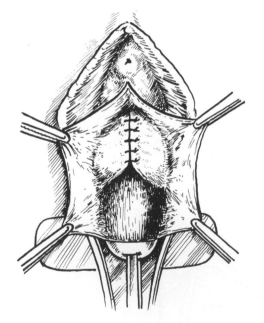

5. Obliteration of the cystocele completed.

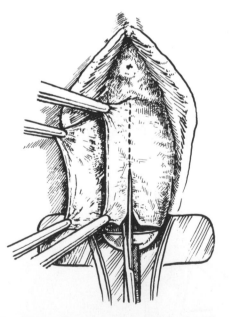

6. Removing redundant vaginal wall. This is followed by closure with interrupted absorbable sutures.

MANCHESTER REPAIR

This involves at the least some shortening of the transverse cervical ligaments and usually amputation of the elongated supravaginal cervix. It is often done in conjunction with anterior and posterior repairs.

1. The cystocele has been repaired. The cervix is being stripped of vaginal wall.

2. Posterior vaginal wall being stripped back.

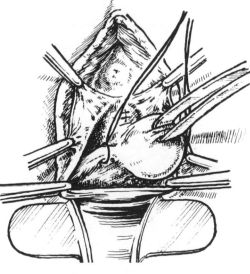

3. Elongated transverse cervical and uterosacral ligaments are sutured and divided.

247

MANCHESTER REPAIR

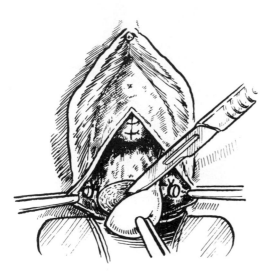

4. Amputation of cervix.

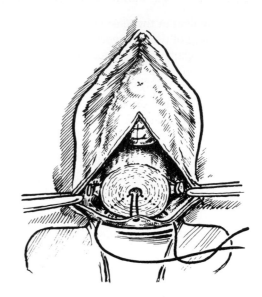

5. Covering the posterior stump with vaginal wall.

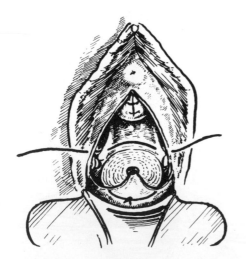

6. Tying the transverse cervical ligaments in front of the cervix and so shortening them and raising the uterus. (This is the so-called Fothergill suture: sometimes two are put in.)

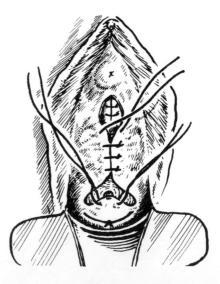

7. Covering cervical stump and closing the vaginal wall. On release of the cervical stump the uterus returns to the pelvis.

POSTERIOR COLPOPERINEORRHAPHY (INCLUDING REPAIR OF RECTOCELE)

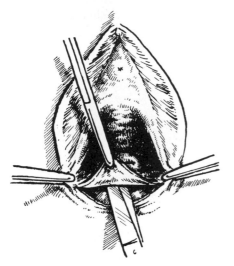

1. Mobilisation of the posterior vaginal wall.

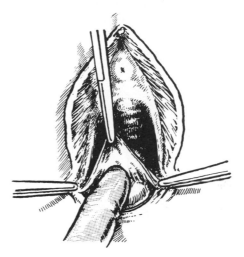

2. Separating rectocele from posterior vaginal wall.

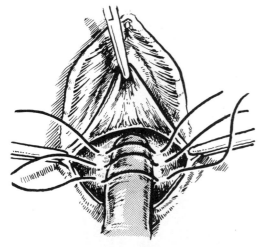

3. Obliterating the rectocele by tightening the fascial layer (cf. obliterating the cystocele.)

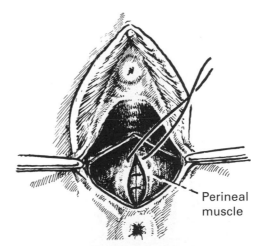

Perineal muscle

4. Excess vaginal skin is removed. The perineal muscles are sutured over the obliterated rectocele. The skin and vagina are closed as in perineorrhaphy (p.180).

REPAIR OF ENTEROCELE

An enterocele is a prolapse of the Pouch of Douglas peritoneum in between the upper vagina and rectum, and must be distinguished from a rectocele. Repair of enterocele is usually combined with repair of uterine prolapse which is not shown here.

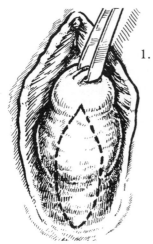

1. Dotted lines show the area of vaginal wall which will be removed.

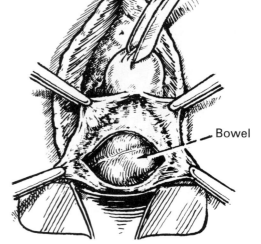

Bowel

2. The enterocele sac is identified and opened.

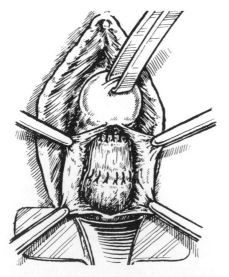

3. Once the sac is mobilised the neck is sutured up as far as possible to obliterate the enterocele. The sac is then sutured to the neck of the cervix. Alternatively a high purse-string suture may be employed.

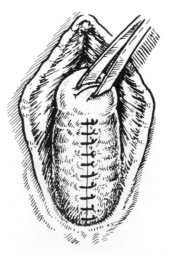

4. The vaginal wall is closed in the usual way.

250

VAGINAL HYSTERECTOMY

Indications

1. When the prolapse is complete. In such cases the ligaments are very attenuated and a better result may be obtained by removal of the uterus.

2. When there is some non-malignant uterine condition — small fibroids, menorrhagia.

Some surgeons will always remove a uterus rather than leave it, when doing a repair. It may be difficult to remove the ovaries by the vaginal route.

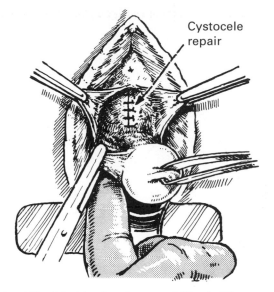

Cystocele repair

1. The bladder has been mobilised. The uterine ligaments are put on the stretch and divided.

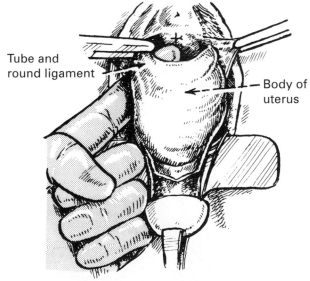

Tube and round ligament

Body of uterus

2. Utero-vesical pouch has been entered. Broad ligament structures are put on the stretch and divided. The uterus is then removed.

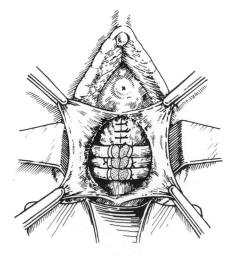

3. The lateral pedicles are sutured together to support the Pouch of Douglas. The vaginal vault is closed. A posterior repair may be performed.

VAGINAL HYSTERECTOMY

OPERATIVE AND POST-OPERATIVE COMPLICATIONS

Selection of patients

1. Neither youth nor age are contraindications but the patient must be reasonably fit, with adequate cardio-respiratory and renal function. Oestradiol vaginal cream may be used to treat atrophic vaginitis prior to surgery.

2. The prolapse should be symptomatic.

3. Beware of causing dyspareunia or apareunia by performing a tight repair, especially in a younger woman.

During operation

1. Bleeding pedicles are more difficult to control than during abdominal surgery. The parametric structures should be clamped, divided and ligated in small rather than large bites.

2. With the uterus gone, there is a risk of distorting the ureters if the bladder fascia is tightened too much during repair of the cystocele.

After operation

There is a tendency to vault haematoma which may become infected and ultimately discharges per vaginam.

LATE COMPLICATIONS

1. Recurrence of Prolapse

(a) **Due to continuing extension of fibrous supports.** This may be a congenital weakness or a result of excessive intra-abdominal pressure as from chronic bronchitis in a fat woman. (Cf. recurrence of inguinal hernia due to imperfect healing.)

(b) **Faulty Technique**

Vaginal repair operations call for some experience. An unsuspected and unlooked for enterocele may appear.

2. Stress Incontinence

Sometimes this appears for the first time after a repair operation, or it is not specifically complained of and ignored during operation.

3. Dyspareunia

The surgeon must enquire before the operation about the patient's sexual activity and must be careful to leave a functional vagina where this is required (even although this may make support of the prolapse more difficult). Occasionally dyspareunia may be caused by vaginal adhesions.

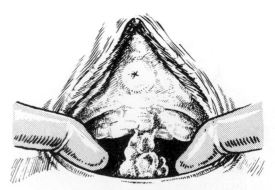

Vaginal wall adhesions

CHAPTER 13

DISEASES OF THE OVARY AND FALLOPIAN TUBE

CLINICAL FEATURES OF OVARIAN TUMOURS

Symptoms due to Size

Because of the lack of any specific symptoms, ovarian tumours are often large by the time the doctor is consulted. Menstrual function is seldom upset, and any irregularity is attributed to the patient's 'time of life'. She may have noticed that her clothes are getting tight and attributed this to weight gain or, if the abdominal swelling has coincided with amenorrhoea, she may believe herself to be pregnant.

Pressure Symptoms

These are commonly increased frequency of micturition, gastro-intestinal symptoms and a dull pain in the lower abdomen. Very large tumours may cause respiratory embarrassment and oedema or varicosities in the legs, and a characteristic 'ovarian cachexia' develops, due perhaps to interference with alimentary function.

Very large tumours are in one sense reassuring, since they are less likely to be malignant. In the time taken to achieve such size, an ovarian cancer would as a rule have already declared itself by some other sign such as ascites or pain.

CLINICAL FEATURES OF OVARIAN TUMOURS

Small tumours remain in the pelvis
and will only be detected on bimanual
examination or by ultrasound.

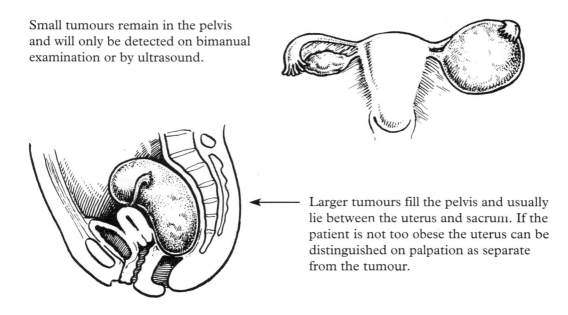

Larger tumours fill the pelvis and usually
lie between the uterus and sacrum. If the
patient is not too obese the uterus can be
distinguished on palpation as separate
from the tumour.

A tumour occupying the abdomen causes a midline swelling and is usually tense.

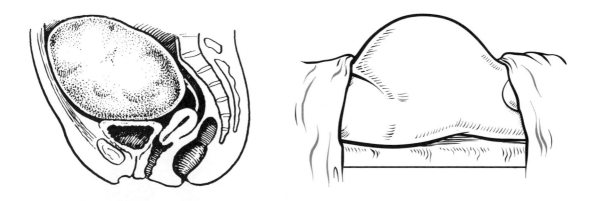

Little can be done at this stage to classify the tumour or exclude malignancy; but very large
tumours are likely to be benign; a primarily malignant tumour would have killed the patient
before reaching such a size.

255

CLINICAL FEATURES OF OVARIAN TUMOURS

If the patient is very thin, irregularities may be palpated and sometimes two tumours may be suspected.

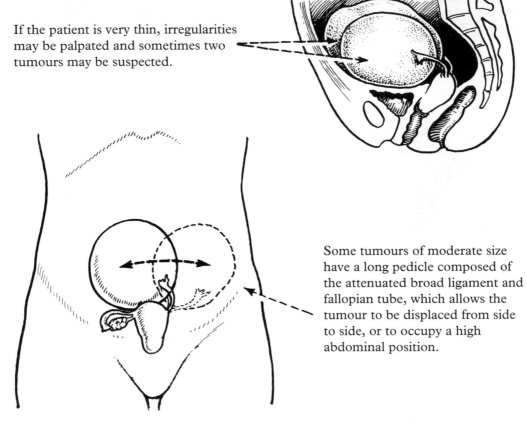

Some tumours of moderate size have a long pedicle composed of the attenuated broad ligament and fallopian tube, which allows the tumour to be displaced from side to side, or to occupy a high abdominal position.

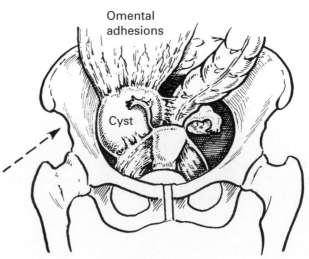

Omental adhesions

Cyst

The upper pole can usually be distinguished and the lower pole can be palpated per vaginam. Adhesions, inflammation and displacement of pelvic organs may all exist along with a tumour and confuse the examiner.

DIFFERENTIAL DIAGNOSIS

An experienced examiner will recognise an ovarian tumour mainly because ovarian tumour is, in the circumstances, the most likely diagnosis. All abdominal swellings should be subjected to ultrasound and X-ray examination.

Two very obvious mistakes must be avoided.

1. The midline swelling due to a full bladder.

2. The 16-week pregnancy. The gravid uterus at this stage has a very soft isthmic region which can resemble the pedicle of a cyst.

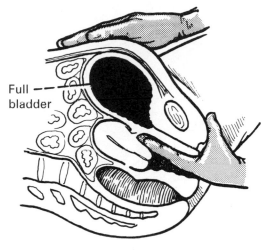

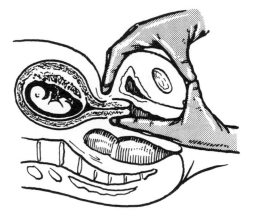

ASCITES

A fluid thrill may be elicited from an ovarian cyst, and ascites and tumour may coexist; but as a rule the distinction should be easily made.

(See 'Shifting Dullness', page 78).

With Ascites
The bowel floats on the fluid. The percussion note is resonant over the top of the swelling and dull over the flanks.

With ovarian cyst
Percussion note is dull over the top of the swelling and resonant in the flanks.

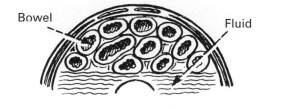

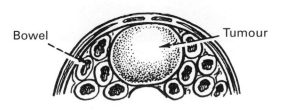

DIFFERENTIAL DIAGNOSIS

Uterine Fibroids

A large midline intramural fibroid (p.213) may be impossible to distinguish from a solid ovarian tumour until the abdomen is opened and an entirely different surgical problem encountered.

An ovarian tumour will displace the uterus forwards or downwards where it may sometimes be made out separately on vaginal examination.

An intramural fibroid will obscure the uterus. The cavity is often elongated.

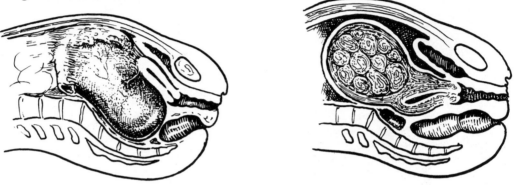

Ultrasound examination should be able to distinguish between fibroid and ovarian cyst; but many ovarian tumours are solid, and some fibroids undergo cystic degeneration. Vaginal ultrasound gives a more detailed picture of the pelvic contents and more precise diagnosis.

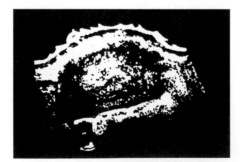

Scan of fibroid

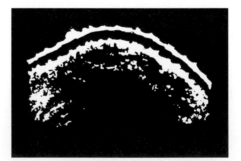

Scan of cyst

DIFFERENTIAL DIAGNOSIS

Pelvic Inflammation

The swelling palpated *per vaginam* may be due to an adherent mass of uterus, tubes, 'chocolate' ovarian cysts, and bowel.

A pyosalpinx, tuberculous or otherwise, may give the same sensation.

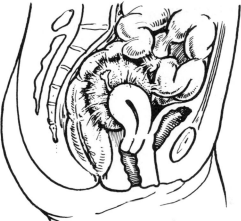

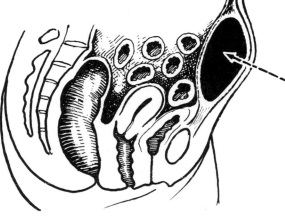

Rectus Sheath Haematoma

This rare condition presents as a fixed abdominal mass, accompanied by pain; and usually follows sudden exertion such as severe coughing. It should be thought of when the pelvis is found to be empty of any tumour.

The Atonic Abdominal Wall

This is seen in old women who display a tense and distended abdomen. There is however resonance to percussion in every area.

Fluid Retention Syndrome

This may cause considerable abdominal distension, particularly in the evening or pre-menstrually.

The Obese Abdominal Wall

The obese patient may be convinced she has a tumour although she is only putting on weight (phantom tumour). Palpation is difficult; but the percussion note in the lower half of the abdomen will be resonant.

Mesenteric Cyst
Hydatid Cyst
Pancreatic Cyst
Large Hydronephrotic Kidney
⎫
⎬
⎭
These are all rarities in the U.K. but must be considered if the physical signs are equivocal and especially if the swelling is not in the midline.

DIFFERENTIAL DIAGNOSIS

Broad Ligament Cysts
The distinction is not likely to be made before laparotomy, when the intact ovary is observed on the back of the swelling.

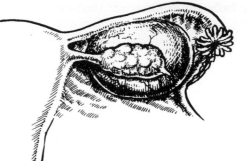

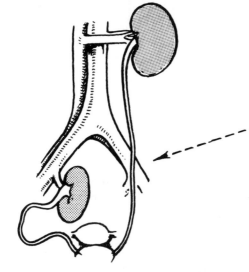

Ectopic Kidney or Spleen
These abnormalities are rare but as they are usually detected for the first time on bimanual examination they must be borne in mind. The ectopic kidney can lie anywhere in the pelvis and derives its blood supply from the iliac vessels. The ureter often runs a tortuous course.

Retroperitoneal Tumours
Retroperitoneal in the surgical sense means behind the peritoneum of the posterior abdominal wall. Such tumours are rare but may arise from any connective tissue, lipoma being the commonest. Examination reveals a fixed tumour; but the lipoma may be deceptively fluctuant. The tumour may displace the ureter and is in close relation to large vessels.

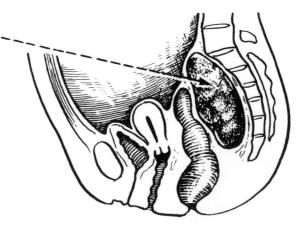

TORSION OF THE PEDICLE

Complications of Ovarian Tumours

TORSION of the PEDICLE
(Axial rotation)

This is the commonest complication and may occur with any tumour except those with adhesions. The thin-walled veins of the pedicle are obstructed first while the arterial supply continues. As a result there is haemorrhage into the tumour and into the peritoneum, and if not treated gangrene will occur. Very rarely the pedicle atrophies and the tumour obtains a new blood supply through its adhesions to surrounding viscera (parasitic tumour).

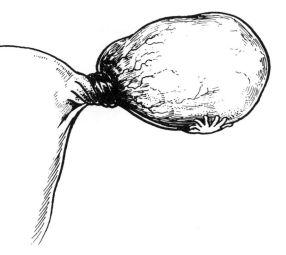

Clinical Features

Subacute
The patient complains of recurrent abdominal pain which passes off as the pedicle untwists. There is a rise in pulse and temperature during the bleeding; and over a period anaemia develops.

Acute
The signs and symptoms are those of an acute abdominal condition. The problem becomes one of differential diagnosis to exclude those conditions in which laparotomy is not needed and laparoscopy may be useful.

Pain tends to be intense and continuous.

Differential Diagnosis
'Surgical Conditions' (i.e. those conditions commonly seen and dealt with by a general surgeon.)

> Acute appendicitis
> Meckel's diverticulitis
> Obstruction of bowel
> Diverticulitis

Ruptured Cyst
This may occur alone or in conjunction with torsion. Rupture is not particularly upsetting to the patient unless the contents are irritant.

TORSION OF THE PEDICLE

Differential Diagnosis

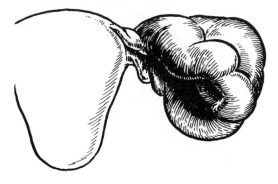

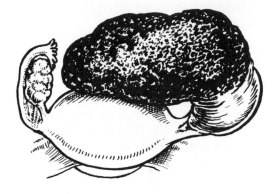

Acute Pelvic Inflammation with tubo-ovarian abscess.

Signs of infection are more marked. A cyst which has undergone rotation is usually larger than the diffuse swelling of pelvic inflammation.

Ectopic Pregnancy
The swelling is usually small although extremely tender and the history usually suggestive; but in a young woman this condition must always be considered.

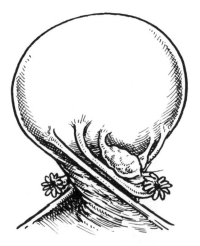

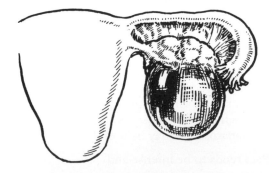

Torsion of a Fibroid
Normal organs very rarely if ever develop axial rotation, but a uterus enlarged by a fibroid may do so.

Ovulation Bleeding
If the ovulation bleeding is greater than usual the woman may show quite marked signs of peritonism. The corpus luteum may thereafter become exaggeratedly cystic and mislead the examiner.

RUPTURE OF OVARIAN CYST

Rupture may be either traumatic or spontaneous.

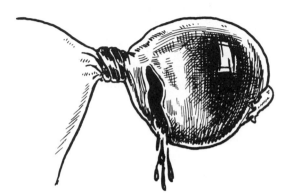

1. Following torsion of a pedicle.

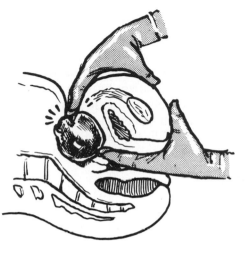

2. During bimanual examination.

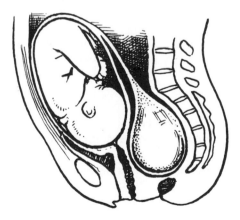

3. During labour when the cyst is impacted in the pelvis.

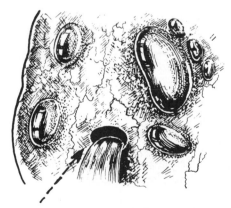

4. Spontaneous rupture. This is not uncommon, especially with malignant cysts, when the epithelial tissue outgrows the connective tissue.

RUPTURE OF OVARIAN CYST

PSEUDOMYXOMA PERITONEI
This rare condition occasionally but not inevitably follows the rupture of a mucinous cystadenoma (page 266). The epithelial cells implant on the peritoneum and continue to secrete a gelatinous pseudomucin which is not absorbed, or secretion is faster than absorption. The abdominal cavity is eventually filled with the jelly, while the secreting cells spread over the parietal and visceral peritoneum. A reactive peritonitis with adhesions is a sequel and the patient must be operated on at intervals for removal of as much of the exudate as possible. The disease develops slowly over several years, but will eventually cause the patient's death from cachexia or obstruction. The 5-year survival rate is about 50% and 10-year survival falls to around 20%. A similar condition is reported chiefly in males, from a ruptured mucocele of the appendix vermiformis.

ASCITES
Ascites (Gk. askos: a wine skin) means free fluid in the peritoneal cavity and its presence in association with an ovarian tumour is strongly suggestive of malignancy. The cause is unknown, but any large tumour may be accompanied by ascites (cf. the small quantities of free fluid sometimes seen at caesarean section).

ASCITES and HYDROTHORAX
The fluid may track via the lymphatic system from the peritoneal to the pleural cavity. Hydrothorax may accompany ascites due to any cause, or may occur as an accompaniment of a lung tumour. The so-called Meigs' syndrome describes the specific condition of ascites and hydrothorax in conjunction with a benign ovarian fibroma.

Features suggestive of malignancy
1. *Age.* If the patient is over 50 the chance of malignancy is over 50% as opposed to less than 15% in premenopausal women. Tumours in childhood are usually malignant.
2. *Rapid growth.*
3. *Ascites* (almost pathognomonic).
4. *Solid tumours*, especially when bilateral.
5. *Multilocular cysts with solid areas.* (At least 10% of cysts are malignant).
6. *Pain.* Pressure pain can occur with any tumour; but referred pain suggests malignant involvement of nerve roots.
7. Tumour markers, such as CA125, may be measured in the blood, but a normal level does not exclude malignancy.

OVARIAN TUMOURS

Ovarian tumours may arise at any age, but are commonest between 30 and 60. Their clinical significance is threefold:

1. Ovarian tumours are particularly liable to be or to become malignant.
2. In their early stages they are asymptomatic and painless.
3. They may grow to a large size and tend to undergo mechanical complications such as torsion and perforation.

Histological Classification
Most tumours arise from the ovarian stroma and germinal epithelium. The embryonic coelom from which that epithelium develops also gives rise to the Müllerian duct from which develop the structures of the genital tract, and it is this common origin which explains the great variety of epithelial patterns which are met with.

PRIMARY EPITHELIAL TUMOURS

1. Mucinous cystadenoma or cystadenocarcinoma (cf. cervical epithelium).
2. Serous cystadenoma or cystadenocarcinoma (cf. tubal epithelium).
3. Endometrioma or Endometrioid carcinoma (cf. endometrium).
4. Clear cell carcinoma.
5. Brenner tumour.

STROMATOUS TUMOURS GERM CELL TUMOURS

1. Fibroma or sarcoma.
2. Dysgerminoma.
3. Teratoma.
4. Gonadoblastoma.
5. Yolk sac tumour.
6. Carcinoid
7. Thyroid tumour Choriocarcinoma } Hormone-producing

HORMONE-PRODUCING TUMOURS

Oestrogen-producing:
1. Granulosa cell tumour.
2. Thecoma.

Androgen-producing:
3. Sertoli-Leydig cell tumour (Arrhenoblastoma).
4. Hilar cell tumour.
5. Lipoid cell tumour.

There is one well-known secondary tumour of the ovary, the Krükenberg tumour, a secondary of a stomach carcinoma.

It is now recognised that all ovarian tumours may secrete hormones, especially oestrogens.

MUCINOUS CYSTADENOMA

A unilocular or multilocular cyst of ovary lined by tall columnar epithelium resembling that of the cervix or large intestine. It is usually large and may reach immense proportions, occupying the whole peritoneal cavity and compressing other organs. It may occur at any age.

The surface of the cyst is completely smooth and round but may be slightly nodular due to projecting loculi.

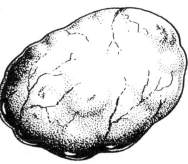

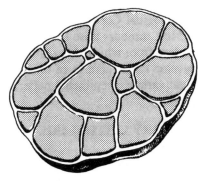

The cut surface of the cyst is multilocular and has a mosaic pattern.

Microscopically the tumour has an outer fibrous capsule from which extend septa supporting the walls of the cysts. The latter are lined by tall columnar epithelium with basal nuclei and contain a gelatinous glycoprotein or mucin.

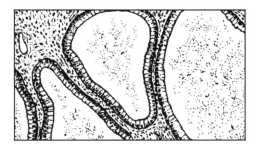

The signs and symptoms are those generally associated with any non-functioning ovarian tumour. Rupture may occur and seeding of the epithelium on the peritoneal surface may cause pseudomyxoma peritonei.

MUCINOUS CYSTADENOCARCINOMA
This is only a third as common as the serous variety. Malignancy in a mucinous cyst is characterised by the formation of areas of solid carcinoma in the wall. The cells are columnar, show mitoses and tend to form glandular structures.

SEROUS CYSTADENOMA

A unilocular or multilocular cyst lined by epithelium similar to the fallopian tube. They are the most common benign epithelial tumours and form 20% of all ovarian neoplasms. In 10% of cases they are bilateral. It is uncommon to find them larger than a fetal head. They show one of three structures:-

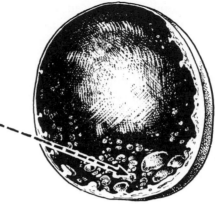

(1) A simple cystic form with smooth surface and smooth lining.

(2) A cystic structure with intra-cystic papillary formations. The latter may be sessile buttons or pedunculated frond-like projections.

(3) An adenomatous form where many of the loculi are small and papillary structures are solid and complex.

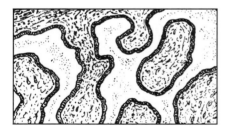

Microscopically the tumour has a fibrous capsule. Septa support the cysts which are lined by cubical epithelium and contain thin serous fluid.

They present no distinctive symptoms.

If rupture occurs papillary structures may land on the peritoneal surface where they may grow or lie dormant for years.

SEROUS CYSTADENOCARCINOMA

This is by far the commonest primary carcinoma, accounting for 60% of all cases, and in over half the cases it is bilateral. The cysts are always of papillary type and the epithelium burrowing through the capsule produces papillary processes on the serous surface. Extension of the growth to the pelvis and adjacent organs fixes the tumour. Ascites is always present.

The papillomata are always more fleshy than in the simple cysts and microscopically the epithelial cells are several layers thick and show numerous mitoses. When they invade the capsule they frequently take an acinar form.

CARCINOMA OF THE OVARY

In developed countries, women have a lifetime risk of developing ovarian cancer of about 1.4%, which is slightly greater than the risk of cervical or endometrial cancers, but well below the 7% average risk of breast cancer.

Genetic factors are sometimes involved, as in the Lynch Syndrome of familial breast, colorectal and ovarian cancer. Ovulation induction with Clomiphene over more than a year carries a 10-fold increased risk of ovarian cancer. Long-term oral contraceptive use reduces the incidence of ovarian cancers.

Nearly 25% of all ovarian neoplasms are malignant. Approximately 80% of them are primary growths of the ovary, the remainder being secondary, usually carcinomata.

Primary Carcinoma of the Ovary   80% of all cases of primary carcinoma of the ovary arise in serous or mucinous cysts. These cysts may however be malignant from the outset. Reference has already been made to these forms of malignancy.

Solid Carcinoma of the Ovary   This accounts for 10% of primary carcinoma. It is commonly bilateral but one tumour is usually larger than the other. The ovarian shape is retained for a time and there is a well-marked pedicle but soon the tumours become fixed, secondary deposits occur in the omentum and ascites develops.

Microscopically the growth may take the form of an adenocarcinoma but more commonly it shows solid alveoli or anaplastic epithelial cells in a fibrous stroma.

Endometrioid Carcinoma of the Ovary   It is now recognised that carcinoma of the ovary may be of endometrial type, sometimes arising in endometrioma. Attacks of pain, unusual with ovarian cancer, are common. Sometimes there is uterine bleeding in post-menopausal cases.

Usually the lesion is cystic and chocolate brown in colour. If such a cyst ruptures spontaneously, malignancy should be suspected. The histology varies as in uterine carcinoma. It may be a well-differentiated adenocarcinoma, an adeno-acanthoma, mucinous adenocarcinoma or clear-celled carcinoma.

Clear Cell Carcinoma   It is doubtful if this exists as a distinct entity. Clear cells may be seen in almost any variety of ovarian carcinoma, but occasionally a carcinoma, usually solid, consists almost entirely of polygonal cells with clear cytoplasm. It behaves in the same way as any other solid carcinoma and has the same prognosis.

Secondary Carcinoma of the Ovary   The ovary may be the site of secondary deposits from growths arising in other parts of the genital tract. These are usually overshadowed by the clinical manifestations of the primary growth.

Ovarian metastases from extra-genital tumours are not uncommon. The commonest sites of primary growth are breast, stomach and large intestine. They usually occur in functioning ovaries and their importance lies in the fact that the metastatic growths reach a large size while the primary growth is small and gives rise to no clinical manifestations. They usually reproduce the histological characteristics of the primary cancer. Owing to their rapid growth they tend to be friable and haemorrhagic giving rise to blood-stained peritoneal exudate.

BRENNER TUMOUR

A benign tumour mainly solid and most common in the 6th decade, composed of fibrous and epithelial elements in varying proportions. It forms 2% of all solid ovarian neoplasms.

It is usually solid and resembles a fibroma. Occasionally there may be microcysts or even an associated large mucinous cyst. Microscopically it is composed mainly of fibrous tissue with small islands of clear epithelial cells of squamous appearance. Sometimes the islands become cystic and the epithelial cells become mucinous.

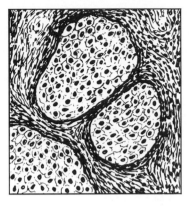

FIBROMA

This is composed of fibrous tissue and resembles fibromata found elsewhere. It is most common in the elderly and accounts for 4–5% of all ovarian neoplasms.

The fibroma is believed by many to be a thecoma which has undergone fibrous transformation. It is sometimes associated with Meig's syndrome.

GERM CELL TUMOURS

There are four main types of germ cell tumour:-

(1) Dysgerminoma;
(2) Tumours of tissues found in the embryo or adult — the teratomata;
(3) Tumours of dysgenetic gonads — commonly a gonadoblastoma;
(4) Tumours of extra-embryonic tissues such as choriocarcinoma or yolk sac tumour.

DYSGERMINOMA

This is the only solid ovarian tumour of characteristic appearance. Usually ovoid with a smooth capsule, it is of rubbery consistency and greyish colour. It is commonest in younger age groups, under 30 years as a rule, and is often bilateral. Sometimes it is found in cases of intersex.

GERM CELL TUMOURS

Dysgerminoma *(contd)*

Microscopically it consists of masses of large clear epithelial cells with large nuclei, resembling primitive germ cells, in cords or alveoli. Fine connective tissue infiltrated by lymphocytes separates the bundles of epithelial cells. The malignancy varies but many appear to be relatively benign and do not recur. Those in children tend to be more malignant.

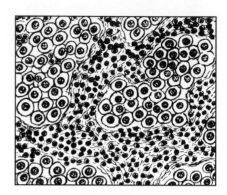

TERATOMATA

These are broadly divided into (a) cystic and (b) solid forms.

(a) Cystic teratoma or dermoid

This is one of the commonest ovarian tumours and is usually diagnosed during the child-bearing period but may be found at any age and is frequently bilateral.

It is ovoid and unilocular with on one aspect a rounded eminence from which hairs grow and on or in which teeth may be found. The wall consists of dense fibrous tissue lined by stratified squamous epithelium. The eminence may contain sebaceous glands, teeth, hair, nervous tissues, cartilage, bone, respiratory and intestinal epithelium and thyroid gland tissue. Thick yellow sebaceous material fills the cyst.

They are particularly liable to have a long pedicle and easily undergo torsion or interfere with the movement of the pregnant uterus.

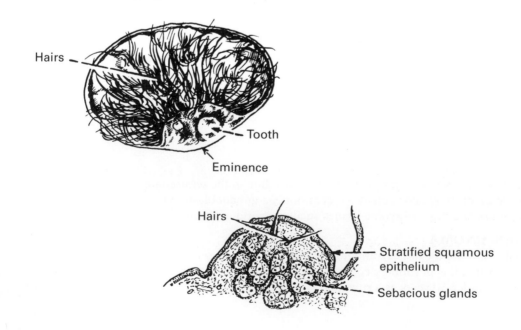

GERM CELL TUMOURS

(b) **Solid teratoma**

These occur at an earlier age than dermoids, often in childhood. They are solid and may contain any tissue from the three germinal layers, mixed in a completely disorderly fashion. They are particularly liable to undergo malignant change, the malignancy arising in any one of the tissues present.

Gonadoblastoma

This is a tumour associated with dysgenetic gonads, usually streak gonads. The patient is an apparent female and may have a diminutive uterus, tubes and vagina, but usually there is a sex chromosome anomaly such as XO/XY.

The tumour is composed of two types of cell: (a) a large primitive germ cell and (b) small cells of granulosa cell type. Call-Exner bodies (small rosettes) may be seen in the latter. These two types of cell form epithelial islands in a stroma which may contain Leydig-like cells. Sometimes the germ cells may undergo rapid proliferation and give rise to a dysgerminoma. Some of the dysgerminomata in children probably arise in this way. Choriocarcinoma may also take origin in a gonadoblastoma. There are frequently some signs of masculinisation and 17-ketosteroid excretion may be raised.

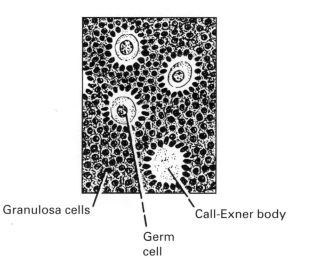

Granulosa cells · Germ cell · Call-Exner body

Yolk sac tumour

This is a rare tumour found in children and young adults. It has a variable histological structure and is highly malignant. The main interest lies in the fact that it produces alpha-fetoprotein and the blood levels can be used as a diagnostic test and as a means of monitoring response to treatment.

Choriocarcinoma is mentioned in the succeeding part dealing with hormone-producing tumours.

KRUKENBERG TUMOUR

This is a secondary carcinoma of the ovary. It is remarkable for its characteristic histological appearance and the fact that the primary growth, usually in the stomach, less commonly in the large intestine, is often clinically silent. The ovarian tumours are bilateral, of equal size, smooth and lobulated. They remain freely mobile with no adhesions. Being firm and fibrous in appearance they are frequently mistaken for fibromata, but these are usually unilateral. The patient is usually between 30 and 40 years of age, younger than the usual gastric carcinoma patient.

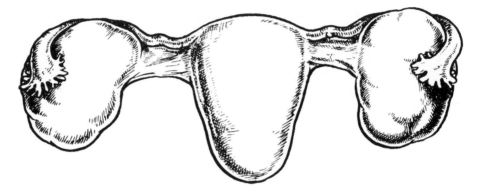

Histologically they have a well-defined appearance. There is a very cellular stroma, resembling a sarcoma, in which are large epithelial cells lying singly or in alveoli. These epithelial cells have a clear cytoplasm with a crescentic nucleus pushed to one side giving a signet-ring appearance which is typical. The cytoplasm is full of mucin.

The majority of patients with this tumour succumb within 1 year of diagnosis.

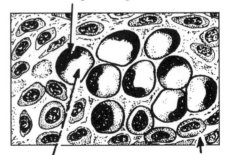

Nucleus of 'signet-ring' cell

Clear mucin-filled cytoplasm

Cellular stroma

HORMONE-PRODUCING TUMOURS

AMENORRHOEA and OVARIAN TUMOURS

Disturbance of menstruation is unusual with the commoner forms of ovarian tumour such as cystadenomas. Amenorrhoea is much more likely to occur in cases of functioning tumours producing steroids.

HORMONE-PRODUCING TUMOURS

The commonest tumours of this kind are steroid-producing, particularly sex steroids. Both androgenic and oestrogenic effects have been described with every histological variety but certain tumours of well defined histological structures are commonly associated with the production of one type of steroid.

OESTROGEN-PRODUCING TUMOURS

These belong to the granulosa-theca cell group and are found at all ages. They account for 3% of all solid tumours of the ovary.

Oestrogen excess causes:

1. Hyperplasia of myomctrium → enlarged uterus.
2. Hyperplasia of endometrium → irregular bleeding. Occasionally amenorrhoea occurs if the production of oestrogen does not fluctuate.
3. Hyperplasia of mammary gland tissue → enlargement, tenderness of breasts.
4. Oestrogenic vaginal smear.

In childhood there is accelerated skeletal growth and appearance of sex hair.

5% occur in children → precocious puberty.
60% occur in child-bearing years → irregular menstruation.
30% occur in post-menopausal women → post-menopausal bleeding.

Diagnosis

Granulosa cell tumour in childhood is the usual cause of female precocity and diagnosis is obvious. In child-bearing and post-menopausal years diagnosis is difficult owing to the multiplicity of causes of irregular vaginal bleeding. Laparoscopy and ovarian biopsy may be useful.

Pathology

These tumours vary very much in function. Large tumours may be virtually functionless. In childhood and early adult life the tumours are composed mainly of granulosa cells. In later life they are usually thecomata. The granulosa cell type of growth should be considered as carcinoma. Recurrence may occur many years after removal of the primary growth. It is not possible to correlate accurately malignancy with histological appearances. In 14% of cases endometrial hyperplasia becomes atypical and carcinoma develops.

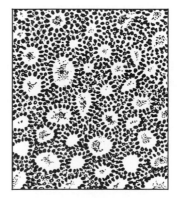

ANDROGEN-PRODUCING TUMOURS

Three distinct types of masculinising ovarian tumour are recognised: (a) Sertoli-Leydig cell tumour (Arrhenoblastoma), (b) Hilar cell tumour, (c) Lipoid cell tumour. All three cause amenorrhoea.

SERTOLI-LEYDIG CELL TUMOUR (Arrhenoblastoma)

This is a rare tumour and forms much less than 1% of all ovarian tumours. It occurs in young adult females. Clinically two stages are recognised:

1. **Period of defeminisation**   2. **Period of masculinisation**

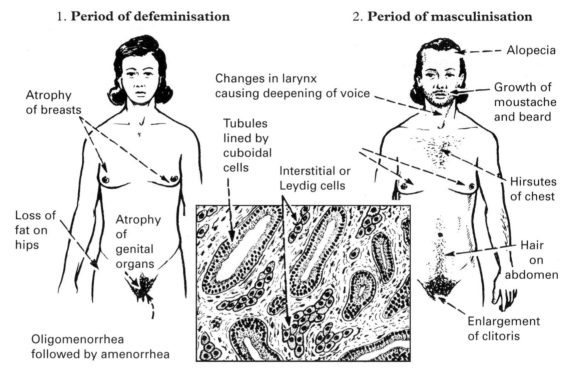

Atrophy of breasts

Loss of fat on hips

Atrophy of genital organs

Oligomenorrhea followed by amenorrhea

Changes in larynx causing deepening of voice

Tubules lined by cuboidal cells

Interstitial or Leydig cells

Alopecia

Growth of moustache and beard

Hirsutes of chest

Hair on abdomen

Enlargement of clitoris

Pathology

Usually appears as a small white or yellowish tumour within the ovarian substance. Cystic degeneration may occur. These tumours are usually of only low-grade malignancy.

Histologically it consists of primitive tubules surrounded by Leydig cells which contain crystalloids of Reinke. These are rod-shaped structures in the cytoplasm of Leydig cells and said to be diagnostic of these cells.

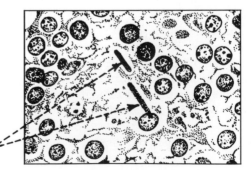

Crystalloids of Reinke

ANDROGEN-PRODUCING TUMOURS

SERTOLI-LEYDIG CELL TUMOUR *(contd)*

Biochemistry

The symptoms are due to the secretion of testosterone. The quantities are small and therefore the output of metabolites such as 17-ketosteroids is within the normal range. Direct estimations of blood testosterone can be made. Some of these tumours secrete oestrogens. Removal of the tumour results in regression of symptoms in the same order as their appearance. Menstruation returns within a month or two. Voice changes tend to be permanent.

HILAR CELL TUMOUR

This is a very rare tumour found in post-menopausal women. Defeminisation occurs but signs of virilism are usually mild, consisting of hirsutes, alopecia and enlargement of the clitoris.

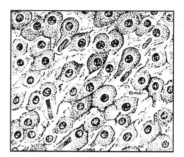

Pathology

Hilar cell tumours are small, brown, simple tumours in the ovarian hilum consisting of polyhedral Leydig cells. Crystalloids of Reinke are occasionally present. 17-ketosteroids are usually within the normal post-menopausal range. Small quantities of androgen are produced.

LIPOID CELL TUMOUR (ovoblastoma, masculinovoblastoma, adrenal-like tumour)

This is also a rare tumour causing masculinisation and producing symptoms and signs of hyper-corticoidism such as skin striae, obesity, polycythaemia, a diabetic glucose tolerance curve and hypertension.

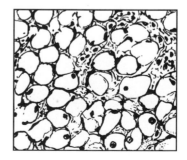

Pathology

The tumour consists of cells with a high content of lipoid and is commonly large and yellowish.

Unlike other virilising tumours the 17-ketosteroid output is greatly increased and the excretion of 17-hydroxycorticosteroids is also raised. ACTH or chorionic gonadotrophin will cause a further increase, but dexamethasone does not diminish the output, thus helping to differentiate the condition from virilism of adrenal origin.

OTHER HORMONE-PRODUCING TUMOURS

CARCINOID (Argentaffinoma: serotonin-producing tumour)

This tumour arises in association with cystic teratoma of the ovary from cells related to respiratory or intestinal epithelium sometimes found in these cysts.

It may give rise to a typical carcinoid syndrome with patchy cyanosis, flushing, diarrhoea, intestinal colic, oedema and cardiac failure due to tricuspid valve lesion. Sometimes the syndrome does not appear until the tumour has metastasised to the liver.

Thyroid Tumour (Struma Ovarii)

Small foci of thyroid tissue are common in ovarian teratomata but large amounts are rare and functioning thyroid tissue is still more rare. When the thyroid tissue actually proliferates and forms a tumour 5-10% become malignant.

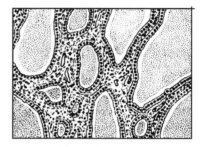

CHORIOCARCINOMA of the Ovary

This is an extremely rare tumour of the ovary. Most commonly it is associated with dysgerminoma and both in turn may be derived from germinal cells in a dysgenetic gonad. Syncytiotrophoblast is always present, but sometimes cytotrophoblast is also formed. The hormones produced are those normally associated with chorionic tissue — chorionic gonadotrophin, oestrogens, etc. Metastases may occur as in any choriocarcinoma.

HORMONE-PRODUCTION by NON-FUNCTIONING TUMOURS

Occasionally the presence of tumour growth in the ovary induces a thecal transformation of the ovarian stroma which in turn produces steroids, sometimes androgenic but more commonly oestrogenic. This has been reported in association with benign and malignant cysts, Brenner tumours, fibroma and secondary carcinoma of ovary. The secretion of steroids results in menstrual upset and in the case of androgens, virilism.

SURGICAL TREATMENT OF OVARIAN TUMOURS

Benign ovarian tumours over 10 cm in diameter must be removed, but clinically and ultrasonically diagnosed cysts under 10 cm (the size of a lemon) in women under 35 years may be reviewed in a few months if there is no suspicion of malignancy. A follicular or luteal cyst may resolve spontaneously.

1. **Resection:** A portion of the ovarian cortex is removed. This procedure is restricted to some cases of polycystic ovary disease.

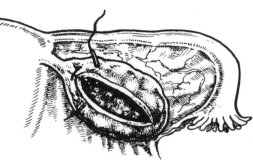

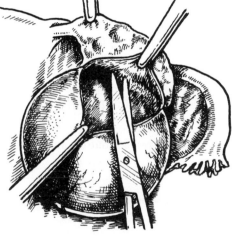

2. **Cystectomy:** Enucleation of the tumour from its capsule of ovarian tissue, which is then rolled into a little bundle and held together with sutures, thus preserving ovarian function.

   Indications:
   A tumour apparently benign in a woman under 35 years of age.
   This operation would not be feasible in the case of a very large tumour, or where there had been previous inflammation.

3. **Ovariotomy:** Removal of an ovary containing a tumour. (Removal of an ovary not containing a tumour is called oöphorectomy.)

   Indications:
   (a) Malignancy.
       (The uterus and other ovary are also removed.)
   (b) The patient is over 35, declines hysterectomy and the other ovary is normal.

4. **Laparoscopy:** This may be diagnostic or therapeutic — small benign cysts may be removed.

TREATMENT OF OVARIAN CANCER

Much attention is being directed towards the treatment of epithelial ovarian cancer which is now the most frequent cause of death from gynaecological malignancy. The principles of treatment are:

1. Ovarian carcinoma is staged surgically, so laparotomy is an essential part of management for most patients.
2. Surgical removal of as much malignant tissue as possible, even if this should call for resection of structures outside the normal field of the gynaecologist.
3. Follow-up with intensive chemotherapy, using various combinations of antineoplastic drugs. Taxanes, probably combined with platinum compounds, are an appropriate first choice.
4. A 'second look' laparotomy or laparoscopy operation (SLO), to determine the actual effectiveness of the chemotherapy and to decide whether it should be stopped does not affect prognosis, so should *only* be performed with informed consent in clinical trials.

It will be seen that treatment of this intensity is beyond the scope of the general gynaecologist working on his own. Co-operation with a general surgeon may be necessary for the first operation but referral to a specialised gynaecological oncologist for the initial laparotomy is in the patient's best interests. Experience in the field of chemotherapy lies mainly with the oncologist or radiotherapist. Treatment by radiotherapy itself is probably of use only in palliation, or in specific circumstances such as a localised malignant deposit.

SPREAD of OVARIAN CANCER
It is essential to know the direction of spread of ovarian cancers, so that the true extent of the disease may be recognised.

1. Direct
The first spread is directly into neighbouring structures — peritoneum, uterus, bladder, bowel and omentum.

2. Transcoelomic
Cancer cells are carried across the peritoneum and along paracolonic gutters by the serous fluid, and achieve widespread seeding. The prognosis is much worse where rupture of a tumour capsule has occurred *prior* to surgery as opposed to rupture during operation. The tumour marker CA125 is usually raised in advanced ovarian cancer and is used to assess response to chemotherapy. No tumour marker sufficiently sensitive to use as a screen for ovarian cancer exists.

3. Lymphatics
Ovarian drainage is to the para-aortic glands, but sometimes to the pelvic and even inguinal groups. Cells seeded on to the peritoneum are drained via the lymphatic channels on the underside of the diaphragm into the subpleural glands and thence to the pleura.

4. Blood stream
Blood spread is usually late, to the liver and lungs.

SURGICAL PROCEDURES IN OVARIAN CANCER

The objectives are:
1. To classify the growth according to its extent of spread (staging) as accurately as possible.
2. To remove as much cancerous tissue as possible ('surgical debulking'; 'cyto-reductive treatment').

Incision

A vertical incision which can be extended is essential to allow a full inspection. Reduction of a cyst by tapping and extraction through a suprapubic incision is not acceptable practice.

Inspection

The whole cavity must be palpated, including liver, subdiaphragm, bowel and mesenteries, omentum and aortic nodes. Suspicious areas are biopsied.

Organs removed

These must always include the uterus, tubes, ovaries, appendix and omentum. Partial resection of bladder and bowel may also be required, but epithelial cancer tends to spread over invaded tissue rather than penetrate it, and a plane of cleavage can often be found.

Cytology

Before handling the tumour, take specimens of ascitic fluid or peritoneal saline washings for cytological examination, and a cytology smear from the underside of the diaphragm.

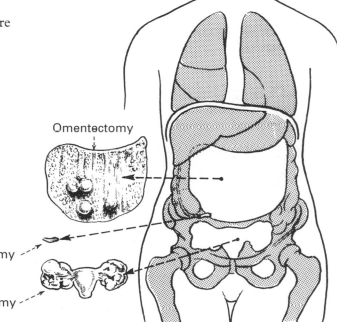

Omentectomy

Appendicectomy

Salpingo-oophorectomy

STAGING OF OVARIAN CANCER

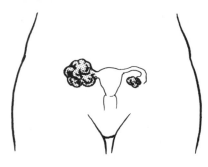

STAGE I Growth limited to ovaries.

Ia. Limited to one ovary. No ascites.

Ib. Limited to both ovaries. No ascites.

Ic. Ascites or positive peritoneal washings also present or tumour on surface of one or both ovaries or capsule ruptured.

Treatment: Surgery alone for Ia and Ib. Add chemotherapy if Ic.

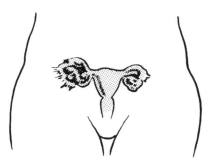

STAGE II Pelvic extension.

IIa. Spread to uterus/tubes.

IIb. Spread to other pelvic tissues.

IIc. IIb with ascites or positive peritoneal washings or tumour on surface of one or both ovaries or capsule ruptured.

Treatment: Surgery and chemotherapy.

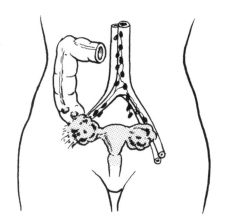

Stage III Extrapelvic intraperitoneal spread and/or retroperitoneal or inguinal positive nodes, or superficial liver metastases.

IIIa Apparent limitation to true pelvis. Nodes negative but proven microscopic seeding of abdominal peritoneum.

IIIb Histologically proven abdominal peritoneal superficial implants < 2 cm diameter.

IIIc Abdominal implants > 2 cm diameter or positive retroperitoneal or inguinal nodes.

Treatment: Surgery as extensive as necessary and possible, followed by chemotherapy.

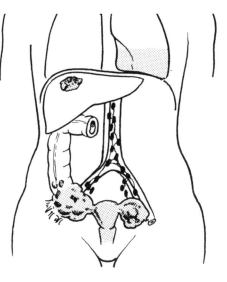

STAGE IV Distant metastases or pleural effusion with positive cytology or parenchymal liver metastases.

Treatment: As much surgical extirpation as possible, perhaps with colostomy, followed by chemotherapy. Palliative radiotherapy may be used here.

ANTINEOPLASTIC DRUGS

Antineoplastic drugs act by inhibiting cell division — both normal and malignant — and thus reducing the number of new cells formed.

TUMOUR GROWTH

Tumour cells multiply at the same rate or more slowly than normal cells, but are not subjected to the same physiological control of numbers of cells, so that a cancer gradually develops.

The Cell Cycle (for both normal and tumour cells)

The time taken for a cell to divide into two daughter cells is between 40 and 80 hours, and the chief variable factor is the initial resting phase (G_1).

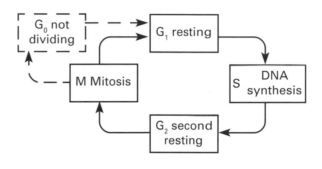

The time taken for a tumour to double its mass is theoretically the same 40–80 hours, but in practice is found to be between 4 and 500 days.

The variable factors in tumour development are the cell-cycle time, the number of cells dividing, and the number lost or incapable of dividing.

	Normal Cells	*Tumour Cells*
Cell-cycle Time	40–80 hours.	40–80 hours. (Tends to be longer than normal cells.)
Cell Loss Factor	100%. Every cell lost is replaced by one cell only and there is no increase in numbers.	Cells are lost through shedding into body cavities, necrosis, immune defences etc. and biologically inadequate cells which cannot divide or only for a few generations ('doomed cells'). Up to 99% may be lost but there is always some growth.
Growth Fraction	Even in normal bone marrow which is a very active tissue only about 20% of the cells (stem cells) are dividing, the remainder being in the G_0 phase.	The growth fraction in tumours varies between 20 and 90%.

PHARMACOLOGY OF ANTINEOPLASTIC DRUGS

ALKYLATING AGENTS

The bivalent alkyl group in these combines with the guanine base in DNA, preventing replication.

    Cyclophosphamide (Endoxana)
    Chlorambucil (Leukeran)
    Melphalan (Alkeran)

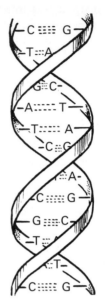

C = Cytosine
G = Guanine
A = Adenine
T = Thymine

ANTIMITOTIC ANTIBIOTICS

They act against human cells by combining with single strands of DNA to prevent protein synthesis.

    Actinomycin D (Cosmegen)
    Doxorubicin (Adriamycin)

ANTIMETABOLITES

Metabolites in this context are the chemical groups required for the synthesis of nucleic acid and protein. An antimetabolite has a similar structure although functionally different and is preferentially taken up by the enzyme system, thus preventing the synthesis of nucleoprotein.

    Methotrexate resembles folic acid.
    5-fluorouracil resembles uracil which is a metabolite of RNA.

VINCA ALKALOIDS

These drugs are derived from the periwinkle plant (vinca) and inhibit growth by interfering with mitosis.

    Vincristine (Oncovin)
    Vinblastine (Velbe)

OTHER NON-ALKYLATING AGENTS

Cis-Platin

Carboplatin is a derivative of Cis-Platin. It is better tolerated than Cis-Platin but is more myelosuppressive.

TAXANES

Paclitaxel (Taxol) and docetaxol (Taxotere) contain the taxane ring structure and block cell division by excessive stabilisation of microtubules. Gemcitabine is a pyrimidine antimetabolite.

TOXICITY

All antineoplastic drugs are extremely toxic when given in effective dosage and there is invariably some depression of the bone marrow and the gastro-intestinal tract. **Cis-Platin** is particularly neurotoxic and nephrotoxic and must be preceded by intravenous hydration and accompanied by mannitol to ensure diuresis. **Doxorubicin** is cardiotoxic and the patient must be given a wig for the resulting alopecia. Other complications include tissue necrosis of the veins and liver failure. Patients taking antineoplastic drugs must be kept under continual supervision, with regular checks on marrow and liver function.

ANTINEOPLASTIC DRUGS

Rationale of Antineoplastic Drug Therapy

It is at present believed that after assault by an antineoplastic drug, tumour cells replace themselves more slowly than normal cells. Treatment is therefore interrupted by rest periods (pulsed therapy) to allow the normal tissues time to recover and increases some patients' life expectancies significantly.

Administration

The drugs are given as the primary treatment when surgery is not feasible and as supportive therapy after adequate extirpative surgery. The alkylating agents are usually given orally, but others such as Cis-Platin and doxorubicin require intravenous infusion with many precautions. Combinations of one or more agents have the merit of increasing the likelihood of response. Cis-Platin based combinations may improve survival. There is an associated increase in toxicity and probably no true synergic effect.

Intraperitoneal chemotherapy with Cis-Platin has a limited role in superficial recurrence or persistence in the peritoneal cavity where higher local concentrations are possible with less toxicity. Paclitaxel (Taxol) may be suitable for this route.

PRESENT PROGNOSIS FOR INVASIVE EPITHELIAL OVARIAN CANCER

Stage	5-year survival
I	60–70%
II	40–50%
III	5–10%
IV	Nil

Borderline epithelial tumours have excellent 5 year survival of 90 to 95% and 15 year survival of 70 to 85% for serous tumours. Mucinous tumours fare 5% or 10% less well. Chemotherapy is effective in the infrequent germ cell tumours.

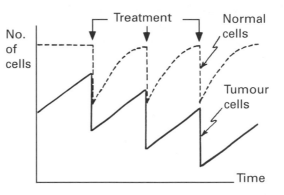

Results of Treatment

Chemotherapy has been used in ovarian cancer for about 30 years, but only relatively recently have mean survival rates beyond 18 months or speculation on cure seemed possible. Taxanes, probably combined with platinum compounds, are the first line treatment, in 1999. Patients showing complete regression could survive $2\frac{1}{2}$ years, partial regression up to 18 months and non-responders perhaps 12 months, depending on the extent of surgery. 'Second look laparotomy' is now regarded as of dubious value.

Paclitaxel shows advantages over existing therapies with a response rate of about 30% in platinum-resistant cases.

Survival in advanced ovarian cancer may possibly be improved by Platinum combination therapy.

Cis-Platin has a dose response curve in advanced (Stages III and IV) ovarian cancer, though with increased toxicity in higher doses. Neuro-toxicity is the principal obstacle to continued use of high dose Cis-Platin.

Median survival:
    114 weeks 100 mg/m² Cis-Platin
    69 weeks 50 mg/m² Cis-Platin
        + 750 mg/m² Cyclophosphamide

Kaye, S.B. et al. *Lancet* (1992), **340**, 329–33.

283

COMPUTERISED AXIAL TOMOGRAPHY (CAT SCANNING)

Patients with presumed ovarian masses should have ultrasound or CT scanning of the abdomen and pelvis. The CAT scanner will demonstrate the presence of lymph node metastases not detectable even by laparotomy, and it will increase the accuracy of staging of ovarian cancer and of assessing the response to treatment.

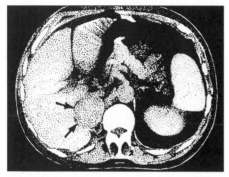

Liver metastasis from ovarian carcinoma

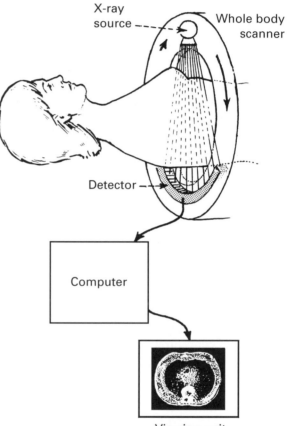

The scanner takes repeated X-ray pictures of a cross-section of the body (nearly 300 pictures within 5 seconds) as the X-ray tube is rotated round the patient.

Some absorption of X-rays takes place according to the density of the tissues through which the X-rays pass. Thus the difference between the amount of radiation entering the body and the amount measured by the detectors is equivalent to the density of the tissues.

These measurements are passed to a computer which performs millions of calculations within a few minutes, and reconstructs from the detector readings a cross-section picture of the viscera.

Magnetic Resonance Imaging (MRI) is also a useful technique, though less widely available.

BROAD LIGAMENT CYSTS

BROAD LIGAMENT CYSTS (Parovarian cysts)

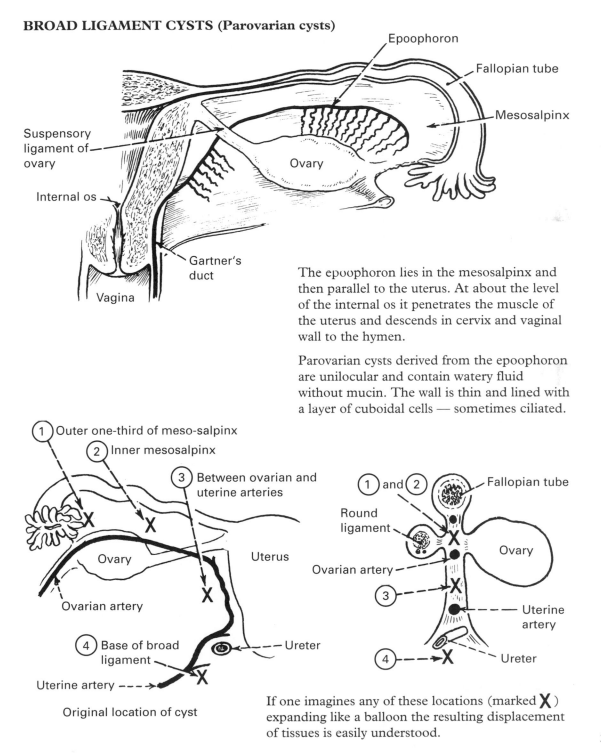

The epoophoron lies in the mesosalpinx and then parallel to the uterus. At about the level of the internal os it penetrates the muscle of the uterus and descends in cervix and vaginal wall to the hymen.

Parovarian cysts derived from the epoophoron are unilocular and contain watery fluid without mucin. The wall is thin and lined with a layer of cuboidal cells — sometimes ciliated.

If one imagines any of these locations (marked **X**) expanding like a balloon the resulting displacement of tissues is easily understood.

285

BROAD LIGAMENT CYSTS

Diagnosis

On palpation, the cyst, which is not mobile, may displace the uterus and is closely related to it. An ovarian cyst with adhesions may feel very similar and it is seldom possible to distinguish between the two before laparotomy.

Operation

Great care must be taken in identifying tissues as the location of the original site of the cyst determines displacement and characteristics.

In the outer third of the broad ligament the cyst tends to develop a pedicle.

In the middle of the broad ligament the tumour is sessile but relatively fixed.

The ovarian vessels are displaced and may be stretched leading to interference with the ovarian blood supply.

It is possible for the ureter and uterine artery to be displaced outwards, but usually they are below and medial to the cyst.

The tumour may increase in size and strip the peritoneum off the pelvic walls and spread laterally and posteriorly obliterating the Pouch of Douglas.

The broad ligament is incised anteriorly where the blood vessels are few and the cyst is enucleated digitally. The oozing area is now exposed and should be obliterated. Care is necessary to avoid damage to blood vessels, ureter and bladder. Redundant broad ligament may require to be excised.

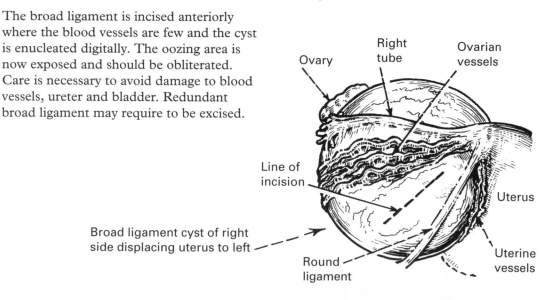

CYSTS of KOBELT'S TUBULES, HYDATIDS of MORGAGNI, FIMBRIAL CYSTS

These are names given to small cysts found in the mesosalpinx and around the terminal portion of the fallopian tubes. They are of indeterminate embryonic origin and are of no clinical significance.

CARCINOMA OF FALLOPIAN TUBES

The fallopian tubes, which are so prone to infection, are extremely resistant to primary malignant change, and the gynaecologist may, in his professional lifetime, expect to see perhaps one case of carcinoma of the tube.

Pathology
The growth is usually an adenocarcinoma of the tubal epithelium which grows inwards and secretes a copious serosanguinous fluid which characteristically discharges per vaginam if the proximal tube remains patent. This classical sign of tubal carcinoma is rare.

Clinical Features
The patient is usually in her fifties and often nulliparous or of low parity. She may complain of postmenopausal bleeding, pain and sometimes watery vaginal discharge. In the absence of definite symptoms the diagnosis is often made rather late. Pelvic signs suggestive of infection in a postmenopausal woman should always be investigated. The differential diagnosis includes carcinoma of the uterus or ovary.

5-year survival rate	
Stage I	40–70%
Stage II	20–40%
Stage III	10–25%

Prognosis depends on the stage of diagnosis and on the degree of differentiation of the tumour.

Overall 5-year survival is only approximately 35%.

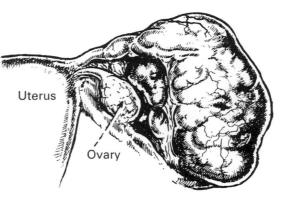

Uterus

Ovary

Aetiology is unknown, since the condition is too rare to attract much attention.

Clinical Staging
Stage I   confined to one or both tubes.
Stage II   pelvic extension.
Stage III spread to other structures (omentum, bowel, etc.), positive retroperitoneal or inguinal nodes or superficial liver metastases.
Stage IV distant metastases (including bladder), pleural effusion with positive cytology or parenchymal liver metastases.

Treatment
Total hysterectomy and bilateral salpingo-oophorectomy should be done as a minimum, followed by external beam radiation. If the surgeon has the experience an extended hysterectomy and lymphadenectomy would be justified, but the disease is usually not diagnosed before laparotomy.

Chemotherapy with cisplatinum increases the survival rate.

STERILISATION

Many women seek sterilisation once they decide that they want no more children, even when still in their early twenties, and the free provision of an operation of such social consequence must inevitably give rise to controversy. The doctor should make certain that his patient knows exactly what the operation involves, its failure rate, its consequences, and the possibilities that may exist for a later recanalisation with no guarantee of success and an increased risk of ectopic pregnancy.

The WOMAN should be as certain as she can be that she wants no more pregnancies, come what may. The decision should be taken with deliberation and not during pregnancy or the immediate post-natal period.

The MALE partner should have a clear understanding of the consequences of the operation, and should if possible be brought to agree.

TECHNIQUES

Occlusion of the fallopian tubes is carried out by the application of ligatures, clips or rings and the object is to traumatise the tube and bring about a permanent blockage by fibrosis. Destruction of a portion of the tube by diathermy is also effective, but has too small an operative safety margin.

1. **Laparotomy and Tubal Ligation** This is the most reliable method but requires several days in hospital and carries the risk of chronic salpingitis.
2. **Occlusion of the tubes by clips or rings under laparoscopic vision** There is virtually no morbidity and hospital stay is short, but the technique is not quite so reliable. Laparoscopic electrocautery carries a risk of thermal trauma to bowel and is less effective. Laser vapourisation carries a higher risk of recanalisation because of minimal fibrosis.
3. **Instillation of chemical substances.** In developing countries with limited facilities and budgets insertion of a pellet of quinacrine, 252 mg, into the uterine cavity through the cervical canal on two occasions 4 weeks apart has proved effective.

POST-STERILISATION SYNDROME

This uncertain entity consists of pelvic adhesions, salpingitis and irregular patterns of menstruation. Women who have been sterilised seem more likely to undergo hysterectomy in later years, especially after tubal ligation, and reductions in plasma progesterone have been shown in such patients. This may be due to interference with the utero-ovarian circulation and would explain the irregular bleeding, as may cessation of oral contraceptive usage.

STERILISATION FAILURE

Laparoscopic techniques have a failure rate about the same as oral contraceptives, probably 1% and tubal ligation rather less.

Failure is more likely when the operation is done at the time of abortion or term delivery and there is a higher than normal risk of ectopic pregnancy. Points of technique are important in sterilisation operations and experience is required.

STERILISATION

TUBAL LIGATION

The easiest way to interrupt the continuity of the fallopian tubes is to tie them with a ligature. The tubes have some powers of resistance (cf. recanalisation of veins) and it is necessary to crush the muscle coat, although the endosalpinx is probably not divided. Failure is very rare (about 1%) and can be due to recanalisation, or to the development of a fistulous opening.

The incision can be small and so placed as to be covered by the pubic hair. If there is any laxity of the vagina and uterine ligaments, it is often possible to reach the tubes through an incision in the posterior fornix.

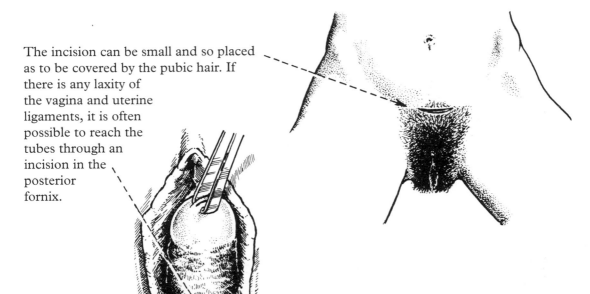

With either route there are small risks of sepsis and embolism. The vaginal route carries a higher complication rate and is rarely employed in the U.K.

A very safe method is to apply two silk sutures and leave the tube uncut.

Type of Ligature

The material used probably does not matter.

In the Pomeroy method, catgut is used and the tube is then cut so that the ends fall apart. In the Madlener method silk is used after crushing the tube. Burial of the proximal end of the ligated tube is also practised, but this technique is no more immune to fistula formation than any other.

LAPAROSCOPIC STERILISATION

The tubes can be occluded by the application of clips or rings under laparoscopic vision. (Two clips are applied to each tube by some operators.)

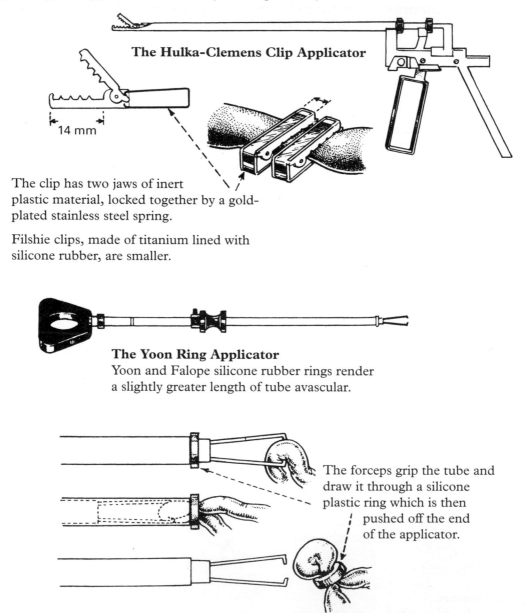

The Hulka-Clemens Clip Applicator

14 mm

The clip has two jaws of inert plastic material, locked together by a gold-plated stainless steel spring.

Filshie clips, made of titanium lined with silicone rubber, are smaller.

The Yoon Ring Applicator
Yoon and Falope silicone rubber rings render a slightly greater length of tube avascular.

The forceps grip the tube and draw it through a silicone plastic ring which is then pushed off the end of the applicator.

These applicators, whether for clips or rings, are passed into the abdominal cavity through a trocar after passage of a laparoscope. The clips should be placed about 1cm from the cornu, and the rings as near that point as possible. Thick and vascular tubes are more difficult to occlude by these methods.

RESTORING TUBAL PATENCY

Once the tube is blocked by infection and adhesions, the chances of restoring patency are poor. There is a tendency for the blockage to recur and tubal function is never as good as in the pristine state. Nevertheless several techniques have been developed.

SALPINGOSTOMY

This is done when the fimbriae have been destroyed, and the artificial opening will not be as effective as the fimbriae. The polyethylene splint should be removed after a week and since splints tend themselves to stimulate fibrosis some surgeons will not use them, but rely on large doses of intraperitoneal hydrocortisone acetate (up to 1.5 g) to inhibit adhesion formation.

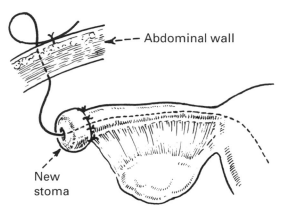

UTEROTUBAL IMPLANTATION

If the interstitial portion of the tube is blocked, the isthmus can be resutured to the cornu after a fresh passage has been made. It is hoped that the passage will become lined with tubal mucosa.

These procedures are now performed laparosopically in some centres.

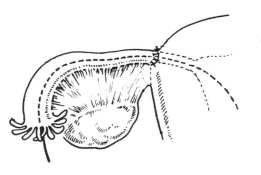

The tube is guided into the uterus and sutured in place.

RESTORING TUBAL PATENCY

This is done by cutting out the occluded and fibrotic portions of tube and anastomosing the ends. The less amount of destruction done to the tube during the sterilisation operation the better, and in this respect the Filshie or the Hulka-Clemens clip, which crushes only 3 mm of tube, has a distinct advantage over other methods. Anastomosis in the isthmic portion gives the best results as the opposing ends of tube are of the same diameter.

TUBAL ANASTOMOSIS

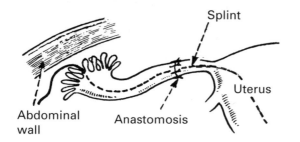

Fibrotic tissue is cut out, and the ends of tube are sutured together over a thin plastic splint, usually an epidural catheter.

This splint should be removed per vaginam a week later.

MICROSURGICAL TECHNIQUES

The use of the operating microscope and suitable instruments for performing tubal anastomosis is becoming more popular but this technique has not yet been shown to be invariably superior to 'macro-anastomosis'. It is particularly recommended when the isthmus has been destroyed and the tubal lumen has to be anastomosed to the cornu.

Under about x20 magnification all fibrotic tissue is removed, bleeding points stopped with fine diathermy, and the lumina anastomosed with very fine multiple sutures

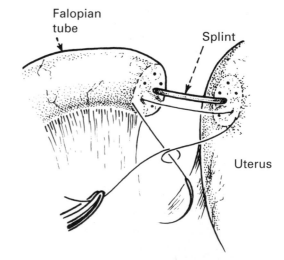

ECTOPIC PREGNANCY

Implantation of the fertilised ovum outside a normal uterine cavity, nearly always in the fallopian tube.

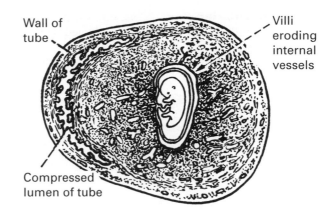

Wall of tube

Villi eroding internal vessels

Compressed lumen of tube

Incidence

It is impossible to compute the number of ectopic implantations per conception, but in practice the incidence seems to be about one case for every 300 deliveries.

Site

The trophoblast can successfully implant on any tissue with an adequate blood supply, but ectopics anywhere other than the tube are a great rarity. The commonest site for an 'ectopic ectopic' is the pelvic peritoneum, but the literature contains accounts of implantation in the liver, the spleen, the lower sac, the stomach and the intestine.

Aetiology

Often unknown, but there are a number of associated factors:

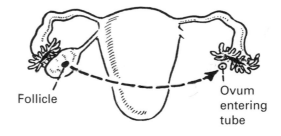

Follicle

Ovum entering tube

1. **Pelvic Inflammatory Disease**
    About half the patients will have signs of salpingitis or a history of infection, including gonorrhea or chlamydia or tuberculosis. This may affect tubal ciliary activity.

2. **Intra-Uterine Devices**
    The IUD may introduce infection or have some unknown effect. Since the probable action of the IUD is to prevent implantation in the uterine cavity, a relative increase in ectopic pregnancy is to be expected as most other pregnancies are prevented.

3. **Migration of the Ovum**
    The corpus luteum is occasionally seen on the side opposite the ectopic and it has been assumed for many years that the ovum, growing as it crosses the pelvis, reaches the stage of implantation while still in the contralateral tube.

4. **Endocrine Causes**
    There is no definite evidence of hormonal causation.

5. **Tubal surgery,** for example reversal of sterilisation, may be a cause.

6. Assisted conception carries an increased incidence of ectopic pregnancy, both with IVF and GIFT.

SITES OF IMPLANTATION

Sites of Implantation

The tubal ampulla is the commonest followed by the isthmus, but the developing ovum can implant anywhere in or out of the uterus.

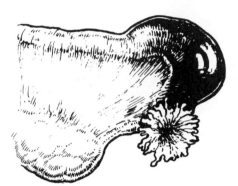

Ampullary implantation. Note the thinning of the tube wall.

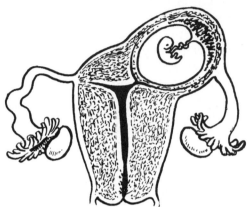

Interstitial implantation is very rare but very dangerous because rupture is accompanied by bleeding from uterine arteries.

Effect on the Uterus

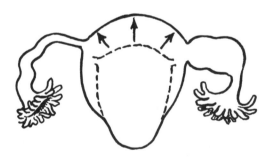

In the first 3 months the uterus enlarges almost as if the implantation were normal. This is a source of confusion in diagnosis.

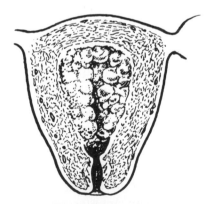

Decidua grows abundantly and degenerates and bleeds when the ovum dies. Rarely is it expelled entire as a decidual cast.

RUPTURE OF THE TUBE

The muscle wall of the tube has not the capacity of uterine muscle for hypertrophy and distension and tubal pregnancy nearly always ends in rupture and the death of the ovum.

RUPTURE into LUMEN of TUBE
Tubal Abortion

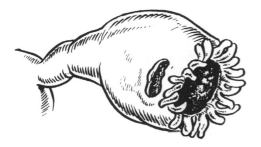

This is usual in ampullary pregnancy at about 8 weeks. The conceptus is extruded, complete or incomplete, towards the fimbriated end of the tube, probably by the pressure of accumulated blood. There is a trickle of bleeding into the peritoneal cavity, and this may collect as a clot in the Pouch of Douglas. It is then called a pelvic haematocele.

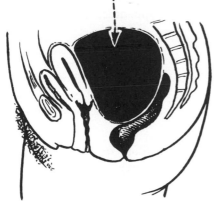

RUPTURE into the
PERITONEAL CAVITY

This may occur spontaneously, or from pressure (such as straining at stool, coitus or pelvic examination) and occurs mainly from the narrow isthmus before 8 weeks, or from the interstitial portion at 12 weeks. Haemorrhage is likely to be severe.

Tube lumen ___

Tube wall (muscular tissue) ___

Point of rupture ___ ___

Blood clot collecting ___ ___
in broad ligament

Sometimes rupture is retroperitoneal between the leaves of the broad ligament — broad ligament haematoma. Haemorrhage in this site is more likely to be controlled.

DIAGNOSIS OF TUBAL PREGNANCY

Tubal pregnancy can present in many ways and misdiagnosis is common.

PAIN in the lower abdomen is always present and may be either stabbing or cramp-like — 'uterine colic'. It may be referred to the shoulder if blood tracks to the diaphragm and stimulates the phrenic nerve and may be so severe as to cause fainting. The pain is caused by distension of the gravid tube, by its efforts to contract and expel the ovum and by irritation of the peritoneum by leakage of blood. More than 50% of ectopics present as chronic rather than acute episodes.

VAGINAL BLEEDING occurs usually after the death of the ovum and is an effect of oestrogen withdrawal. It is dark brown and scanty ('vaginal spotting') and its irregularity may lead the patient to confuse it with the menstrual flow. In about 25% of cases tubal pregnancy presents without any vaginal bleeding.

INTERNAL BLOOD LOSS will, if gradual, lead to anaemia. If haemorrhage is severe and rapid (as when a large vessel is eroded) the usual signs of collapse and shock will appear. Acute internal bleeding is the most dramatic and dangerous consequence of tubal pregnancy but it is less common than the condition presented by a slow trickle of blood into the pelvic cavity.

PELVIC EXAMINATION in the conscious patient will demonstrate extreme tenderness over the gravid tube or in the Pouch of Douglas if a haematocele has collected. If the pregnancy is sufficiently advanced and rupture has not occurred, a cystic (and very tender) mass may be felt in the fornix; but often tenderness is the only sign elicited.

PERITONEAL IRRITATION may produce muscle guarding, frequency of micturition, and later a degree of fever, all leading towards a misdiagnosis of appendicitis.

hCG PREGNANCY TESTS are positive early in pregnancy. A negative result almost completely excludes a diagnosis of ectopic pregnancy.

SIGNS and SYMPTOMS of EARLY PREGNANCY must be expected, all of which can confuse the clinical picture. When implantation occurs in the isthmus, tubal rupture may occur before the patient has missed a period and pregnancy tests may be negative until the 40th day.

ABDOMINAL EXAMINATION will demonstrate tenderness in one or other fossa. If there has been much intra-peritoneal bleeding there will be general tenderness and resistance to palpation over the whole abdomen.

ULTRASOUND may demonstrate an intra-uterine pregnancy but this does not totally exclude a co-existant ectopic pregnancy, especially following IVF/GIFT.

DIAGNOSIS OF TUBAL PREGNANCY

Differential Diagnosis

This includes salpingitis, abortion, torsion of the pedicle of a cyst or rupture of a cyst and perhaps appendicitis.

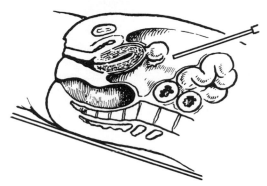

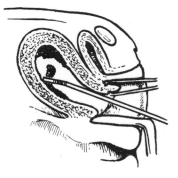

1. **Laparoscopy**

   This is the most useful method of diagnosis in doubtful cases, and is especially useful in excluding tubal pregnancy.

2. **Curettage**

   If products of conception are obtained, a co-existing tubal pregnancy is very unlikely. Decidua alone means an ectopic but the histological report must be awaited. Marked decidual reaction with absence of chorionic villi suggests ectopic pregnancy. This is known as the Arias-Stella phenomenon.

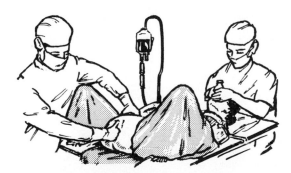

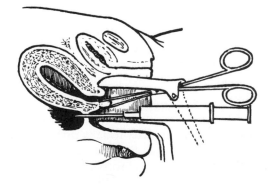

3. **Examination under Anaesthesia**

   This is not likely to yield more information than in the conscious patient. It should always be done in theatre because of the risk of starting haemorrhage.

4. **Culdocentesis**

   The passing of a wide-bore needle through the posterior fornix. Old blood is very suggestive, but the absence of blood does not exclude an ectopic pregnancy.

TREATMENT OF TUBAL PREGNANCY

1. Haemorrhage and shock must be treated but if there is delay in obtaining blood the operation should be proceeded with. The patient's condition will improve as soon as internal bleeding is controlled.

2. Salpingectomy or even salpingo-oophorectomy may be necessary to control the bleeding. The risk of conservation is of course the theoretically increased chance of another ectopic; but if there are no obvious signs of infection in the intact tube, and if the affected tube is not too damaged by haemorrhage and oedema, then conservation may be attempted. These procedures may be performed laparoscopically, unless the patient is shocked.

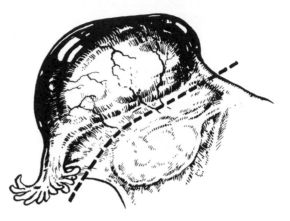

3. Conservative management without surgery is an option when the diagnosis has been made in an asymptomatic patient with hCG levels below 2,000 IU/l in a situation with permanent access to theatre. Progressive decrease in hCG levels indicates resolution. Methotrexate as an alternative to surgery is not recommended.

Natural History of Ectopic Pregnancies

Rupture or abortion is almost inevitable in tubal pregnancy but absorption must very occasionally occur and 40 years ago it was common practice to encourage natural resolution by vaginal drainage of a pelvic haematocele.

Abdominal pregnancies usually present as obstetrical problems, but in such cases the fetus may also be absorbed or passed per rectum or present as a bizarre gynaecological problem with lithopaedion formation.

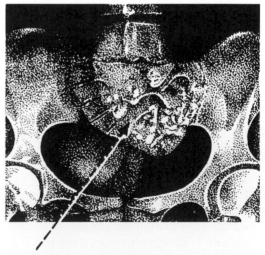

Lithopaedion is the name given to calcification of the fetus. This X-ray picture shows a lithopaedion which took $4^{1}/_{2}$ years to develop.

OTHER VARIANTS OF ECTOPIC PREGNANCY

CERVICAL PREGNANCY

This is a rare variant of ectopic pregnancy, which carries a considerable risk of severe bleeding.

Clinical Features

The patient is likely to be misdiagnosed as a case of inevitable abortion.

1. The cervix is dilated and thin-walled and contains products of conception.

2. A small firm uterine corpus can be palpated, resting on the swollen cervix.

3. Attempts at evacuating the 'abortion' cause increased bleeding.

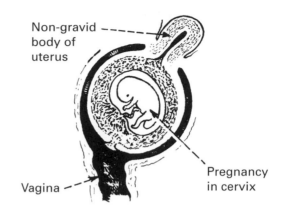

Non-gravid body of uterus

Vagina

Pregnancy in cervix

Management

This is a dangerous condition. The choice is between hysterectomy and local excision, and the former is strongly indicated if the bleeding is heavy and not controllable, especially if the maturity is beyond 8 weeks.

If local excision is attempted, the cervix must be clamped laterally to occlude the lateral vessels. After the pregnancy is dissected out, any cervical tears must be repaired and the vagina should be packed.

OVARIAN PREGNANCY

Implantation of the fertilised ovum in the ovary makes up 1% of all ectopics. The symptoms and course of the condition are much the same as for other ectopics, but the ovarian tissue is perhaps less likely to rupture than is the muscular wall of the tube. An enlarged ovary is found at operation and if an ectopic is suspected, the tumour should be excised. It should be possible to preserve the ovary.

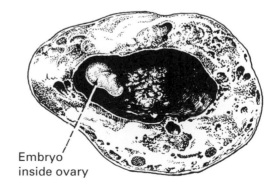

Embryo inside ovary

CHAPTER 14

THE URINARY TRACT IN GYNAECOLOGICAL PRACTICE

THE URETERS

The ureter enters the pelvis retroperitoneally by crossing over or near the bifurcation of the common iliac artery.

The ureter is itself crossed by the ovarian vessels and is near the fold of peritoneum which forms the infundibulopelvic ligament.

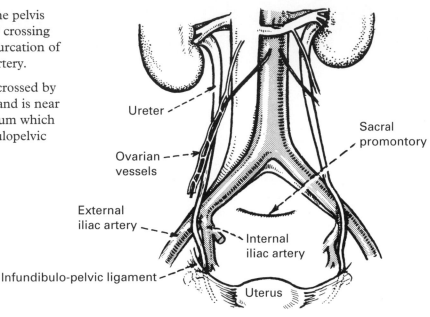

It passes down and medially behind the ovarian fossa and is in close relation to the internal iliac artery. In the healthy subject its shape can be made out beneath the peritoneum and peristatic movements observed (vermiculation).

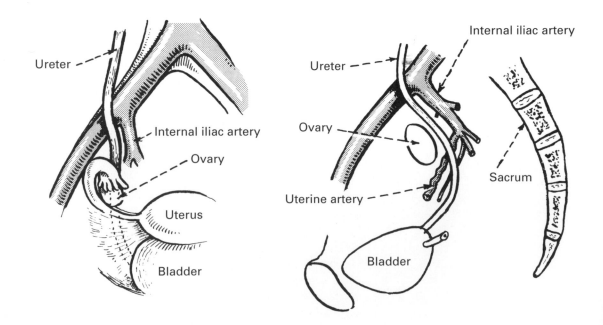

THE URETERS

The ureter then passes beneath the base of the broad ligament, through the transverse uterine ligament and into the bladder. In this parametrial part of its course it lies alongside the vaginal fornix and passes under the uterine artery.

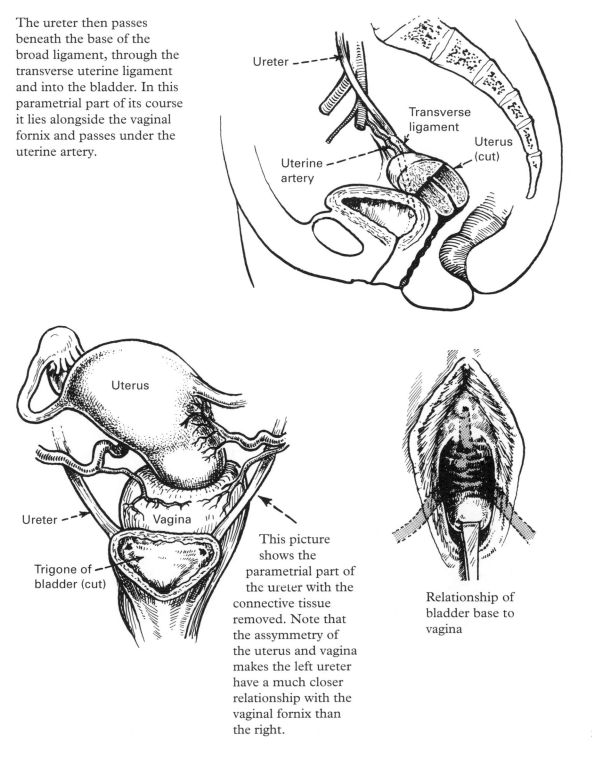

This picture shows the parametrial part of the ureter with the connective tissue removed. Note that the assymmetry of the uterus and vagina makes the left ureter have a much closer relationship with the vaginal fornix than the right.

Relationship of bladder base to vagina

303

THE URETERS

BLOOD SUPPLY OF THE URETER

The ureter is supplied by branches from the main arteries with which it is in relation, principally the renal and ovarian arteries. The pelvic vessels are variable, and because the blood enters mostly at the upper and lower ends the peri-ureteric anastomoses are important.

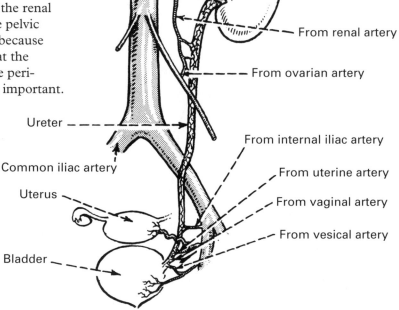

From renal artery

From ovarian artery

Ureter

From internal iliac artery

Common iliac artery

From uterine artery

Uterus

From vaginal artery

From vesical artery

Bladder

HISTOLOGY OF THE URETER

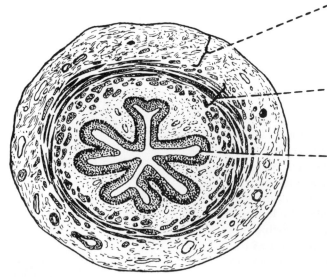

The Adventitia is a fibrous sheath containing the peri-ureteral arterial network, the autonomic nerves and the lymphatics.

The Muscularis consists of two or three layers of smooth muscle irregularly arranged.

The lumen is lined by plicated transitional epithelium on a loose areolar stroma. This arrangement allows for distension of the ureter as required (cf. the fallopian tube).

INJURY TO THE URETER

The ureter will occasionally be damaged no matter how much skill and care are exercised.

1. The ureter is not easily demonstrated or dissected where it is in closest relationship to the genital tract; and not always easily palpated.

2. The ureter's course is to some extent variable, and under pressure it will gradually change its position in the pelvis. A large tumour filling the pelvis will displace it laterally. A tumour in the broad ligament may displace the ureter outwards and upwards. Double ureters are occasionally met with.

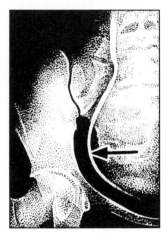

IVP showing lateral displacement

Ureter displaced by a fibroid which has occupied the broad ligament.

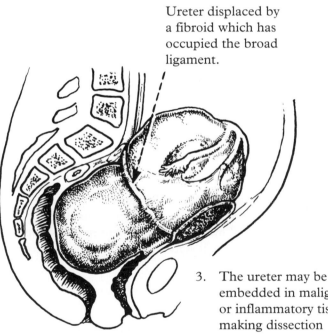

3. The ureter may be embedded in malignant or inflammatory tissue, making dissection almost impossible.

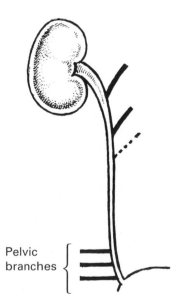

Pelvic branches

4. Radical surgery may destroy so much of the pelvic blood supply that the pelvic ureter becomes ischaemic, leading to fibrotic narrowing or fistula. Damage to the blood vessels may also be produced by pelvic irradiation.

MANAGEMENT OF URETERIC INJURY

Ureteric injury should be managed in consultation with a urologist, or a gynaecologist with subspecialty training in urogynaecology.

1. **Ureteric injury identified at operation.**

   a. Crush injury from clamp or ligature. The clamp or ligature should be removed, and a ureteric stent inserted.

   b. Ligation of the ureter
   Ligation of the ureter should be treated by end to end anastomosis, reimplantation of the ureter into the bladder or by uretero-ureteric anastomosis into the opposite ureter.

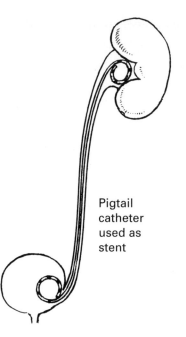

Pigtail catheter used as stent

2. **Ureteric injury identified post operatively.**

Clinical features

The signs and symptoms relate to leakage of urine in ureteric fistulae, and to ureteric obstruction when the ureter has been ligated. If a ureteric fistula is present, urine leakage may be observed into an abdominal drain, or from surgical incisions. The patient may develop lower abdominal pain and pyrexia. If the ureter has been ligated, the patient may develop loin pain and pyrexia.

Investigations

1. Ultrasound.
   If ureteric obstruction is suspected, ultrasound may be a useful initial test to identify hydronephrosis.

2. Intravenous urography
   Intravenous urography (IVU) is useful in the investigation both of ureteric fistulae and of ureteric obstruction. The urinary tract is outlined by radio-opaque dye and the site of leakage or obstruction of urine identified. Small fistulae may not be identified by this approach.

MANAGEMENT OF URETERIC INJURY

3. Percutaneous nephrostomy followed by antegrade pyelography.

    This manoeuvre is both therapeutic and diagnostic. Percutaneous nephrostomy is carried out under ultrasound or X-ray control. Using local anaesthesia, a catheter is passed through the skin and into the renal pelvis or ureter (percutaneous nephrostomy). This allows drainage of the kidney, and prevents further renal damage. Contrast medium can be injected through the catheter (antegrade pyelography), and gives further information about ureteric damage.

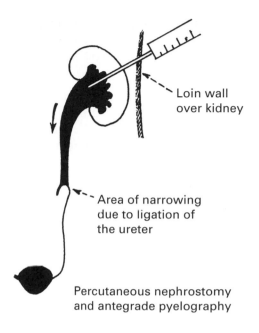

Loin wall over kidney

Area of narrowing due to ligation of the ureter

Percutaneous nephrostomy and antegrade pyelography

Treatment of ureteric injury

When ureteric injury is diagnosed, the principle of treatment in the first instance is to relieve ureteric obstruction, thus preventing back pressure on the kidney and renal necrosis. Clearly if both ureters have been damaged, and renal compromise is already apparent, consideration should be given to renal dialysis. The following manoeuvres may be useful in the short term:

1   Percutaneous nephrostomy (see above)
2. Cystoscopy and retrograde insertion of ureteric stents.

In the longer term, formal repair of the ureter is necessary, and may be achieved using one of the techniques outlined above. It should be emphasised again that these techniques are outwith the expertise of most gynaecologists.

PHYSIOLOGY OF MICTURITION

The involuntary voiding of small amounts of urine is very common in women. It is known, perhaps wrongly, as 'stress incontinence' and its treatment calls for an understanding of bladder and urethral physiology.

Intravesical Pressure

The bladder displays the phenomenon of adaptation to increased urinary volume. Pressure remains below 10 cm H_2O until over 500 ml of urine are contained.

Intra-urethral Pressure

Urethral pressure is maintained by the 'internal sphincter' made up of longitudinal and circular plain muscle and elastic tissue; and an 'external sphincter' which contributes striated muscle.

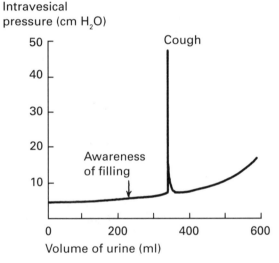

Intravesical pressure (cm H_2O)

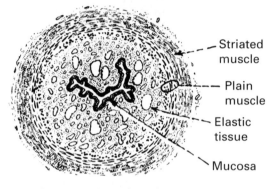

Cross section of urethra

A 'urethral pressure profile' shows the changes in pressure along the length of the urethra. This is normally much greater than the intravesical pressure, thus ensuring continence.

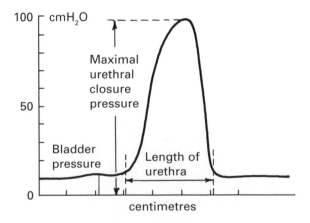

PHYSIOLOGY OF MICTURITION

Innervation of Bladder and Urethra
There is an intercommunicating sympathetic, parasympathetic and somatic supply. The parasympathetic stimulates detrusor contraction, and the sympathetic fibres (chiefly through the alpha receptors) stimulate contraction of the bladder neck and urethra. There is thus some degree of reciprocal activity, but the precise function of each type of nerve and the exact control of the mechanism of bladder neck opening are not yet known.

The striated muscle has been shown to have a dual autonomic/somatic supply via the pelvic plexus, and the long-held concept of pudendal innervation is being questioned. In normal urethral closure all the components of the sphincter mechanism must function together and the striated muscle has more to do than merely contract voluntarily when the desire to micturate must be resisted.

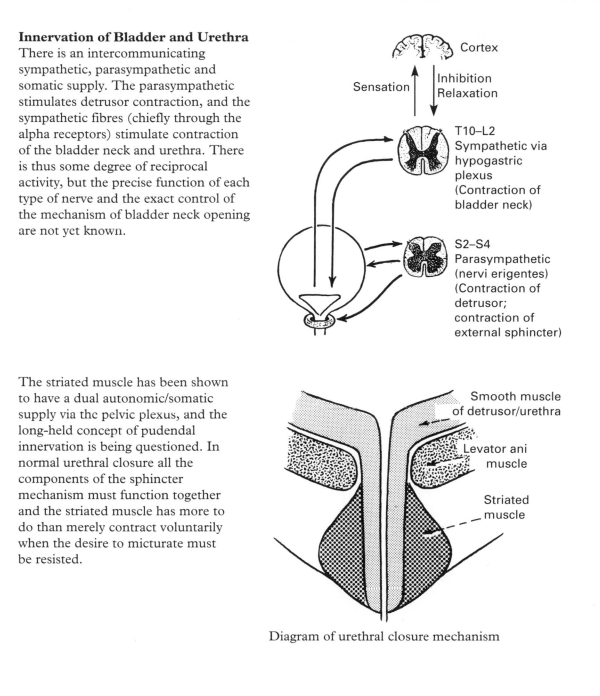

Diagram of urethral closure mechanism

MECHANISM OF VOIDING

Cystometry recording demonstrates the timing of events.

1   Intra-abdominal pressure increase. (Measured per rectum.)

2. Detrusor contracts. (Intravesical pressure increase).

3. Sphincter relaxes. (Electromyogram of anal sphincter.)

4. Urine flow begins.

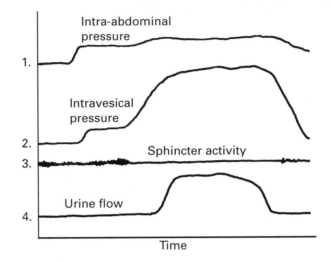

The urethra and bladder neck are maintained in the closed state by the trigonal condensation of muscle (the base plate) and the urethral sphincter (plain and striated muscle).

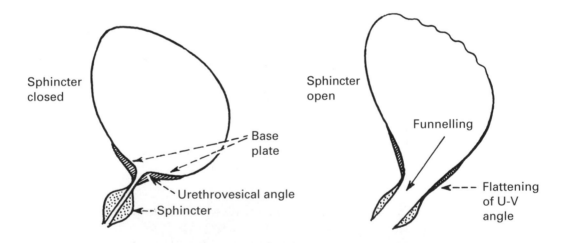

When cortical inhibition is withdrawn the detrusor contracts and the bladder neck relaxes (funnelling). The sphincter also relaxes and urine is voided. As the flow continues, the bladder neck moves downwards and backwards and the urethrovesical (UV) angle is obliterated.

DETRUSOR INSTABILITY

Detrusor instability

The loss of the ability to inhibit detrusor contractions when they are provoked by filling of the bladder, or standing erect or coughing and straining. This may also cause involuntary incontinence, but the mechanism is altogether different from that of genuine stress incontinence.

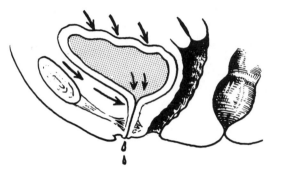

Symptoms

The patient experiences an irresistible and sudden desire to micturate (urgency). Detrusor instability is the commonest cause, but it may also be due to inflammatory disease of the bladder without detrusor contraction. All forms of bladder pathology must be considered including calculus and carcinoma. There is usually an associated complaint of frequency.

GENUINE STRESS INCONTINENCE

Symptoms

When a sudden increase in intravesical pressure is caused by a contraction of the detrusor muscle or by an increase in intra-abdominal pressure as by coughing or straining, the stimulus is usually applied to the intra-abdominal urethra as well, and there is no leakage of urine. If urine does escape, the symptom is called *stress incontinence*.

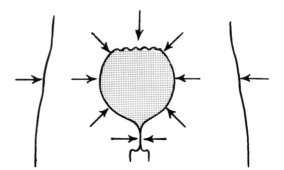

Genuine stress incontinence

(alternatively named urethral spincter incompetence)

Involuntary leakage occurring in the absence of a detrusor contraction. This leakage is attributed to some displacement of the bladder neck so that it cannot respond normally to a sudden increase in intra-abdominal pressure. The cause is likely to be a pelvic floor weakness as a result of parturition and/or oestrogen deficiency. Less commonly, the condition is due to fibrosis after bladder neck surgery, trauma, or congenital conditions such as epispadias.

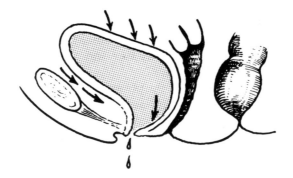

OTHER INCONTINENCE MECHANISMS

Fistula Incontinence is described on page 323 et seq.

Overflow Incontinence

Sudden retention is rare in women except after pelvic floor operations. Spasmodic detrusor contractions force a little urine into the urethra and the stretched muscle takes several days to regain its tone.

When obstruction to outflow occurs gradually, as from pressure by a pelvic tumour or an incarcerated retroverted gravid uterus, the detrusor has time to hypertrophy and for a time forces urine out; but eventually the bladder become atonic and painless and urine dribbles out only when the intra-abdominal pressure is raised.

Neurological Disease

Failure of detrusor inhibition is the commonest symptom and is the cause of senile incontinence. It is also a symptom, although not usually the presenting one, of multiple sclerosis. Full sensation is present, but the incontinence is of the urgency type and cannot be resisted.

Failure of bladder sensation is a result of diseases which interrupt the posterior columns of the cord, e.g. tabes, syringomyelia, occasionally multiple sclerosis. Chronic overdistension leads to an atonic bladder and overflow incontinence, and infection is a common complication.

OTHER SYMPTOMS AND SIGNS ASSOCIATED WITH INCONTINENCE

Frequency

Increased frequency of micturition is defined as the passage of urine seven or more times during the day, and twice or more during the night. It may arise from any source of irritation including infection, detrusor instability, tumour or incomplete emptying. It is usually diurnal — during waking hours only — but in severe cases will awaken the patient from her sleep. It is one of the earliest symptoms of pregnancy.

Urgency

This is defined as a desire to void urine before the bladder contains 50 ml of urine. True urgency occurs in the absence of a detrusor contraction, and is often associated with infection. Severe urgency leads to 'urge incontinence'.

Dysuria

This means pain associated with micturition and indicates either an infection of the bladder and urethra, or of the vulval and perineal epithelium which is irritated by the dribbling of urine.

Nocturia

Requiring to pass urine during the night.

THE URETHRAL SYNDROME

The urethral syndrome includes complaints of frequency, dysuria, urgency and a sensation of incomplete emptying in a patient in whose urine no evidence of infection can be demonstrated. The cause is not known and there are several views.

Urinary infection is strictly defined as being present only when 10^4 or more typical urinary pathogens are grown per ml of freshly voided mid-stream urine and it may be that the urethral syndrome is simply a condition caused by fewer than the usual number of organisms, or by organisms which cannot be cultured in the media used for conventional organisms. Clinically these patients must be regarded as suffering from a urinary tract infection and investigation must be persevered with. Even if no evidence of infection is obtained some empirical treatment will have to be given.

INVESTIGATION OF INCONTINENCE

It is necessary to distinguish between genuine stress incontinence and detrusor instability since their treatment is different and this cannot be done with certainty on the history and clinical examination alone.

Incontinence due to:

1. Genuine Stress Incontinence	**2. Detrusor Instability**
Gradual onset after one or more pregnancies.	History of a weak bladder even before pregnancies if any.
Urine appears only after effort (stress) such as coughing, laughing, running for a bus.	History of enuresis especially in childhood.
Only small quantities of urine are passed, whether the bladder is full or not.	Complaints of urge incontinence and frequency, especially at night (nocturia).

Stress incontinence combined with urgency incontinence due to bladder infection or cystocele is quite common. Continuous incontinence suggests fistula (page 323).

The degree of severity is indicated by the extent to which the patient feels socially restricted.

Examination
Signs of infection (urethritis) and scarring from previous surgery are looked for, and the usual bimanual and speculum examinations are made (pages 80–82).

Demonstration of Stress Incontinence
The patient is asked to strain and cough and, if stress incontinence is present, small amounts of urine will be observed escaping from the urethral meatus. Unfortunately this test is really valid only in the erect position when observation of the meatus becomes almost impossible.

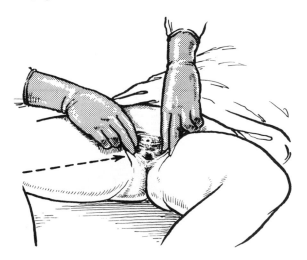

URODYNAMIC INVESTIGATION OF BLADDER FUNCTION

This means an investigation of bladder movements and tensions during different levels of filling, and involves measurement of bladder activity (cystometry) and urethral flow (uroflowmetry). Modern apparatus is sophisticated and expensive.

Cystometry

The bladder pressures are continuously recorded as the bladder is filled. In twin channel cystometry, the rectal pressure which represents intra-abdominal pressure is simultaneously recorded by a transducer in the rectum. The detrusor pressure is calculated by subtracting abdominal pressure from intravesical pressure.

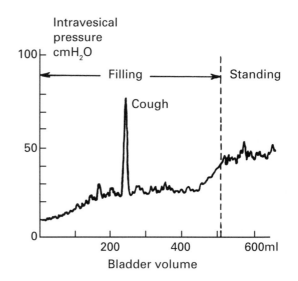

Abnormal cystometry

If detrusor contractions which cannot be suppressed by the patient are seen in the filling phase (up to 400 ml infused into bladder), a diagnosis of detrusor instability can be made.

In stress incontinence, leakage on coughing etc. occurs in the absence of a rise in detrusor pressure.

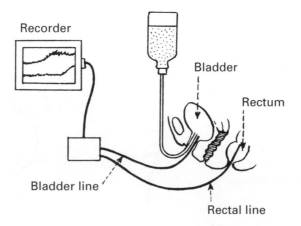

INDICATIONS FOR URODYNAMIC ASSESSMENT

Indications for Urodynamic Assessment

These investigations are invasive and expensive, but their application would be justified in the presence of the following indications:

1. Continuing difficulty in distinguishing genuine stress incontinence from detrusor instability.
2. After failure of surgery to relieve a complaint of incontinence.
3. Where there are other complicating factors such as neurological disease.
4. Where difficulty in voiding urine is complained of or is suspected. Such a condition may be met with after pelvic surgery and leads to incomplete emptying and perhaps retention overflow.
5. Enthusiasts would advocate urodynamic assessment prior to surgical treatment for stress incontinence.

OTHER INVESTIGATIONS

Bacteriological Culture of Urine

This must be carried out in every case.

Fluid balance chart

The patient is asked to record the volume of oral fluid intake and urine output over the course of a week. Recordings of urine production should include the volume and the time of each micturition. Any episodes of incontinence should also be recorded. This procedure is useful for identifying the patient with an excessive oral intake. An estimate of the patient's normal bladder capacity can also be made.

Neurological Disease

This possibility must always be borne in mind and the gynaecologist should test for reflexes in the usual manner. The integrity of the sacral reflexes is demonstrated by contraction of the anal sphincter in response to a perineal skin prick. Where there is doubt, the patient must be referred to a neurologist.

Endocrine Diseases

Diseases such as diabetes mellitus and insipidus may present with frequency and hormonal assays may be required.

TREATMENT OF STRESS INCONTINENCE

General measures:

The following should be treated if present:

1. Chronic urinary tract infection
2. Obesity
3. Chronic cough and dyspnoea.

Conservative treatment of stress incontinence.

1. Physiotherapy — pelvic floor exercises.

   Pelvic floor exercises may be of value, especially in the puerperium. These include repeated pressing together of the buttocks and thighs and the stopping of the urine stream during micturition. The patient also may practise contracting the vaginal sphincter over her two fingers. Lead cones are available which may be placed temporarily in the vagina and retained by contracting the perineal muscles.

2. Mechanical devices to occlude urethra or support the bladder neck.

These are now commercially available. Efficacy ranges from 40–80%. Urinary tract infection and patient discomfort may be a problem with some devices.

New surgical developments in the treatment of stress incontinence

1. Periurethral injections.
   Substances such as collagen or subcutaneous fat are injected around the urethra using a vaginal approach. This procedure is suitable for frail patients. Cure rates of up to 80% have been reported.

2. Artificial urinary sphincters
   Implantation of an artificial urinary sphincter may be considered as a last resort in the treatment of stress incontinence.

SURGICAL TREATMENT OF STRESS INCONTINENCE

All operations attempt to elevate the bladder neck above the pelvic floor and behind the symphysis so that increases in intra-abdominal pressure will compress the urethra and not force it downwards. There are 3 conventional methods, each with several variations.

1. **Anterior colporrhaphy**
    (See p.245). This procedure may be useful in women with coexisting anterior vaginal wall prolapse, but the rate of objective cure for stress incontinence is less than 60%.

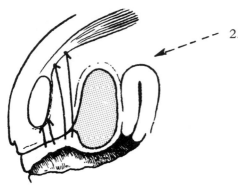

2. **Urethropexy**
    The bladder neck is approached through a suprapubic incision and elevated by suturing the paraurethral tissues to adjacent structures such as the rectus sheath or the ilio-pectineal ligament.

    These operations are more difficult than vaginal urethroplasty, especially in obese women. Some operators employ a laparoscopic technique.

3. **Urethral Sling Operations**
    A sling of synthetic material, sutures or tendon is passed under the urethra and attached to the rectus muscles or adjacent ligaments. This requires a combined vaginal-suprapubic approach and is the most difficult of the 3 methods.

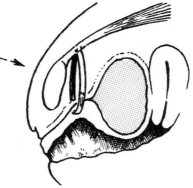

The urethropexy operations are probably most likely to be successful when the incontinence is due to urethral inadequacy and not detrusor instability.

MARSHALL-MARCHETTI-KRANTZ URETHROPEXY

The urethrovesical junction is made to adhere firmly to the anterior vaginal wall by suturing the vaginal tissue to the back of the symphysis pubis.

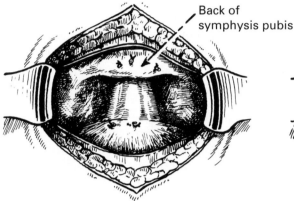

Back of symphysis pubis

1. The urethrovesical junction is exposed in the space of Retzius. Adhesions are divided and all bleeding points picked up. The urethra must be dissected to within 1 cm of the external meatus.

2. A Foley's catheter in the bladder helps to identify the urethrovesical junction. Silk sutures pick up vaginal tissue on either side and suture it to the pubic periosteum.

    Closure is with a Redi-Vac drain for 48 hours in case of urinary leakage or haematoma formation. Haematuria is common and continuous catheterisation is required for 7 days.

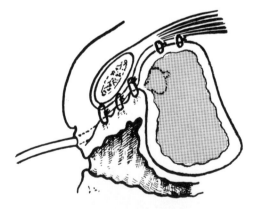

3. Additional sutures are added between bladder muscle and rectus muscles. (This step is sometimes unnecessary.)

Periosteitis is sometimes a late complication and the operation is difficult in the presence of excessive obesity. If too acute an angle is produced, the patient may have difficulty in emptying her bladder.

BURCH'S COLPOSUSPENSION OPERATION

This operation elevates the anterior vaginal wall, bringing the urethra up with it.

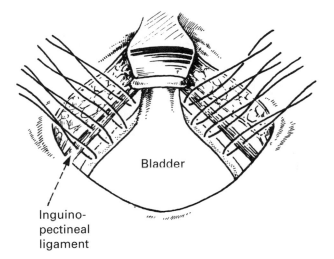

1. Through a suprapubic incision the bladder neck area is mobilised from the paravaginal fascia. This procedure is accompanied by a good deal of bleeding which must be controlled by tightening the sutures.

2. The paravaginal fascia (and some vaginal tissue as well) is sutured on each side to the inguino-pectineal ligaments, using four or five Dexon sutures.

The wound is closed with Redi-Vac suction drainage as for the Marshall operation, and the possible complications are similar. Suprapubic operations can be difficult when the patient is very obese. This procedure may now be performed laparoscopically by appropriately trained surgeons.

STAMEY COLPOSUSPENSION OPERATION

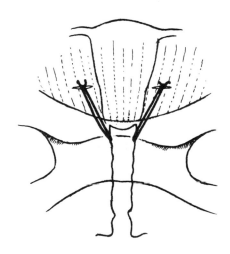

This is a less invasive procedure, where a long Stamey needle is passed through a small incision above the pubis on each side, *behind the pubic bones*, into the vaginal lumen. A nylon suture is attached to the vaginal wall and tied to the rectus sheath, to elevate the vagina and bladder base.

A cystoscope is passed to ensure that the needle has not entered the bladder after each pass of the Stamey needle.

TREATMENT OF DETRUSOR INSTABILITY

BLADDER RETRAINING

This may be done as an inpatient or an outpatient, although inpatient treatment is more effective. The patient is instructed to void only at defined intervals (to start with this is normally 1.5 h). When the patient can achieve continence between scheduled voiding, the interval is increased gradually. A normal fluid intake should be allowed. Support and enthusiasm from medical and nursing staff is required for this procedure to be effective.

DRUG TREATMENT

Antimuscarinic agents (oxybutynin, flavoxate, tolterodine). These agents act by blocking parasympathetic stimulation of the detrusor muscle. Improvement is seen in 70% of patients who can tolerate the drug. Non compliance is common, due to the anticholinergic side effects of dry mouth, blurred vision, tachycardia, drowsiness and constipation. Oxybutynin has more side effects than flavoxate but is more effective. Tolterodine is a new antimuscarinic agent with a lower incidence of side effects.

Tricyclic antidepressants (imipramine)

These drugs are useful if nocturia is a significant complaint. Anticholinergic side effects may be a problem.

Oestrogen

Although few trials have formally evaluated the efficacy of oestrogens, they appear to have a role in post menopausal women.

URINARY FISTULA

(L. *fistula*: a pipe) A pathological connection between the urinary tract and an adjacent structure through which urine escapes. A fistula between the bladder base and the vagina is the condition most often seen.

Aetiology

1. The exposed bladder wall is torn or penetrated during a vaginal operation, or during total abdominal hysterectomy. This is the commonest cause in this country.

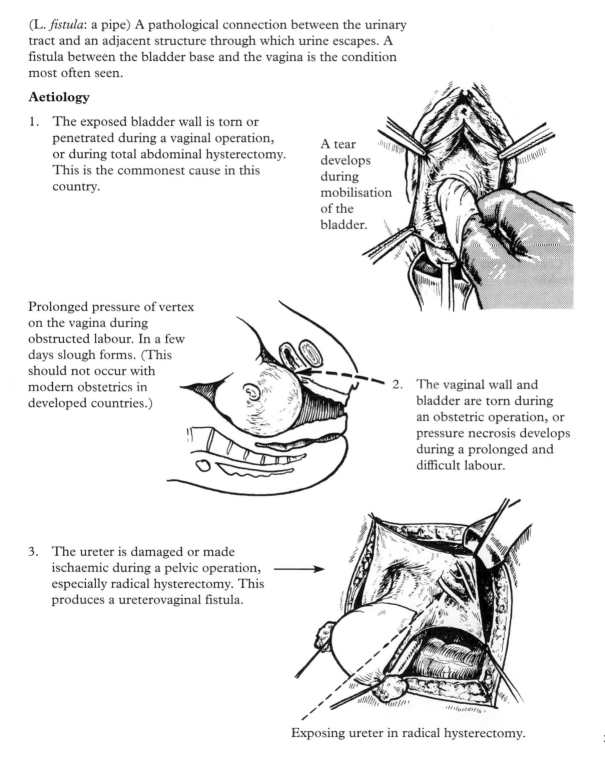

A tear develops during mobilisation of the bladder.

Prolonged pressure of vertex on the vagina during obstructed labour. In a few days slough forms. (This should not occur with modern obstetrics in developed countries.)

2. The vaginal wall and bladder are torn during an obstetric operation, or pressure necrosis develops during a prolonged and difficult labour.

3. The ureter is damaged or made ischaemic during a pelvic operation, especially radical hysterectomy. This produces a ureterovaginal fistula.

Exposing ureter in radical hysterectomy.

URINARY FISTULA

Aetiology *(contd)*

4. Radiation burns following treatment for carcinoma of the cervix. This fistula may appear several years after treatment.

5. Untreated or recurrent cancer of bladder or genital tract. (This may also be complicated by radiation effects.)

6. Chronic tuberculosis or syphilis. Fistula may complicate surgical treatment of pelvic tuberculosis.

7. Congenital fistula. An accessory ectopic ureter may open into the vagina. This condition should be recognised in childhood.

Symptoms

Incontinence may immediately follow the injury, but usually the patient has several days of dysuria and haematuria with symptoms of urinary infection. A discharge appears followed by sloughing, and the patient finds her vulva and perineum are constantly wet. This is soon followed by excoriation of the skin accompanied by a strong ammoniacal smell and incrustation of vulva and vagina with urinary salts. The area becomes extremely tender.

Diagnosis

This is usually easy, but if the patient says she also passes urine normally, two conditions must be considered.

1. **A very small fistula.** Most of the urine is retained in the bladder and passed per urethram. Sometimes quite large quantities of urine may be held temporarily in the vagina while the patient is resting, and she will say that she seems to be dry at night. Small 'pinhole' fistulae may persist for years and be mistaken for stress incontinence.

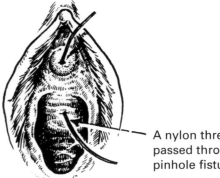

A nylon thread passed through a pinhole fistula

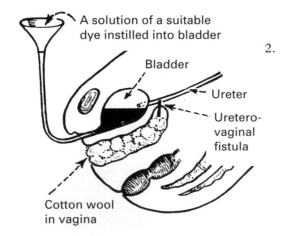

A solution of a suitable dye instilled into bladder

Bladder

Ureter

Uretero-vaginal fistula

Cotton wool in vagina

2. **A ureterovaginal fistula** produces a constant trickle of urine, but the bladder is still intact and will continue to function. The usual test is to instill a solution of a suitable dye into the bladder. Cotton-wool in the vagina will not be stained if the fistula is ureteric. During cystoscopy the dye is injected intravenously to identify the ureteric openings, and cotton-wool in the vaginal vault will then be stained. An intravenous pyelogram will show contrast medium leaking into the vagina.

CHAPTER 15

VENOUS THROMBOSIS

DEEP VEIN THROMBOSIS (DVT)

Aetiology

1. Any abdominal or pelvic floor operation. When contemplating hysterectomy, especially if other aetiological factors are present, it should be remembered that the risks of thrombo-embolism are greater with the abdominal than with the vaginal operation. An 80% risk of DVT and up to 10% risk of fatal pulmonary thomboembolism has been suggested for major pelvic surgery in the absence of prophylactic measures.
2. Chronic venous insufficiency (varicose veins, phlebitis). (Crude odds ratio 6:3.)
3. Obesity. (Crude odds ratio 9:5.) Diabetes. (Crude odds ratio 3:4.)
4. Immobility leading to circulatory stasis.
5. Oral contraceptives. Hormone replacement therapy (first year of use only).
6. Thrombophilia defects, especially antithrombin III deficiency, the presence of factor V Leiden or several concurrent defects.

Curiously, cigarette smoking increases the risk of myocardial infarction but does not seem to predispose to DVT.

Pathology

The theory embodied in 'Virchow's Triad' is still clinically useful:

1. Changes in the vessel wall.   2. Changes in the rate of flow.   3. Changes in the blood.

1. Changes in the vessel wall

Damage to the endothelium allows platelets to adhere to the exposed collagen tissue and then to release substances which will cause further platelet aggregation. Fibrin and leucocytes then adhere to the platelets. Research now suggests that a balance is maintained between different groups of prostaglandins.

Prostaglandin (PGI) is an *anti-aggregatory* substance secreted by intact endothelium. It also causes vasodilatation.

Thromboxane (TXA) is a *pro-aggregatory* substance released by platelets. It also causes vasoconstriction.

2. Changes in the rate of flow

Venous flow in the legs is much reduced in the post-operative period as a result of inactivity and poor muscle tone.

3. Changes in the blood

Platelet count, platelet 'stickiness' and fibrinogen levels are all increased. Fortunately there is a compensating increase in fibrinolytic activity so that nearly all thrombi are naturally broken down.

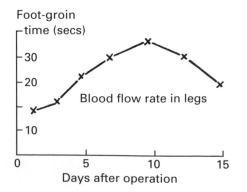

Blood flow rate in legs

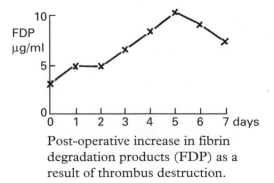

Post-operative increase in fibrin degradation products (FDP) as a result of thrombus destruction.

VENOUS THROMBOSIS

SITES OF THROMBUS FORMATION

1. Calf veins, extending to popliteal.

2. Long and short saphenous veins, especially lateral to the knee.

3. Ilio-femoral segment, extending to vena cava.

4. Superficial thrombosis in veins.

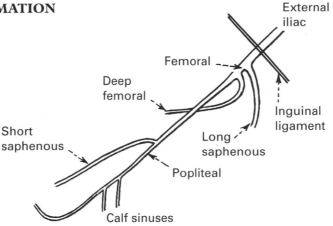

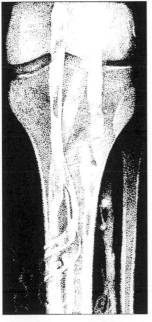

Phlebogram showing thrombi in calf veins and extending up the popliteal.

FORMATION OF THROMBUS

Some endothelial lesions allow the platelets to come in contact with the subendothelial structures to which they adhere. In the process of aggregation various substances are released, including adenosine diphosphate (ADP), which increase adherence. Liberated thromboplastins initiate the formation of fibrin clot. The vessel wall also liberates a substance, prostacyclin, which inhibits platelet adherence, and activator, which initiates fibrinolysis. If the local concentration of these substances is inadequate, thrombus formation continues and an embolus may break off into the blood stream.

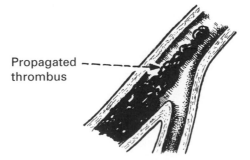

Propagated thrombus

CLINICAL FEATURES OF DVT

There is very often no complaint, but silent thrombosis is now known to be a common post-operative complication and clinical signs should be looked for. Predisposing factors are thrombophilia defects, previous thrombosis, age, obesity, a history of oral contraception, HRT commenced within the previous year, sepsis and immobility.

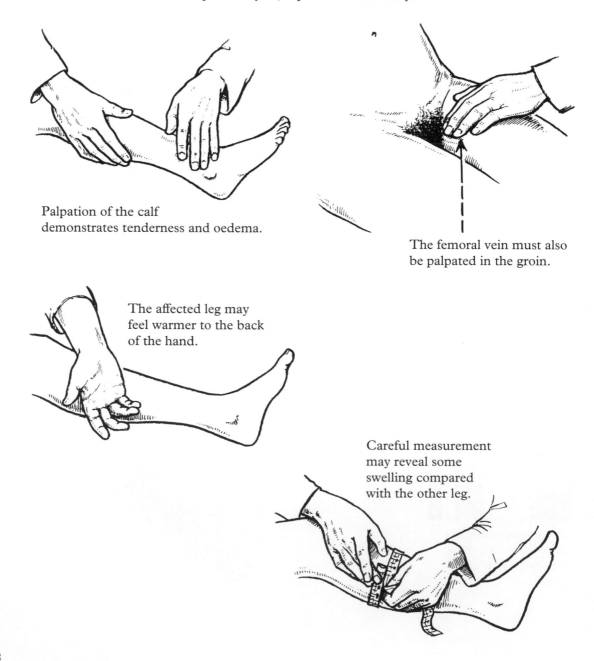

Palpation of the calf demonstrates tenderness and oedema.

The femoral vein must also be palpated in the groin.

The affected leg may feel warmer to the back of the hand.

Careful measurement may reveal some swelling compared with the other leg.

SCREENING TESTS FOR DVT

PHLEBOGRAPHY

This is the most reliable method of demonstrating thrombi in veins, but it is time consuming and requires experience. The contrast medium may aggravate the phlebitis.

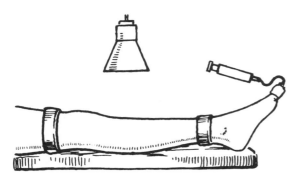

Contrast medium is injected into a vein near the big toe. Two inflated cuffs force it into the deep veins where its progress can be watched on image intensification apparatus.

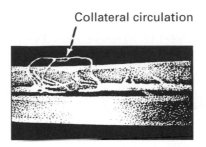

Collateral circulation

A filling defect indicates the site of thrombosis. Note the opening of the collateral circulation.

ULTRASONIC DIAGNOSIS

The flowing movement of blood produces characteristic sounds when picked up by an ultrasonic transducer held over the vessel. The frequency and amplitude of the sounds are increased when the flow is accelerated by squeezing the calf.

The transducer is placed over the femoral vein in the groin, and the thigh or calf compressed with an inflatable cuff. Absence of any increased sound suggests that flow is impeded by a thrombus.

This method is less reliable than isotope scanning and will not detect small thrombi.

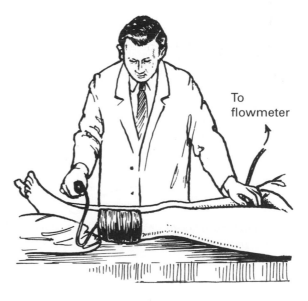

To flowmeter

PREVENTION OF DVT

When DVT occurs the immediate risk is pulmonary embolism, but there is also a likelihood of permanent damage to the veins, producing what is called the 'post-phlebitic syndrome' of swelling, bursting pain, varicose veins, ulceration. In modern surgical practice there now exists an obligation to take some form of prophylactic measure. The Royal College of Obstetricians and Gynaecologists Working Party on Prophylaxis against Thromboembolism (1995) recommended individual assessment of thromboembolism risk and appropriate prophylactic measures.

PHYSICAL MEASURES TO PREVENT STASIS

1. Early Ambulation

All patients however frail should be 'walked round the bed' on the day following the operation, and they should be encouraged as they gain strength to walk about the wards.

2. Post-operative Physiotherapy

This is particularly valuable but is time consuming and expensive. The physiotherapist encourages the patient in deep breathing and in exercises to restore muscle tone.

3. Compression bandaging

This reduces the pooling of blood in the leg veins. A crepe bandage can be used or, more effectively, an elastic stocking.

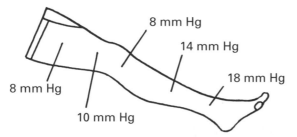

Graduated static compression stockings exert a greater pressure at the ankle than at the thigh.

4. 'Pneumatic Stockings'

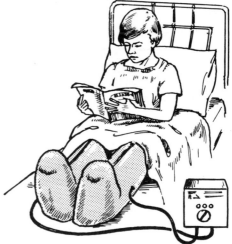

Inflatable gaiters exercise an intermittent pneumatic pressure to the legs during operation and afterwards. They are rather cumbersome, get in the way of nursing, and have to be taken off for ambulation and then reapplied.

PREVENTION OF DVT

LOW DOSE HEPARIN

Dosage: 0.2 ml (5000 IU) is injected subcutaneously, avoiding injection sites near the site of any proposed wound, 3 times daily starting before operation and continuing for a week. There is a slight increase in wound haematoma but no laboratory control is required. This system of treatment is rather uncomfortable for the patient.

Low molecular weight heparin, dosage as per the individual manufacturer's intsructions, has the advantage of less frequent administration and does not require monitoring.

Rationale: Low dose heparin increases the activity of antithrombin III, the most important inhibitor of blood clotting. In high doses it directly inhibits thrombin.

OTHER DRUGS MODIFYING PLATELET BEHAVIOUR

Dipyridamole ('Persantin') is a coronary vasodilator which also inhibits platclet aggregation.

Sulphinpyrazone ('Anturan') was introduced for the treatment of gout and has been found to impair platelet aggregation.

Aspirin has been found to inhibit the release of thromboxane from the platelets. However, it also inhibits prostacyclin synthesis.

None of these drugs has yet found a place in the routine prophylaxis of DVT.

TREATMENT OF DVT

ANTICOAGULANT DRUGS

These are indicated in all but the most minor and superficial degrees of thrombosis, which may be treated by elevation of the leg and tight bandaging. The patient must be encouraged to walk about as soon as she is free of pain.

HEPARIN is a mucopolysaccharide extracted from the lungs and intestines of cattle. It combines with antithrombin and in large doses interrupts the coagulation process at almost every step. The object is to prevent the further growth of a thrombus by preventing the manufacture of fibrin.

Administration of Heparin   Continuous infusion is the most effective at the rate of 30,000 IU in 24 hours. If the necessary supervision is not possible 10,000 IU may be given intravenously every 8 hours.

Side-effects   The only serious side-effect is bleeding from the operation site. This can be severe and may occur even when coagulation tests are normal. The anticoagulant action is reversed by 5 ml protamine sulphate and this may take up to an hour to be effective. Prolonged heparin therapy can cause osteoporosis.

Control of Dosage   The simplest method is the in vitro clotting time which should not go beyond 20 minutes. A more precise monitoring is achieved by the activated partial thromboplastin time (APTT) which should be 1.5 to 2.5 times the control.

Duration of Treatment   Usually Warfarin treatment is begun about the 5th day, and heparin can then be discontinued after about 4 days.

WARFARIN, a derivative of the coumarin series, is given orally. This drug acts as a vitamin K antagonist and reduces the plasma concentrations of Factors II (prothrombin) VII, IX and XI.

Administration of Warfarin   A loading dose of 25 mg is given orally and maintenance is about 5 mg every second day. The drug is started either at the same time as the heparin infusion or after 5 days of heparin, and the therapeutic level is reached in about 48 hours with the dose being adjusted to keep the International Normalised Ratio (INR) between 2.0 and 3.0. Heparin can then be discontinued.

Side-effects   The danger is bleeding, and microhaematuria is the rule. Gastric haemorrhage, skin bruising and rectus sheath haematoma may occur with varying severity. The antidote is vitamin K, 5–30 mg, which will take 24 hours to be effective. If anticoagulation is to be maintained it is better to give fresh frozen plasma to replace deficient factors.

PHENINDIONE (DINDEVAN) is a derivative of indanedione, and an alternative oral anticoagulant. It has the same action as Warfarin and the loading dose is 200 mg daily. It turns the urine pink or orange.

Control of oral anticoagulants   The prothrombin time is estimated against the standard British Comparative Thromboplastin (BCT) or by the 'Thrombotest' reagent. The therapeutic test time is 10% of normal which is near the bleeding level.

Duration of Treatment   depends on the severity of DVT but should extend for at least a week after complete disappearance of symptoms and not less than 4 weeks altogether, though some prefer 3 months.

EXAMPLE OF ANTICOAGULANT TREATMENT OF DVT

Day 1. Begin heparin 10,000 units 6-hourly. Control by clotting time or thrombin time. Alternatively infuse by pump at 40,000 units in 24 hours, monitoring every 4 hours. If the thrombin time exceeds 60 seconds, give 2 mg of protamine sulphate. Give a loading dose of 30 mg of Warfarin. Some would delay this for a few days.

Day 2. Stop heparin when the therapeutic level is reached with Warfarin.

Day 3 et seq. Adjust Warfarin dosage by thrombotest.

By the 10th day, Warfarin dosage should be stabilised with the INR between 2.0 and 3.0. Urine should be tested daily for haematuria.

DRUGS INTERACTING WITH ORAL ANTICOAGULANTS

ENHANCEMENT	Mechanism
Butazolidine, Indomethacin, Alcohol.	Interfere with liver catabolism.
Salicylates, Sulphonamides.	Compete with drug at binding sites.
Broad spectrum antibiotics.	Decrease bowel synthesis of Vit.K.
INHIBITION Barbiturates, Oral contraceptives.	Induce liver enzyme activity.

CONTRAINDICATIONS TO ORAL ANTICOAGULANT THERAPY

Cardiovascular
Malignant hypertension,
Retinopathy,
Endocarditis,
Non-embolic cerebral haemorrhage.

Haematological
Pre-existing haemostatic defect.

Renal
Renal impairment of severe degree.

Long term oral anticoagulant therapy requires good patient co-operation, and is contraindicated in mental defectives and alcoholics.

PULMONARY EMBOLISM

An embolism arises from a thrombus which is non-occlusive in the vessel in which it was formed and is therefore symptomless. It has long been recognised that clinically florid venous thrombosis is unlikely to give rise to embolism; the danger is from the clinically silent thrombus that may be floating in the vein of the other leg.

PERIPHERAL PULMONARY EMBOLISM

Small emboli are lysed rapidly and are symptomless unless infarction occurs. They often precede a major embolism unless treatment is given.

Symptoms	Signs
1. Fever 2. Tachypnoea 3. Pleural pain 4. Haemoptysis (40%)	1. Pyrexia 2. Pleural rub 3. Crepitations 4. Perhaps opacity on lung X-ray

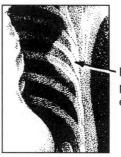

Peripheral pulmonary emboli

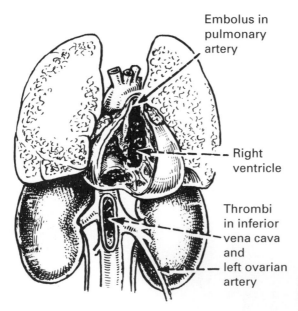

Embolus in pulmonary artery

Right ventricle

Thrombi in inferior vena cava and left ovarian artery

CENTRAL PULMONARY EMBOLISM

A large embolus impacting in the main pulmonary artery will be immediately fatal, but if a little more peripheral, circulatory obstruction will be incomplete and there is a chance of survival.

Symptoms	Signs
1. Collapse 2. Faintness 3. Respiratory distress 4. Pain.	1. Shock — vasoconstriction — hypotension 2. RV failure — distended neck veins — Gallop rhythm 3. Cyanosis.

The cardiac output drops at once and there is intense reflex vasoconstriction, leading to tachycardia, hypotension, and syncope if the patient is sat up. The respiratory distress is very severe, and the pulmonary cyanosis may be aggravated by a right-to-left shunt through the patent foramen ovale which exists in 25% of individuals.

PULMONARY EMBOLISM

INVESTIGATIONS

ECG changes consistent with right heart change will occur but last only a few hours.

SQT waves all show inversion.

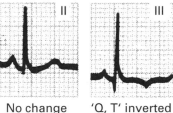

'S' inverted   No change   'Q, T' inverted

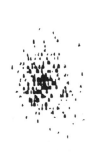

Only the upper lobe arteries are seen. The embolism has lodged at **X**.

PULMONARY ANGIOGRAPHY

Contrast medium is injected through a catheter in an arm vein. This investigation is only necessary in cases of suspected massive embolism in a very ill patient.

PERFUSION SCANS

These require special facilities. Technetium-labelled albumin is injected and the lungs scanned with a gamma camera or scintillation scanner. Different postures are required and this is not for the seriously ill patient.

It takes 1–2 hours to perform and, of course, other causes of reduced perfusion such as bronchitis will show a similar picture.

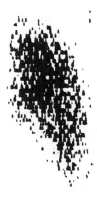

Right lung perfusion much reduced.

PULMONARY EMBOLISM

IMMEDIATE RESUSCITATION

The patient should be transferred to an intensive care unit as soon as possible, but some resuscitative measures are called for. The longer the period of survival, the better the ultimate prognosis.

Reducing the Degree of Obstruction

External massage may move the embolus onwards so that it is less obstructive.

Heparin, 15,000 units intravenously, is given as a serotonin antagonist as well as an anticoagulant, and may reduce pulmonary vasoconstriction and bronchospasm.

Improving Venous Return to the Heart

Keep the patient lying flat and expand the blood volume with Dextran.

Oxygenation

Give oxygen by mask and inject bicarbonate 5 m.eq. to combat the inevitable acidosis.

DIFFERENTIAL DIAGNOSIS

Minor (Peripheral) Embolism	
Pneumonia Acute and chronic bronchitis Other causes of haemoptysis and pleural effusion.	Recent surgery and sudden onset are highly indicative. The legs will show a positive scan.
Major (Central) Embolism	

1. Other causes of collapse:
    Myocardial infarction,
    Cardiopulmonary oedema,
    Septic shock.
 	
2. Other causes of acute dyspnoea:
    Pneumothorax,
    Asthma.
 	
3. Minor embolism with existing
    cardiopulmonary disease.
	With the exception of angiography in massive embolism, there is no specific confirmatory test for pulmonary embolism and any or all of the expected signs and symptoms may be absent.

TREATMENT OF PULMONARY EMBOLISM

USE OF THROMBOLYTIC AGENTS
This is an effective but dangerous treatment which would be resorted to only if thrombi or emboli continued to be produced and is contra-indicated within 5 days of surgery.

Streptokinase is an exotoxin derived from haemolytic streptococci. The drug must first overcome the antibodies which everyone possesses against streptococcal infection.

Urokinase is a natural lytic activator manufactured in the kidneys and excreted in the urine. It is very expensive but virtually non-antigenic.

Both these drugs stimulate the conversion of plasminogen to plasmin which then lyses the fibrin in the thrombus. The dosage of streptokinase is 100,000 IU per hour, with a loading dose of 250,000 IU.

PRECAUTIONS WITH THROMBOLYTIC AGENTS

1. Treatment should not last more than 3 days.
2. Severe bleeding can be controlled by anti-fibrinolytic agents such as tranexamic acid 500 mg (Cyklokapron) given 4-hourly.
3. No injections or withdrawals of blood can be carried out during treatment, so there can be no laboratory control.
4. Once treatment has stopped, anti-coagulants should be given.

CONTRAINDICATIONS TO THROMBOLYTIC AGENTS

1. Any operation within 5 days (All fibrin is broken down).
2. Open wound or ulcer.
3. Pregnancy or abortion.
4. Menstruation.
5. Hypertension.
6. Any tendency to be a 'bleeder' or known thrombophilia defect.

INTERRUPTION OF THE INFERIOR VENA CAVA
This is a cardiovascular surgeon's technique and might be indicated in the presence of extensive iliac vein thrombosis, especially if a small non-fatal embolism has already been observed.

Many devices have been described and the most recent is the Kim-Ray Greenfield filter which is introduced under X-ray screening through the internal jugular vein. It consists of an arrangement of steel struts fitted into an apical hub and having small hooked ends which grasp the wall of the IVC and prevent displacement.

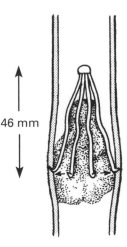

46 mm

PULMONARY EMBOLECTOMY.
This requires cardiac bypass and carries a high fatality rate.

TREATMENT OF PULMONARY EMBOLISM

SUMMARY OF MANAGEMENT

1. Massive embolism.
   Death appears imminent.

   Only embolectomy may be of use here, preferably under cardiopulmonary by-pass. Otherwise only resuscitative and supportive measures can be applied.

2. Major embolism
   with or without shock.

   Treatment of shock should be started along with heparinisation. If the patient continued to produce emboli or if the thrombosis appeared to be enlarging locally, streptokinase treatment would be considered.

3. Minor (peripheral) emboli.

   Heparinisation.

Pulmonary embolism is a catastrophe better avoided, but the patients who are going to die will do so almost at once, and complete resolution can be expected in those who survive the first 2 hours.

CHAPTER 16

ABORTION AND ABNORMALITIES OF EARLY PREGNANCY

ABORTION

The termination of a pregnancy before the 24th week.

THREATENED ABORTION

Technically this refers only to bleeding from the placental site which is not yet severe enough to terminate the pregnancy. In practice any case of bleeding before the 24th week may be classed as a threatened abortion in the absence of any other explanation. The presence of a continuing pregnancy should be confirmed by ultrasound. After the bleeding has diminished, the cervix should be examined.

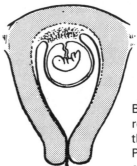

Threatened abortion
Bleeding is slight, not retro-placental and the cervix is closed. Pregnancy is likely to continue.

INEVITABLE ABORTION

Here bleeding is also slight, and the cervix is open. There is usually pain. Clinically the patient presents as a threatened abortion, but bleeding is retro-placental and the ovum is already dead.

Ultrasound shows no fetal heart beat. The pregnancy test may still be positive as hCG is produced by the chorion, not the fetus.

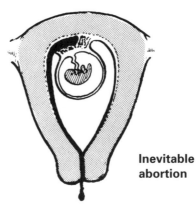

Inevitable abortion

INCOMPLETE ABORTION

The fetus and membranes are expelled but the chorionic tissue remains attached and bleeding continues.

Ultrasound shows debris in the uterine cavity.

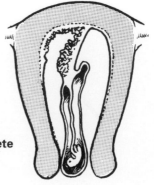

Incomplete abortion

ABORTION

MISSED ABORTION

The retention of a dead fetus for several weeks. The normal reaction of the uterus to the death of the fetus is to expel it, but for some unexplained reason this may not occur. Absence of fetal heart pulsation is detected by ultrasound.

If left alone spontaneous expulsion is likely. However such management carries a small risk of coagulation defect and the patient will usually press for active treatment. Surgical uterine evacuation is safe if the uterus is ≤12 weeks' size, but otherwise the condition is better managed medically (p.347).

THERAPEUTIC ABORTION

A termination of pregnancy carried out under the provision of the Abortion Act of 1967. This Act allows consideration of various social and emotional factors as well as the physical and mental state of the mother and fetus.

SEPTIC ABORTION

Any abortion which becomes infected. Such infection carries a risk of septic shock (p.342).

ANTI-D SERUM

In all Rhesus negative women who bleed during pregnancy it is necessary to administer anti-D serum to prevent Rhesus iso-immunisation. 250 iu anti-D IgG immunoglobulin is given to unsensitised Rh-negative women up to 20 weeks' gestation.

SEPTIC ABORTION

Uterine infection at any stage of an abortion.

Causes

1. Delay in evacuation of the uterus. Either the patient delays seeking advice or the surgical evacuation has been incomplete. Infection occurs from vaginal organisms after 48 hours.

2. Trauma, either perforation or cervical tear. Healing is delayed and infection is more likely to be a peritonitis or cellulitis. Criminal abortions are of course particularly liable to sepsis.

Infecting Organisms

These are usually the vaginal or bowel commensals.

1. Anaerobic streptococcus
2. Coliform bacillus
3. Clostridium Welchii
4. Bacteroides fragilis.

Any of these organisms but particularly the last two may be the cause of septic shock (q.v.).

Clinical Features

Slight bleeding continues with pyrexia and a raised pulse rate. Examination reveals pelvic tenderness and the patient displays anxiety.

Treatment

This should be active to minimise the risk of septic shock. Cervical and high vaginal smears, and several blood cultures are taken and a broad spectrum antibiotic such as cephaloridine and metronidazole exhibited forthwith. Curettage should be carried out as soon as possible; there is nothing to be gained by leaving infected material in utero. Perforation of a septic uterus is easily done, and in a few cases hysterectomy must be resorted to. In the past, septic abortion was a relatively common cause of renal failure following septic shock. Legal therapeutic termination of pregnancy has virtually eliminated this.

INCOMPLETE ABORTION

INCOMPLETE ABORTION — Dilatation and Evacuation

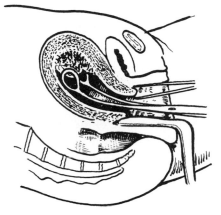

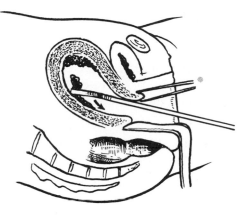

The patient is anaesthetized and the cervix is dilated. Once dilatation is sufficient the bulk of placental tissue may be removed with sponge forceps.

Further tissue is carefully removed with a curette.

The concave side of the curette loop is pressed against the uterine wall and pulled down. A 'clean' uterine wall gives a characteristic sensation to the operating hand.

Some operators prefer to use suction to evacuate the uterus. An Oxytocic agent such as syntometrine is used at the end (some prefer at the beginning) of the procedure to reduce the risk of bleeding.

THERAPEUTIC ABORTION

Indications for Therapeutic Abortion under the Abortion Act (1967), amended 1992.

1. ...the continuance of the pregnancy would involve risk to the life of the pregnant woman greater than if the pregnancy were terminated.

2. ...the termination is necessary to prevent grave permanent injury to the physical or mental health of the pregnant woman.

3. ...the pregnancy has NOT exceeded its 24th week and the continuance of the pregnancy would involve risk, greater than if the pregnancy were terminated, of injury to the physical or mental health of the pregnant woman.

4. ...the pregnancy has NOT exceeded its 24th week and the continuance of the pregnancy would involve risk, greater than if the pregnancy were terminated, of injury to the physical or mental health of the existing child(ren) of the family of the pregnant woman.

5. ...there is substantial risk that if the child were born it would suffer from such physical or mental abnormalities as to be seriously handicapped.

A certificate of opinion is given by 2 medical practitioners before the commencement of treatment for the termination of pregnancy to which it refers.

A single practitioner may give an emergency certificate before termination or, where not reasonably practical, within 24 hours of termination and terminate a pregnancy if it is necessary to save the life of the pregnant woman or to prevent grave permanent injury to her physical or mental health.

Illegal abortion
Since the introduction of the Abortion Act, illegal or criminal abortion is now rarely performed in the UK. Illegal abortion is usually performed in unsterile conditions by operators with little or no medical training. The abortion achieved is often incomplete. Not suprisingly, intrauterine infection is a frequent complication of this procedure and in some women, septic shock and death are the ultimate consequences.

FIRST TRIMESTER THERAPEUTIC ABORTION

1. SUCTION TERMINATION OF PREGNANCY (STOP)

Suction termination of pregnancy can be performed up to 12 weeks' gestation.

The Karman plastic suction curette is commonly used and is less likely to damage the uterus than metal instruments. Plastic curettes are available in diameters from 4 to 12 mm. The cervix is conventionally dilated to a diameter 2 mm less than the gestation in weeks.

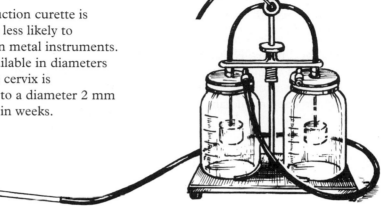

Preoperative cervical ripening

Cervical damage at the time of abortion can be minimised by the use of preoperative cervical ripening agents. Effective agents include:

— gemeprost (prostaglandin E$_1$) given as a vaginal pessary 3 h before surgery
— misoprostol (a prostaglandin analogue) given vaginally 3 h before surgery
— mifepristone (an antiprogesterone) given orally at least 12 h before surgery
— laminaria tents inserted into the external cervical os.

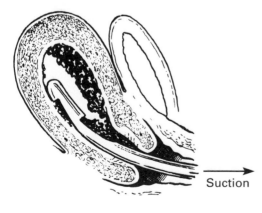

Suction

Complications

1. Incomplete uterine evacuation.
2. Uterine perforation and/or damage to abdominal viscera.
3. Sepsis. Broad spectrum antibiotics have been shown to minimise the risk of post abortal infection.
4. Haemorrhage. Blood loss can be minimised by the use of prostaglandins for preoperative cervical ripening. Bleeding during or after the procedure can be reduced by oxytocic agents such as ergometrine or syntocinon.
5. Rhesus isoimmunisation. Anti D should be administered to rhesus negative women.

FIRST TRIMESTER THERAPEUTIC ABORTION

2. MEDICAL TERMINATION

Mifepristone (RU 486) is an anti-progestogen which offers a medical alternative to vacuum aspiration of early pregnancy, up to 63 days from the first day of LMP or dated by ultrasound. The use of mifepristone is strictly controlled to approved NHS hospitals and premises approved under the Abortion Act.

600 mg mifepristone orally is taken in the presence of the prescribing doctor and the patient observed closely for 2 hours. Unless abortion has already occurred the patient is admitted 36–48 hours later and a 1mg Gemeprost pessary is administered vaginally. Over 95% of pregnancies are aborted completely but curettage may be required for incomplete abortion. Side effects include abdominal pain with up to 20% requiring opiate analgesia following prostaglandin administration. Blood loss is similar to that following suction termination of pregnancy at the same gestation.

Mifepristone is contraindicated in suspected ectopic pregnancy, in smokers over 35 years of age, in chronic adrenal failure, porphyria, corticosteroid therapy, coagulation disorders and in women on anticoagulant therapy.

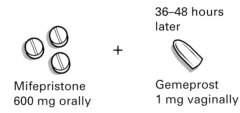

36–48 hours later

Mifepristone
600 mg orally

+

Gemeprost
1 mg vaginally

Modifications

A recent study has shown that the dose of mifepristone can be reduced to 200 mg with no loss of efficacy.

Misoprostol (a prostaglandin E analogue) may be used instead of gemeprost. The oral dose is 600 μg. Alternatively 800 μg may be given vaginally.

SECOND TRIMESTER ABORTION

Surgical methods

1. Dilatation and evacuation (D and C) involves cervical dilatation to a maximum diameter of 20 mm, and removal of the intrauterine contents. This is the method of choice for second trimester termination of pregnancy in the USA but it is not commonly performed in the UK.

Medical methods

2. Mifepristone and prostaglandins.

Mifepristone (200–600 mg) is followed 36–48 h later by 1mg gemeprost administered vaginally. Gemeprost is repeated 6-hourly. Mifepristone significantly reduces the interval from induction (prostaglandin administration) to abortion so that the vast majority of patients abort within 24 h.

3. Extra-amniotic abortion

This method may be used if mifepristone and gemeprost are unavailable.

PGE2 is very slowly instilled into the cervix through a Foley catheter at a rate not exceeding 2.5 ml/hour. After 6–8 hours of PGE2 the cervix will be soft enough to allow the action of oxytocin given intravenously in gradually increased dosage up to 150 mU/minute to cause abortion to occur.

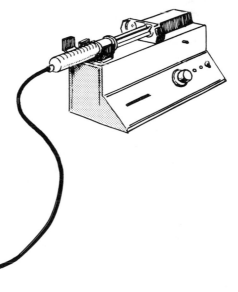

Curettage may be required in up to 30% of patients undergoing second trimester abortion using medical methods.

COMPLICATIONS OF THERAPEUTIC ABORTION

IMMEDIATE

Major complications (2%)
e.g. haemorrhage, thrombo-embolism, operative trauma, infection.

Minor complication (10%)
e.g. lower abdominal pain, bleeding, PID.

Incomplete abortion (≤5%).

Mortality

In the UK, the mortality related to induced abortion is 2.2 per million maternities, which is significantly less than that associated with continuing the pregnancy, namely 55.7 per million maternities.

Late complications

1. Infertility
   If abortion is complicated by post abortal infection there is a risk of tubal occlusion and subsequent infertility. If women are screened and treated for genital tract pathogens prior to abortion, the risk of post abortal infection is significantly reduced. With modern methods, the risk of infection related to therapeutic abortion is very small.

2. Effect on future pregnancies
   Several well designed studies have shown no adverse effects on a future pregnancy from a single therapeutic abortion.

3. Psychological sequelae
   Although an abortion is a potentially traumatic procedure, several studies have shown an improvement in psychological wellbeing 3 months after abortion compared with before the procedure.

4. Rhesus isoimmunisation
   This can be minimised by administering anti-D to rhesus negative women. 250 iu of anti-D is required in women up to 20 weeks' gestation.

RECURRENT MISCARRIAGE

This condition is present when a woman has had 3 consecutive miscarriages.

Aetiology and investigation:

1. Genetic factors
   Karyotyping of both partners will reveal parental chromosomal anomalies where present.

2. Anatomical factors
   Uterine anomalies (10–15%).
   Cervical incompetence.
   Hysteroscopy ± hysterosalpingography will delineate abnormalities such as an intrauterine septum.

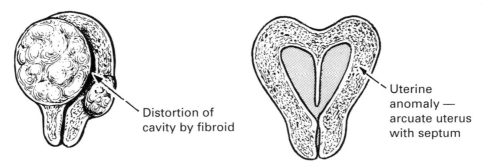

Distortion of cavity by fibroid

Uterine anomaly — arcuate uterus with septum

3. Endocrine problems
   Elevated follicular phase LH levels.
   e.g. as in polycystic ovarian disease (see p.94).

4. Immunological factors
   Recurrent miscarriage is commoner in couples with similar HLA types. Since no effective treatment exists, HLA analysis is not normally performed.

   Recurrent miscarriage is also commoner in women with the 'antiphospholipid antibody syndrome'. This syndrome is characterised by some or all of the following: recurrent miscarriage, thrombosis, thrombocytopenia, poor obstetric history. Anticardiolipin antibodies and lupus anticoagulant levels are often abnormal.

5. Maternal disease
   e.g. SLE, renal disease.

   Maternal thrombophilia is increasingly recognised as a cause of recurrent miscarriage. Screening for protein C and protein S deficiency is indicated.

6. Environmental factors
   e.g. smoking and alcohol.

RECURRENT MISCARRIAGE

Treatment of recurrent miscarriage

Even after careful investigation, the majority of women have no obvious cause for recurrent miscarriage. Notwithstanding, the prognosis is generally good, with a mean probability of a live birth in the next pregnancy of around 70%.

Treatment of specific causes is as follows:

1. Genetic factors

    No treatment available. If a future pregnancy is successful, consideration should be given to karyotyping the fetus to exclude an abnormality.

2. Anatomical factors

    Uterine anomalies
    Uterine surgery may correct the abnormality, but may not necessarily improve the prognosis. These procedures may cause adhesions and therefore reduce fertility and should not be entered into lightly.

    Cervical incompetence
    Cervical cerclage may be of benefit.

    Diagnosis of this condition is made on a history of late abortions and by palpations or occasionally by hysterography.

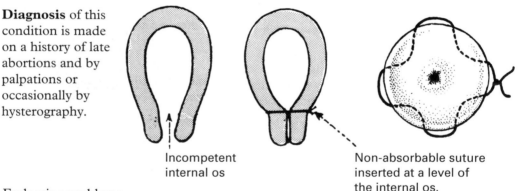

Incompetent
internal os

Non-absorbable suture
inserted at a level of
the internal os.

3. Endocrine problems
    No effective treatment.

4. Immunological factors
    In women with the anticardiolipin antibody syndrome, treatment with low dose aspirin and heparin has been shown to improve the outcome in future pregnancies.

5. Maternal disease
    If protein C and protein S deficiency are found, thromboprophylaxis should be considered. Few well conducted trials exist for the treatment of these conditions, although there is a rationale for low dose aspirin therapy.

6. Environmental factors
    All women wishing to become pregnant should be advised to stop smoking and to minimise their alchohol intake.

HYDATIDIFORM MOLE

This is a peculiar condition of the placenta showing apparent degenerative changes in the stroma of the villi combined with varying degrees of neoplastic activity of the chorionic epithelium. The incidence varies in different countries, being relatively common in some equatorial regions and rather rare in the northern hemisphere. It is frequently associated with abortion and usually there is no fetus.

The true incidence is unknown in all countries since the degree of change is not constant and the aborted conceptus may be discarded as a simple abortion. The following are reported figures:

UK	1 in 1200 to 1 in 2000 pregnancies.
USA	1 in 1000 to 1 in 2500.
Russia	1 in 330.
Mexico	1 in 200.
Philippines	1 in 173.
Formosa	1 in 120.

Pathology

Five forms of the disease have been described.

1. Complete Hydatidiform Mole

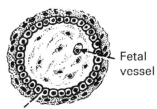

Fetal vessel

Chorionic epithelium

Normal villus

In complete hydatidiform mole the villi are grossly swollen and are likened to 'bunches of grapes.'

There is no embryo.

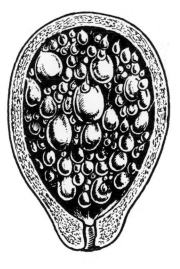

HYDATIDIFORM MOLE

Microscopically, the villi are enormously distended. Hyperplasia of both syncytiotrophoblast and cytotrophoblast can be observed.

Fetal vessels are absent and the interior of the villi is occupied by relatively acellular myxoid stroma. Occasionally so-called 'cisterns' are present in the interior. These may be mistaken for vascular channels but they contain no cells.

The ovaries in all types of hydatid change tend to be enlarged and often contain theca lutein cysts. This is due to the activity of the high serum hCG.

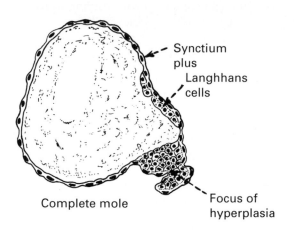

Synctium plus Langhhans cells

Complete mole

Focus of hyperplasia

2. **Partial Mole**

In this case there are two populations of villi. Some are of normal size and configuration, containing fetal vessels while others show the typical grape-like appearance of hydatidiform change, and fetal vessels are absent. Frequently an embryo is present indicating that some degree of utero-placental circulation has been established. Trophoblast hyperplasia is very focal and usually confined to the syncytio-trophoblast.

3. **Placental site trophoblast tumour**

This is a rare lesion in which few villi are formed. The bulk of the tissue consists of chorionic epithelium, much of which has not properly differentiated into the usual 2 types. Although generally benign, occasionally it can undergo malignant change and prove fatal.

HYDATIDIFORM MOLE

4. Invasive mole

This is a condition in which molar tissue burrows through the decidua and into the myometrium and associated blood vessels. It may result from complete or partial hydatidiform mole.

Perforation of the uterus may occur, resulting in invasion of the parametrium.

Sometimes parts of villi may form emboli and reach the lungs but only in some cases does true malignant transformation occur.

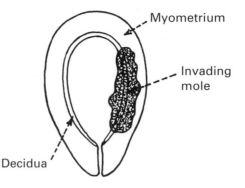

5. Chorio-carcinoma

This is a rare condition especially in Caucasian peoples (1 in 14000 pregnancies). It is said to be commoner in Asiatic countries but exact figures are not available.

The growth may be malignant from the very beginning but at least 50% arise from a molar condition. One of the disturbing features is that the carcinoma may arise many months after the mole has been evacuated, hence the reason for extended follow-up in all types of mole. Only about 2% of moles give rise to chorio-carcinoma but the risk is 1000 times greater than the risk after normal delivery.

The gross appearance of the uterus containing chorio-carcinoma is of a large haemorrhagic mass showing a ragged invasion of most of the uterine wall.

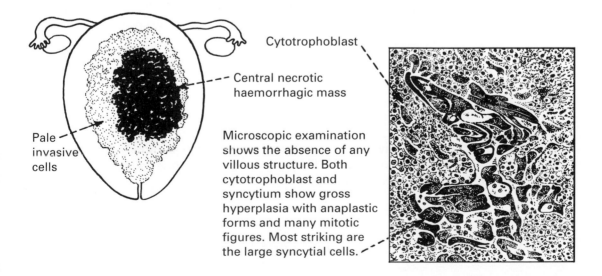

Microscopic examination shows the absence of any villous structure. Both cytotrophoblast and syncytium show gross hyperplasia with anaplastic forms and many mitotic figures. Most striking are the large syncytial cells.

HYDATIDIFORM MOLE

Epidemiology of hydatidiform mole
The following features are associated with hydatidiform mole:

1. The peaks of incidence are known, related to age. These occur in women under 20 and over 45.

2. The rarity of the condition in Caucasian women and its commoner occurrence in Asians. The reported differences in incidence may be related to selection bias in hospital based studies, rather than a true racial difference.

3. Previous molar pregnancy. After one molar pregnancy, the risk of a second is up to 3%. After two molar pregnancies, the risk of a third is up to 28%.

Genetics of hydatidiform mole

1. Complete mole

The karyotype of complete mole is 46XX but all of the chromosomes are of paternal origin. The pronucleus of the ovum fails to develop properly and disappears. However the empty egg is fertilised by a haploid 23X sperm which duplicates its chromosomes without cell division (less commonly) or by two different sperm. Why the ovum should fail to contribute to the process is not known. Since complete moles are more likely to become malignant, the karyotype of every mole should be determined.

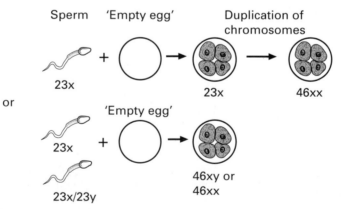

2. Partial mole

In partial mole fetal tissue of some type is present and the karyotype is entirely different. Usually it is triploid — 69XXX or 69XXY. This is due to fertilisation of the egg by two sperm. Partial moles are less likely to undergo malignant change.

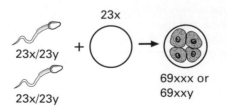

HYDATIDIFORM MOLE

Clinical course

Usually the first sign is bleeding. 50% of cases are admitted with pain and bleeding and the condition is assumed to be an ordinary abortion. The blood loss, however, is frequently high and this should raise suspicions, since a coagulation abnormality may arise.

Simple abortion usually occurs around the 10th to 12th week of pregnancy but examination will show that the uterus in a molar condition is larger than expected for the dates in 60 to 80% of patients and has a 'doughy' feel.

Questioning of the patient is likely to reveal that nausea and vomiting have been excessive.

The ovaries are enlarged and may equal the uterus in size. Fctal parts cannot be palpated. There may be signs of pre-eclampsia — high blood pressure and proteinuria.

A few hydatid vesicles may be passed per vaginam and confirm the diagnosis.

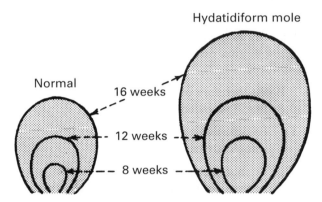

If not, the following examinations should be made:

1. Ultrasound

   This will reveal the absence of fetal parts. The shadow of the mole shows an irregular mass with speckled surrounding areas.

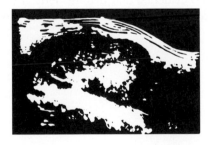

2. If ultrasound is not readily available an ordinary X-ray will show the absence of fetal parts.

3. Ordinary auscultation will reveal absence of fetal heart sounds but this often proves difficult and examination with the Doppler flowmeter will confirm the absence of a fetal heart.

Differential diagnosis

A mole can mimic two common complications of early pregnancy — hyperemesis and threatened abortion — and the enlarged uterus may give rise to suspicions of twins or tumour.

HYDATIDIFORM MOLE

Treatment of molar conditions

Treatment of hyatidiform mole

- vacuum aspiration to empty the uterus

- registration with national mole follow-up service (UK)

- appropriate follow up.

Follow up of hydatidiform mole

- serum or urine hCG measurements
  biweekly until below the limit of detection
  then monthly until 1 yr. postuterine evacuation
  then three-monthly until 2 yr. postuterine evacuation.

(More limited follow up may be appropriate if hCG levels fall rapidly postuterine evacuation, e.g. to normal by 56 days postuterine evacuation — the risk of abnormal sequelae in these patients is minimal).

Controversies

1. The use of the oral contraceptive pill
    The prevention of pregnancy is essential during mole follow-up. Some studies suggest that the use of the COCP before hCG levels have fallen to normal may increase the risk of requiring chemotherapy.

2. Prophylactic chemotherapy
    There is no good evidence that prophylactic chemotherapy reduces the risk of recurrence. It may be appropriate if close follow-up is not possible.

PERSISTENT DISEASE

Persistent disease is suggestive of invasive mole or chorio-carcinoma. A histological diagnosis is not necessary. Persistent disease should be treated with chemotherapy. Surgery should be avoided if possible. The major risk is of haemorrhage from tumour in the uterus or metastasis in lung, liver, brain etc. CT scanning should be considered to identify distant metastases.

Indications for chemotherapy
The WHO recommend chemotherapy in the following instances:

1. A high level of hCG more than 4 weeks after uterine evacuation (serum level >20 000 IU/L; urine levels > 30 000IU/L).

2. Progressively increasing hCG values at any time after uterine evacuation.

3. Histological identification of chorio-carcinoma at any site or evidence of central nervous system, renal, hepatic or gastrointestinal metastases, or pulmonary metastases >2 cm in diameter or >3 in number.

4. Persistent uterine haemorrhage with an elevated hCG.

An X-ray of the lung fields should always be carried out if invasive mole is suspected. There may be one large shadow (Cannon-ball metastasis) or numerous emboli ('Snowstorm'). These metastases are abolished by chemotherapy.

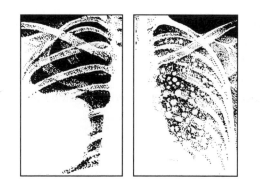

CHEMOTHERAPY FOR CHORIO-CARCINOMA

Prognostic variables which help determine which chemotherapeutic regimen is the most appropriate are shown below. This system has been adopted by the World Health Organisation.

Prognostic factors	Score			
	0	1	2	4
Age (years)	<39	>39		
Antecedent pregnancy	Hydatidiform mole	Abortion	Term	
Interval*	4	4–6	7–12	12
hCG (IU/l)	$<10^3$	10^3–10^4	10^4–10^5	$>10^5$
ABO groups (female x male)		$0 \times A$ $A \times 0$	B AB	
Largest tumour, including uterine tumour		3–5 cm	>5 cm	
Site of metastases		Spleen, kidney	Gastrointestinal tract, liver	Brain
Number of metastases identified		1–4	4–8	>8
Prior chemotherapy			Single drug	2 or more

The total score for a patient is obtained by adding the individual scores for each prognostic factor.
Total score: <4=low risk; 5–7 = middle risk; >8= high risk.
*Interval time (in months) between end of antecedent pregnancy and start of chemotherapy.

Chemotherapy

Low risk (score 5 or less)

Methotrexate and folinic acid on alternating days for 8 days. Several courses may be required.

Medium / high risk
EMA/CO: a cocktail including course of etopside, methotrexate, folinic acid and actinomycin followed by vincristine and cyclophosphamide.

CHORIO-CARCINOMA

Side-effects of chemotherapy

Bone marrow — Leucopenia, anaemia, agranulocytosis.

Gut — Stomatitis, glossitis, nausea, vomiting, diarrhoea.

Liver — Jaundice.

Kidney — Proteinuria, renal impairment. Methotrexate is excreted unchanged and can damage the kidney tissue directly. Make certain that fluid intake is adequate.

Skin — Alopecia, rashes.

Tests to be carried out during therapy

1. Full blood count including platelets every other day during therapy.

2. Estimation of liver transaminase level prior to beginning therapy and every 2 days during treatment.

3. Test urine regularly for protein.

PREGNANCY AFTER CHEMOTHERAPY

Methotrexate can be retained in the body for up to 8 months and the theoretical risk is of cytotoxic damage to oocytes resulting in an increased incidence of fetal abnormality. However this does not seem to be borne out in practice, although patients are advised to delay conception for a year. Post treatment, fertility is high with 86% of patients who wished to conceive being successful in one series.

CHAPTER 17

SEXUALITY AND CONTRACEPTION

PHYSIOLOGY OF COITUS

Response to sexual stimulation is primarily an autonomic nervous reflex which is reinforced or inhibited by psychological and social factors. These factors are infinitely variable; but as a generalisation it may be said that the female responds to the consciousness of being desired as a whole person, while the satisfaction of the male depends to a greater extent on visceral sensation.

EXCITEMENT PHASE

This takes most of the time needed for coitus and, in the male, becomes longer with experience, while the female learns to respond in a shorter time.

Female:
Vasodilatation and vasocongestion of all erectile tissue. Breasts enlarge, the vaginal ostium opens and secretion from the vestibular glands and vaginal exudations cause 'moistening'.

Male:
Penile erection occurs and may be transient and recur if this stage is prolonged. Scrotal skin and dartos muscle contract and draw testes towards the perineum.

INTROMISSION

The couple assume the chosen coital position and the penis is inserted into the open vagina. Although this is the irrevocable commitment to intercourse, it is still in the excitement phase until thrusting begins, and the male still has some control over the timing of orgasm.

PLATEAU PHASE

The pulse rate is doubled and blood pressure and respiratory rate are beginning to rise. Both partners make involuntary thrusting movements of the pelvis towards each other.

Female:
Vasocongestion increases, and contraction of the uterine ligaments (which contain muscle) lift the uterus and move it more into alignment with the axis of the pelvis. The cervix dilates. There is engorgement of the lower third of the vagina and ballooning of the upper two thirds.

Male:
The intensity of penile erection increases and the testes are enlarged by congestion. Seminal fluid arrives at the urethra as a result of sympathetic nervous stimulation of the vas deferens, seminal vesicles and prostate. There is some pre-ejaculatory penile discharge which may contain sperm.

PHYSIOLOGY OF COITUS

ORGASM

Pulse and respiration rate are at double the resting rate and blood pressure may reach 180/110. Pelvic and genital sensations are completely dominating, and there is a noticeable reduction in sensory awareness in other parts of the body. The pelvic floor contracts involuntarily, with rhythmic contraction of vagina, urethra and anal sphincter.

Female:
Climactic sensations appear to be caused by spasmodic contractions of uterine muscle but orgasm is reported after hysterectomy. The female is potentially capable of repeated orgasm.

Male:
Strong contractions pass along the penis causing ejaculation of seminal fluid. The greater the volume of ejaculate (after several days' continence) the more intense the sensations of orgasm.

POSTCOITAL PHASE or RESOLUTION PHASE

Pulse, respiratory rate and blood pressure rapidly return to normal and there is marked sweating. Vasocongestion recedes over about 5 minutes and there is complete relaxation of all muscles and detumescence of erectile tissue. In the male, but less so in the female, there occurs a refractory period which varies with individuals, from a few minutes to several hours when there is no response to further stimuli.

SEXUAL PROBLEMS AFFECTING THE FEMALE

FAILURE TO ACHIEVE ORGASM

It is common in gynaecological practice to meet women who profess never or seldom to have experienced orgasm and yet appear to enjoy sexual fulfilment. This is never the case with the male. The psychological gratifications of coitus must never be underestimated in the female, but the physical elements dominate and orgasm is the natural response of the female to adequate erotic stimulation. Many women require stimulation of the clitoris or other erogenous zones to achieve orgasm.

The cause of anorgasmia is therefore failure of stimulation, either to receive it or to respond to it.

FAILURE TO RECEIVE STIMULATION

This is theoretically the more easily dealt with since its correction requires 'only' some education and instruction of the male. However the barriers to communication are formidable and a deficiency in the male (premature ejaculation for example) may arise from some deficiency in the female.

FAILURE TO RESPOND TO STIMULATION

Primary Failure	**Secondary Failure**
Early psychological trauma.	Puerperal depression.
Early inculcation of social or religious taboos.	Fear of another pregnancy.
	Marital stress.
Profound defect of personality.	Dyspareunia (q.v.).
Lesbian tendency, unrecognised or undisclosed.	Endocrine disease.
	Any debilitating illness.

FRIGIDITY

This term, now outmoded, implies a failure by the woman to provide a satisfying coitus for the man, and it embodies an attitude to woman's sexuality which is not now acceptable. Women will, in consultation, declare a condition which might be described as frigid: 'I have no interest in my partner; I wouldn't mind if I never had sex, but I go through with it to keep him happy'. Such women are conscious of and resent the absence of physical satisfaction and are far better regarded as suffering from failure to achieve orgasm. The male's attitude may well be at fault, but he may fail to be aware of, or admit to, this.

Loss of libido sometimes responds to testosterone, 50 or 100 mg implanted subcutaneously at 6 month intervals. Post-menopausal women may notice an improvement in libido on HRT.

ANORGASMIA

MANAGEMENT OF ANORGASMIA

Mechanical and Clinical Causes

Conditions such as puerperal depression, fear of pregnancy and local vaginal lesions can usually be diagnosed and treated by the gynaecologist in the appropriate manner.

Psychological and Personality Causes

These must be correctly identified and treated by a clinical psychologist. Ideally both parties should attend.

TREATMENT

If the treatment indicated is basically a matter of achieving communication and confidence between sexual partners and gradually allaying their apprehensions, the gynaecologist or the general practitioner may have to function as a therapist and, for such work, experience both sexual and therapeutic is essential.

The couple must face the situation and discuss it in detail without inhibition, much as in the manner of the alcoholic. They must accept that the object of treatment is to provide *both* parties with a satisfying and affectionate copulatory relationship *as an end in itself*, and once free communication is achieved the couple proceed gradually to give and receive pelvic and genital stimulation, the female learning to welcome arousal, the male to control his own response. Progress must be discussed in detail with the therapist and it will be appreciated that this intensive treatment requires a properly motivated couple, a dedicated and experienced therapist, and a good deal of time and patience.

DYSPAREUNIA

DYSPAREUNIA (Painful coitus)

SUPERFICIAL DYSPAREUNIA

Vaginal pain during intromission of the penis. It is usually a genuine complaint and not simulated with the intention of avoiding coitus.

Causes include:

1. Vulvovaginitis (especially infection by trichomonas or candida).

2. Vaginal cysts. Small ones are usually symptomless.

3. Infection of Bartholin's gland.

4. Post-menopausal shrinkage.

5. Rarely there is a congenital smallness of the ostium or a thick hymen.

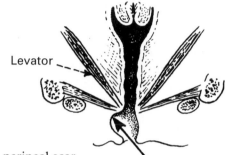

Levator

6. Painful perineal scar.
   This may be due to an inflamed or fibrous scar following childbirth, or to an imperfectly repaired episiotomy or tear which allows the formation, by attempts at coitus, of a small very tender 'blind alley' just inside the vagina below the levator muscle.

DEEP DYSPAREUNIA

Pain is due to penile pressure on an area of tenderness near the vaginal vault. The cause is often difficult to identify and there may be no obvious disease. If the pain complained of cannot be reproduced by the examining fingers the gynaecologist should consider the possibility of a functional complaint.

Causes include:
1. Retroverted uterus with prolapsed ovaries, the 'ovarian entrapment' syndrome.
2. Chronic pelvic infection.
3. Endometriosis.
4. Pelvic tumours including ectopic pregnancy.
5. Removal of a cuff of vaginal vault at hysterectomy or scarring at the vaginal vault.

PELVIC CONGESTION

Some women complain of congestive pain developing after coitus and lasting several hours. It has been suggested that this is a result of sexual frustration following failure to achieve orgasm and there is often some functional element to be identified. No specific treatment is widely recognised but pelvic venous congestion may be diagnosed by venography and treated by the interventional radiographic technique of embolisation.

VAGINISMUS

VAGINISMUS

A partly voluntary contraction of the pelvic muscles which takes place when introduction of the penis is attempted, making coitus impossible.

Mild Vaginismus

The patient has erotic desires, takes part in preliminary love play and is aroused by manual stimulation of the genitals. Vaginismus occurs only when intromission is attempted.

Severe Vaginismus

No touching of the vulva is allowed and attempts are met with an arching of the back and strong apposition of the thighs. Some reluctance or tenseness is usually apparent in the preliminary love play.

Causes are those of other forms of sexual dysfunction. Mild degrees are usually the result of apprehension, severe degrees may relate to some profound disturbance of personality.

Treatment

1. An examination under anaesthesia should be carried out to exclude organic causes and to reassure the patient that there is no anatomical abnormality.

2. Male and female should be interviewed together and the use of vaginal dilators of graduated sizes explained. The purpose is not to dilate a narrow vagina but to give the patient confidence that her vagina can easily accommodate the penis. Once the patient can use them up to the largest size, the male partner should be instructed in their insertion in the vagina and from there the couple should achieve intromission.

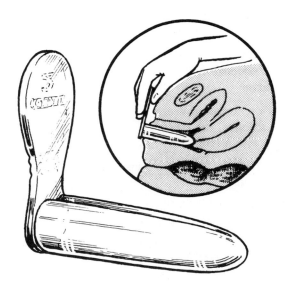

Failure of this treatment is an indication for more extensive psychiatric investigation. Mild vaginismus usually responds well to these simple measures, but in severe cases the results are poor.

The clinical psychologist and the medical hypnotist can often be helpful in treating vaginismus.

SEXUAL PROBLEMS AFFECTING THE MALE

The gynaecologist is not normally called upon to deal directly with the male, but he must be aware of these sexual problems and know something of their management.

PREMATURE EJACULATION

The male ejaculates before or immediately after intromission. If this prevents the female from achieving orgasm, it must be regarded as a disability.

Certain behavioural patterns seem to be associated:

1. Inexperience, producing undue haste and an inadequate excitement phase.

2. Pre-marital conditioning to rapid response — clandestine intercourse under fear of discovery, intercourse with prostitutes.

3. Any display of disinclination on the part of the female.

Treatment

If both partners genuinely seek improvement and can be induced to discuss the problem without inhibitions, treatment is generally successful. The male must be allowed to gain the confidence to prolong foreplay, and the female learns to respond more readily.

The 'squeeze technique' of Masters and Johnson

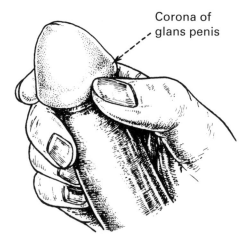

Corona of glans penis

If the female squeezes the penis for a few seconds, the erection will decrease a little with a temporary loss of the stimulus to ejaculate. This can be repeated several times, extending the excitement phase and accustoming the male to delay ejaculation.

Perhaps the greatest advantage of this technique is the complete communication and awareness that develops between male and female.

Drug Treatment

Reserpine (Serpasil) 0.1 mg taken in the evening is said to retard the ejaculatory reflex, and sedative drugs such as diazepam (Valium) 2 mg act by reducing the level of erotic response. When the nervous system is intact, drugs should not really be required in the treatment of this condition.

EJACULATORY FAILURE

EJACULATORY FAILURE

Inability to ejaculate although there is no loss of erotic drive, and erection and intromission are normal.

The ejaculatory reflex requires intact pathways in both autonomic and somatic systems. Somatic nerves receive the sensory stimuli of coitus and pass impulses to the sympathetic nerves which stimulate the delivery of seminal fluid to the urethra by the vasa deferentia, seminal vesicles and prostate, and prevent retrograde ejaculation into the bladder by causing contraction of the internal urinary sphincters. Sympathectomy from T12 to L3 will abolish ejaculation without affecting erectile ability or the sensations of orgasm, producing a phenomenon known as 'dry sex'.

Aetiology is nearly always psychological, although some drugs are known to cause the condition.

Psychological Factors
1. Influence of repressive religious teaching on a susceptible personality. Coitus comes to be regarded as an act of sin.
2. Excessive maternal domination. There may be a subconscious oedipal conflict.
3. Some traumatic episode such as a humiliating sexual rejection; or the discovery of infidelity by the female partner.
4. Fear of pregnancy.
5. Dislike of the female partner.
6. Repressed homosexuality.

Drugs
Any drug with psychotropic action or which interferes with the autonomic system may cause impotence. Ejaculatory failure alone is known to occur with thioridazine (Melleril) and guanethidine (Ismelin) and especially with Indoramin, an alpha-adrenergic blocking agent.

Treatment
A complete analysis of the problem, involving both partners, must be made and this requires the skills of the psychotherapist.

If there is no serious psychological inhibition, treatment becomes essentially a matter of restoring the male's confidence, like the treatment of premature ejaculation in reverse. The female must manipulate the penis in the manner which is most acceptable to her partner, until extravaginal ejaculation occurs. Thereafter it becomes possible by degrees to achieve ejaculation after intromission.

Intercourse with another woman (a 'replacement partner') may well be more effective if the female has no interest in her partner's ejaculation or if her sexual approach is inadequate, but such single-minded therapy would, of course, introduce other problems.

IMPOTENCE

IMPOTENCE — Inability to achieve or sustain an erection.

PRIMARY IMPOTENCE

Physical causes due to some form of intersex abnormality are extremely rare, and primary impotence is nearly always due to psychological inhibition arising from abnormal influences in upbringing (medical, religious, homosexual, etc.).

SECONDARY IMPOTENCE

This may have either a physical or psychological basis.

Psychological

1. Developing from ejaculatory failure and having the same causation.
2. Social and domestic stress. The patient is typically successful, overworking and probably overdrinking. He is under stresses which affect his confidence and the harmony of his relationship.

Drugs

1. Alcohol in excess.
2. Hypotensives — beta blockers, methyldopa, guanethidine.
3. Phenothiazines — chlorpromazine.
4. Tricyclic antidepressants — imipramine, amitryptiline.

Endocrine Disease

Pituitary tumour may present as impotence.
Diabetes mellitus commonly causes impotence.

CNS Disease

Multiple sclerosis, paraplegia.

Vascular Disease

Iliac and pudendal thrombosis.

Postoperative sequel

Usually after radical pelvic operations such as abdomino-perineal resection or extended prostatectomy.

Urological Causes

These include congenital abnormalities such as hypospadias, chordee, congenital short urethra and Peyronie's disease, a fibrosis of the erectile tissue or the tunica albuginea. Such conditions are classed as 'mechanical' causes of impotence because the penile deformity gradually makes coitus impossible, but psychological impotence may be superimposed.

IMPOTENCE

TREATMENT OF IMPOTENCE

PSYCHOTHERAPY

This is seldom successful in primary impotence, but in secondary impotence, if a cause can be identified, psychotherapy may be successful. The management of the couple should be in the hands of the psychiatrist and the psychotherapist.

PHYSICAL CAUSES

These may be reversible as in endocrine lesions and drug impotence, or irreversible as in vascular and CNS disease.

Drugs acting on the autonomic nervous system, mainly antihypertensive and psychotropic drugs (including all the major tranquillisers) are recognised causes of impotence or ejaculatory failure.

SEX HORMONES

Simple prescription of male sex hormone is seldom successful and its part in the physiology of erection and ejaculation is not yet known. It seems reasonable to suppose that complete absence of male sex hormone would result in impotence; but castrated males can achieve erections. Sex hormones in such cases are presumably supplied by the adrenal glands.

PAPAVERINE

This is a smooth muscle relaxant. Intracavernosal injection of 7.5 mg initially, increasing to 30–60 mg according to response, is an effective treatment for impotence. Phentolamine 0.25–1.25 mg may be added if the response to papaverine is not adequate.

N.B. Papaverine, and NOT *Papaveretum* (hydrochlorides of alkaloids of opium), must be prescribed and dispensed!

SIDENASIL (VIAGRA)

An oral therapy for erectile difficulties, this does not produce an erection without sexual stimulation to respond to. Unfortunate side effects have been reported in men with cardiovascular problems on cardiovascular medication.

When the gynaecologist is consulted by a female patient about her real or supposed sexual inadequacy, it is essential that he bears in mind the possibility that the cause may lie with her partner. For example, failure of intromission is less likely to be due to a small vaginal introitus than to an imperfect or absent erection, but the female, from embarrassment, loyalty or ignorance, may not raise this possibility.

MEDICO-LEGAL PROBLEMS

RAPE

The doctor may on occasion be asked to examine a victim of alleged rape.

This crime has heavy penalties and examination must be thorough and careful.

The following preliminary notes should be made:
1. Authority for examination.
2. Consent for examination.
3. General appearance of person and clothing.
4. History of circumstances of crime.

Rape is defined as unlawful sexual intercourse with a woman by force and against her will.

Sexual intercourse is described as the slightest degree of penetration of the vulva by the penis and entry of the hymen is therefore not necessary. (Use of vaginal tampons by virgins may confuse the issue.)

The vulva should be inspected for signs of bruising, scratching or tearing. The hymen may be torn and bleeding.

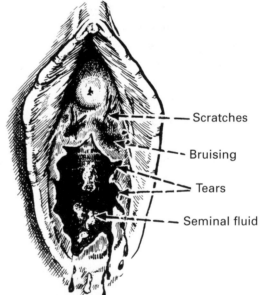

Scratches

Bruising

Tears

Seminal fluid

When the orifice is small or the hymen vestigial, bruising may be present because of the force needed to penetrate against the resistance of the victim. The presence of seminal fluid in the vagina and cervix may be the only sign. This fluid is removed and examined microscopically.

General examination of the patient may show injuries and bruising confirming a story of resistance overcome by violence.

Skin should be swabbed for blood, semen or saliva, using a swab moistened with sterile water, if there is evidence of these fluids, for DNA analysis. Finger nail clippings should be taken if there is blood or debris under them.

Comb the head and pubic hair for hairs from the assailant and cut 10 hairs from each site from the victim for comparison. Blood and urine samples should be taken. These may require to be tested for drugs.

Major police forces have specially trained rape investigation teams whose expertise may be invaluable.

Careful record keeping is essential. Collection, storage and transport of specimens must comply with legal requirements so that their source cannot be challenged.

MEDICO-LEGAL PROBLEMS

SIGNS OF RECENT DELIVERY

Pregnancy and birth have usually been concealed when a medical opinion is sought. The patient is usually primiparous and looks exhausted and pale. The breasts, their veins prominent, are enlarged, tense and knotty and pressure will express milk and colostrum.

The abdomen is lax and there may be fresh striae gravidarum — especially in the flanks.

The uterus is firm and remains 5–6 inches above the pubis in the first day or two, is behind the pubis by the 10th day and in 6 weeks is completely involuted and of normal parous size.

The labia and perineum may be lacerated and bruised.

The cervical os is torn and soft and will admit two fingers for a few days and one finger for another week or so. At 2 weeks the os is closed.

The lochial discharges are of blood and mucus for about 5 days, becoming brown, yellow and finally serous, and drying up in 4 weeks.

A pregnancy test is normally positive for a few days in the puerperium.

CRIMINAL ABORTION

Expulsion of the uterine contents by unlawful means is a crime in Scotland and in England and Wales. If maternal death occurs the crime becomes at least culpable homicide (manslaughter in England and Wales) and may be murder.

The history may help. Examination of the woman is important. The cervix is soft and partly patent with recent abortion. The abortion may be incomplete.

Visual examination of the cervix may show signs of injury, e.g. forceps marks. There may be signs of uterine infection or of peritonitis.

Confidentiality is maintained as far as possible, but if the patient becomes seriously ill, the proper legal authorities must be notified. Careful record keeping is essential.

METHODS OF CONTRACEPTION

FEMALE

Barrier Methods — Diaphragm
— Cervical cap
— Female condom

Hormonal Methods — Oral contraceptive — Combined oestrogen/progestogen
— Progestogen only
— Depot progestogens — Injections
— Subcutaneous silicone implants
— Vaginal — Silicone rings releasing oestrogen and progestogen

Intra Uterine Devices — Inert
— Copper bearing
— Progestogen releasing.

Natural Methods — Rhythm or Billings
— Breast feeding (while baby is totally breast fed)

Spermicides — Creams, Films, Foams, Jellies, Pessaries, Sponges
(All of these are mainly Nonoxynol based.)

Surgical Methods — Laparoscopic sterilisation — Rings
— Clips
— Bipolar diathermy
— Laser
— Tubal ligation
— Intra-uterine quinacrine producing tubal fibrosis,
in developing countries.

Immunological Methods — These are still at an investigative stage.

MALE
Condom
Vasectomy
Male oral contraception with androgens and with cotton seed oil ⎱ Still at investigative
Immunological contraception ⎰ stage.

Relative popularity of methods
(National Opinion Poll, 1990, Schering Healthcare. Women aged 16–44.)

Oral contraception	32%	IUCD	8%
No contraception	22%	Diaphragm/Cap	2%
Condoms	17%	Withdrawal	2%
Female sterilisation	12%	Rhythm/Billings	0.5%
Male sterilisation	12%		

Even the most intelligent, articulate people are often ill-informed about contraception and fears about possible ill-effects, together with problems experienced by friends and relatives, may play a greater role in influencing choice than medical advice and statistics. Many doctors are surprisingly poorly informed and therefore unable to give appropriate advice. Adequate, correct information and counselling are essential, and written details should, ideally, be supplied as well as verbal.

ORAL CONTRACEPTION

About three million women in the United Kingdom are said to be 'taking the pill'. The pill is a mixture of oestrogen and progestogen, or a progestogen alone, and its most serious disadvantage is the increased risk of cardiovascular disease, though this is lower with modern low-dose preparations.

Mode of Action

The pill prevents ovulation. FSH secretion is depressed and the LH peak is abolished. Urinary androgen excretion is much increased and this must add to the contraceptive effect.

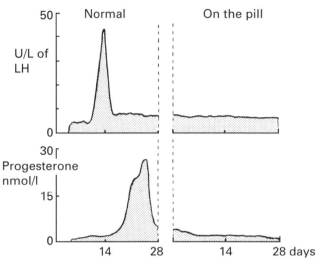

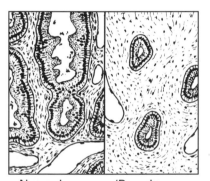

Normal endometrium   'Pseudo-atrophy'

Changes in cervical mucus make sperm penetration less likely.

Absence of a corpus luteum inhibits preparation of an endometrium suitable for implantation, and a 'pseudo-atrophy' develops.

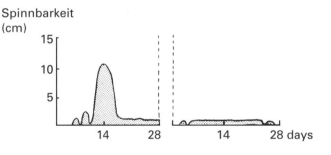

All these effects are the result of synergistic action between the oestrogen and progestogen. Progestogens when used by themselves have varying degrees of oestrogenicity.

On progestogen only oral contraceptives some 50% of women ovulate and menstruate and contraception is probably by effects on cervical mucus and implantation. Some bleed irregularly and around 15% are amenorrhoeic with no follicular development.

ORAL CONTRACEPTION

Constituents

Oestrogens (O)	Progestogens (P)
Ethinyloestradiol	Levonorgestrel
	Norethisterone
Mestranol	Ethynodiol diacetate
(ethinyloestradiol-	Desogestrel
3-methyl-ether)	Gestodene
	Norgestimate

Choice of Pill

There are over 30 brands available, using different drugs in different proportions.

High O, high P
ethinyloestradiol 50 μg
norethisterone acetate 4 mg

Medium O, low P
ethinyloestradiol 30 μg
L-norgestrel 150 μg

Low O, low P
ethinyloestradiol 20 μg
norethisterone acetate 1mg

P only
L-norgestrel 30 μg
norethisterone 350 μg

O/P and triphasic pills are taken from the 5th to the 25th day of the cycle. P only pills are taken every day, at exactly the same time each day.

Triphasic pills
O/P proportions vary roughly according to the phase of the cycle.

		days	1–6	7–11	12–21
	ethinyloestradiol	(μg)	30	40	30
	L-norgestrel	(μg)	50	75	125

1. As a general rule, since both O and P constituents are responsible for unwanted side-effects, use the pill with the lowest amount of steroid drug. None is perfect and several may have to be tried to find one that is acceptable to the patient.

2. P-only and low-O pills are less reliable as contraceptives than those with 50 μg of O, and tend to cause more breakthrough bleeding. P-only pills may be accompanied by depression.

3. O-dominant pills are required for women with greasy skin or acne.

4. Triphasics have the lowest amount of steroid and are indicated in the older age group who have a higher risk of thrombosis than younger women. They are O-dominant and may cause fluid retention and pre-menstrual irritability.

5. Where hirsutism or other androgenic effects are a problem, the anti-androgenic progestogen cyproterone acetetate may be useful. Dianette contains 35 μg ethinyl oestradiol plus 2 mg cyproterone acetate daily for 21 days.

ORAL CONTRACEPTION — RISKS

A great deal of clinical and laboratory research and epidemiological analysis all go to support an association between OCs and myocardial infarction, thrombo-embolism and stroke.

This evidence of association is not universally accepted (a verdict of 'not proven' has been suggested) and there is as yet no readily available and standardised test for hypercoagulability. Nevertheless OCs have been shown to increase many of the factors related to coagulation of the blood and the clinician must take note of the probable risks. Modern low-dose preparations probably carry less associated risk, about half of that pertaining in pregnancy.

THROMBOEMBOLISM
This appears to be due to the oestrogen component and is dose related, hence the introduction of low-dose oestrogen or progestogen-only. Even the low-oestrogen pills are associated with a significantly higher risk in women over 25, and hypertension and obesity are predisposing factors. In 1995 evidence was produced that third-generation pills carried a greater risk of thrombo-embolism but only the UK and Germany issued warnings. The overall risk remains low and the 1995 data has been questioned.

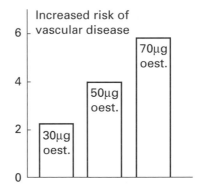

MYOCARDIAL INFARCTION AND STROKE
It has been claimed that OC users run a fourfold risk of these diseases, especially women over 35 who smoke. Arterial disease is attributed mainly to the effects of the progestogens. It has been known for some time that OCs alter the characteristics of lipoproteins in the direction of vascular disease. Low levels of high density lipoprotein-cholesterol (HDL-C) are produced by many of the progestogens used (oestrogens appear to increase HDL-C), and new progestogens have been introduced in which this effect has been reduced. Androgen-derived progestogens reduce lipoprotein 'a' (LP_a), a favourable effect.

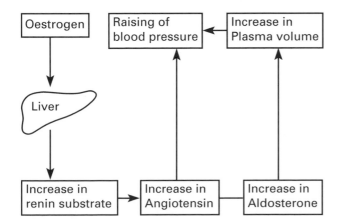

HYPERTENSION
OCs gradually raise the blood pressure, sometimes to the hypertensive range. The blood volume is increased by fluid retention, and the secretion of angiotensin is increased.

ORAL CONTRACEPTION — RISKS

MINOR SIDE-EFFECTS OF OCs

Oestrogen	**Oestrogen and Progestogen**	**Progestogen**
Breakthrough bleeding	Weight gain	Acne
Nausea	Post-pill	Depression
Painful breasts	amenorrhoea	Dry vagina
Headache		Loss of libido
		Insulin resistance
		(This is not a minor
		complication in diabetes.)

ORAL CONTRACEPTIVES AND NEOPLASIA

No causal link has yet been established between OC and any kind of neoplasia, but there has been much epidemiological controversy.

BREAST CANCER

Progesterone stimulates mitotic activity in breast epithelium and evidence has been published which suggests that long-term OC users before age 25, especially with the more potent progestogens, may incur an increased risk of subsequent breast cancer.

CERVICAL CANCER

Evidence has been offered to suggest that long-term OC users run a greater risk of cervical cancer and dysplasia, perhaps because the steroid hormones reduce immunity to antigenic causal factors. Long-term users should certainly have regular cervical cytology examinations.

ENDOMETRIUM AND OVARY

Prolonged OC use depresses mitotic activity in the endometrium and follicular maturation in the ovary, and these effects are considered to offer some protection against cancer of these tissues with ovarian cancer only 20% as common after 10 years of use as in non-users. Japan, where combined oral contraception is not approved, is alone among developed countries in showing no decline in incidence.

CONTRAINDICATIONS

History of cardiovascular disease
Hypertension
Heavy smoking
Obesity
Chronic hepatitis
Endogenous depression
Acute porphyria
Arterial or venous thrombosis
Thrombophilia defects

SPECIAL PRECAUTIONS

Collagen diseases
Otosclerosis
Diabetes mellitus
Sickle cell anaemia
Severe varicose veins
History of depression
Migraine

OTHER ROUTES

VAGINAL RINGS

Silastic ring pessaries have been developed which release either progestogen alone or combined oestrogen and progestogen, absorbed vaginally, thereby avoiding the first pass through the liver with subsequent reduction in dosage.

CONTRACEPTION BY INJECTION OF PROGESTOGEN

Two long-acting compounds are used:
— Medroxyprogesterone acetate (Depo-Provera) 50 mg every 3 months.
— Norethisterone oenanthate (Noristerat) 200 mg

Depo-Provera is now licensed for long-term use in the United Kingdom. It tends to have side-effects such as irregularity of the menstrual cycle, depression and loss of libido, and has induced breast tumours in experimental animals when given in large doses. The only significant metabolic effect appears to be a reduction in HDL-cholesterol which also occurs with oral progestogens. Three-monthly injections offer a simple and effective method of contraception in some circumstances, but in this country they are usually on a short-term basis. Use for 5 years or more is associated with some loss of bone mineral density.

PROGESTOGEN ONLY IMPLANTS

Norplant, comprising 6 silastic rods for subdermal insertion on the inner aspect of the upper arm releases 80 μg levonorgestrel daily initially, gradually falling to 30 μg by 5 years, when they are removed. The mode of action is similar to that of progestogen only pills but irregular bleeding is common. Removal may be difficult and must be performed by someone trained in the procedure.

FAILURE OF THE PILL

The failure rate of the combined pill is very small, between 0 and 1%, and there is often an avoidable factor.

1. The patient may forget to take the pill. Packing by the pharmaceutical firms is ingenious but not foolproof. If one pill is missed, two are taken the next day.

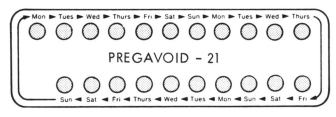

2. Gastroenteritis, perhaps following dietary indiscretion, may impair absorption.

3. Certain groups of drugs such as anticonvulsants, usually phenytoin and phenobarbitone, and the antibiotic rifampicin are known to increase the metabolic activity of hepatic enzymes and increase the rate of excretion of contraceptive steroids. (Cf. the treatment of neonatal jaundice with phenobarbitone.)

4. Several antibiotics including ampicillin are associated with an increase in breakthrough bleeding, and pregnancy has been reported. Oral contraceptives are conjugated in the liver, excreted in the bile, and partly reabsorbed. If gut bacteria are inhibited by antibiotics, reabsorption may not occur, leading to increased bowel excretion but lower circulating levels of steroids.

CONTRACEPTION BY THE INTRA-UTERINE DEVICE (IUD)

An IUD is made of polythene and copper (gold, silver and stainless steel have also been used) and is sufficiently flexible to be drawn into an introducer for insertion into the uterine cavity.

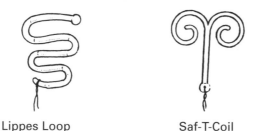

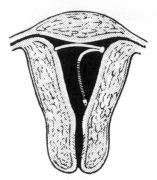

Lippes Loop   Saf-T-Coil   Copper-7 IUD in place

These are polythene ('inert') IUDs, a little bulkier than copper-and-polythene, and therefore perhaps more likely to cause heavy periods. There have been reports of pelvic actinomycosis in association with inert IUDs, and recent results suggest that these inert devices predispose to colonisation with actinomyces-like organisms, especially actinomyces israeli, notably in long-term users. Inert IUDs should be changed every 3 years or so. Most authorities recommend copper containing IUDs.

Copper-containing IUDs incorporate a winding of copper wire which is said to increase contraceptive efficiency. Their thinner diameter makes them easier to insert, and it is claimed that the menstrual loss is smaller.

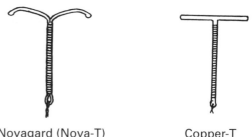

Novagard (Nova-T)   Copper-T

Because of the gradual absorption of copper, these IUDs are renewed every 2 or 3 years. Copper IUDs produce local concentrations of copper salts which apparently give some protection against bacterial contamination.

Some IUDs are licensed for 5 years and there may be devices licensed for 10 years eventually.

The Mirena
This levonorgestrel-releasing (20 μg/24hrs) intra-uterine system is now licensed for 5 years. It is said to be as effective as female sterilisation, but immediately reversible by removal. It reduces menstrual blood flow (time and amount) and markedly reduces blood loss in menorrhagia. It protects against pelvic inflammatory disease.

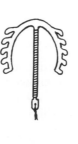

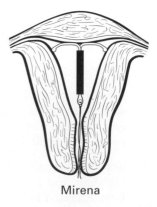

Multiload   Mirena

INTRA-UTERINE DEVICES (IUD)

MODE OF ACTION

This varies in experimental animals, and in the human it is not yet certain whether it prevents implantation or fertilisation. An inflammatory reaction is certainly induced in the endometrium and there is an increase in serum immunoglobulins, suggesting an immune reaction. Endocrine patterns are unchanged, but the luteal phase is often shortened by about 2 days, perhaps because of an increased secretion of prostaglandin. Yet IUDs do not, as a rule, cause dysmenorrhoea. Progestogen releasing intra-uterine systems deliver the progestogen directly to the endometrium, rendering it unreceptive to implantation. Cervical mucus is thickened.

PRINCIPLE OF INSERTION OF IUDS

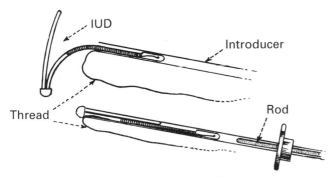

1. The IUD is first of all folded and inserted into a plastic tube called the introducer.

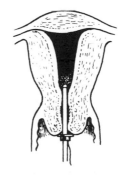

2. The introducer is then inserted into the uterus.

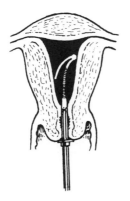

3. The IUD is forced out of the introducer by a rod...

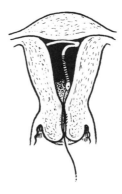

4. ...and takes up its position in the uterus.

INTRA-UTERINE DEVICES (IUD)

TECHNIQUE OF INSERTION

1. The cervix is exposed, swabbed and grasped with a tenaculum forceps.

2. The introducer is inserted and the IUD expelled into the cavity. The thread is then cut, leaving about 2 inches in the vagina.

With very nervous women some sedation or even an anaesthetic may be required.

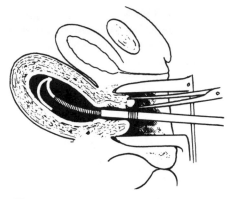

COMPLICATIONS OF IUDS

1. **Increased menstrual loss.**
   The cause may be the increased fibrinolytic activity which occurs round the IUD. It can be minimised by the use of antifibrinolytic agents such as tranexamic acid. Antiprostaglandin agents such as mefanemic acid or diclofenac are also effective. Progestogen releasing devices *decrease* loss.

2. **Infection**
   There is an increased risk of pelvic inflammatory disease, especially during the first year, and inert IUDs are associated with actinomycosis infection if retained for long periods. There is disagreement about how long an IUD should be left if symptomless, but extraction is often more difficult after several years in situ, and changing the IUD at 3-yearly or 5-yearly intervals seems sensible. Progestogen-releasing systems may *reduce* the incidence of infection.

3. **Pregnancy**
   This is about 1 to 1.5 per 100 woman years and is most likely in the first 2 years. It is lower with copper-bearing coils and may be as low as 0.1 per 100 with the Mirena.[†] The risk of ectopic pregnancy is greater in IUD users and has been calculated as 1.2 per 1000 woman years.[*] This increase is greatest with the progesterone-releasing Progestasert IUD and is not present with the Mirena levonorgestrel-releasing IUD.

4. **Expulsion**
   There is a 5 to 10% incidence, usually in the first 6 months.

5. **Translocation**
   The IUD passes through the uterine wall into the peritoneal cavity or broad ligament. It is thought that this begins at the time of faulty insertion, and once diagnosed by X-ray the IUD should be removed at laparoscopy.

[†] Sivin I. et al. *Contraception* (1991)44:473
[*]Vessey M.P. et al. *Lancet* (1979)ii, 501

CONTRAINDICATIONS TO IUD CONTRACEPTION

1. Existing pelvic inflammatory disease.
2. Menorrhagia.
3. History of previous ectopic pregnancy.
4. Severe dysmenorrhoea.

IUDs inserted at or after age 40 do not require to be replaced.
Progestogen releasing IUDs may be used to *treat* menorrhagia.

THE VAGINAL DIAPHRAGM ('DUTCH CAP')

This is a rubber diaphragm which when smeared with spermicidal cream will prevent sperms from reaching the cervical canal. It is less efficient than oral contraceptives or IUDs unless used strictly according to instructions; but it has few side-effects.

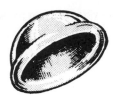

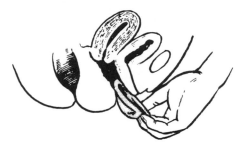

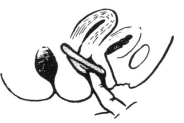

1. The diaphragm is smeared with spermicidal cream round the edges and on both sides, and guided into the posterior fornix.

2. The front end is tucked up behind the symphysis.

The diaphragm must not be removed until 6 hours after intercourse and if intercourse is repeated in that period more cream must first be injected with an applicator.

A female condom, 'Femidom', has recently become available.

VAGINAL SPERMICIDES

Spermicidal agents are inserted into the vagina in the form of creams, pessaries, gels or aerosols. One dose of spermicide must be injected before each act of coitus. The method is simpler in practice than the diaphragm, but probably less reliable.

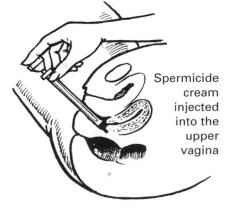

Spermicide cream injected into the upper vagina

THE COLLATEX SPONGE
A disposable plastic sponge is inserted into the vagina and can be left in situ for at least 24 hours. Sponges need no fitting, are comfortable and, when smeared with spermicidal cream, offer an effective barrier.

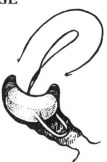

CONTRACEPTION BASED ON TIME OF OVULATION

THE RHYTHM METHOD ('Safe Period')

The woman must take her temperature every morning and watch for the sustained rise which indicates ovulation. Such graphs are not now accepted as being very precise indicators, but women with regular periods can usually identify the peri-ovulatory time with a fair degree of accuracy.

If the evidence suggests ovulation, say between the 12th and 14th days, 24 hours are allowed for ovum survival and 3 days should be allowed for the survival time of sperms in the genital tract, these times being all suppositious. This means that coitus must be avoided from the 9th to the 15th day and a 24 hour safety margin at either end increases the avoidance period from the 8th to the 17th day inclusive.

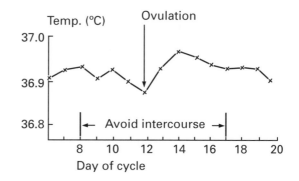

THE OVULATION METHOD (The Billings' Method)

The woman is taught to identify the peri-ovulatory phase by noting the vaginal sensations associated with changes in cervical mucus.

This method provides the same opportunities for coitus as the Rhythm method, but should be more accurate.

In practice, more protection would be afforded by a combination of arbitrary distinction between safe and unsafe days, and a close observation of physical signs and symptoms.

Say 5 days	Menstruation	
2–3 days	'Early Safe Days'	Sensation of vaginal dryness
4–5 days	Moist Days — **Not Safe**	Increasing amounts of sticky mucus
2 days	Ovulation Peak — **Not Safe**	Copious, clear 'slippery' mucus
3 days	Post-ovulation Peak — **Not Safe**	Gradual decrease in secretion
11 days	'Late Safe Days'	Minimal secretion

POSTCOITAL CONTRACEPTION

POSTCOITAL CONTRACEPTION ('Morning After' Contraception; 'Intraception')
Effective postcoital contraception has been sought for many years, usually in the form of douching with various liquids which have been unsuccessful because of the rapidity with which the sperms leave the vagina for the cervical canal and uterus. Modern methods are extremely effective if started early enough.

High Dosage Oestrogens
Ethinyloestradiol 5 mg, or diethylstilboestrol 50 mg taken daily for 5 days in divided doses starting within 72 hours of coitus. These dosages cause nausea and vomiting which may be so severe that the patient cannot continue with treatment and it is possible that levels of antithrombin III may be reduced, contributing to an increased risk of thrombo-embolism.

Method of Action
Corpus luteum function is depressed and the preparation of the endometrium for implantation is prevented.

Double Dose of OC Pill
Two tablets of 50 μg ethinyloestradiol and 500 μg levonorgestrol (Eugynon-50 or Ovran) are taken within 72 hours and repeated in 12 hours. This treatment is very much better tolerated.

Antiprogesterone.
The antiprogesterone RU486 may be more effective, with fewer side effects (Glasier, A. 1993 Postcoital contraception. *Reproductive Medicine Review* 2: 75-84)

Complications of Hormone Treatment
1. Pregnancy may not be prevented and there is a theoretical risk that the embryo may be affected.

2. If pregnancy occurs, there is an increased risk of ectopic pregnancy.

Insertion of IUD
This method is more effective and can be used for up to 5 days after coitus or 5 days after the estimated date of ovulation. It offers the advantage of being free from patient failure and should be offered when hormonal treatment is contraindicated, but like steroid hormones it should not be used if there is a history of previous ectopic pregnancy.

ETHICAL CONSIDERATIONS
The distinction between contraception and abortion depends on the stage at which the individual is considered to have come into existence — at fertilisation or nidation — and whatever method of postcoital contraception is used, there can be no certainty as to the point at which interference with the natural process took place.

FAILURE RATES IN CONTRACEPTION

There are 4 factors affecting the failure rate for any method of contraception:

1. **Inherent Weakness of the Method**
   For example, the rhythm method, which depends on the accurate determination of the time of ovulation, can never be as reliable as OC.

2. **Age**
   With all methods, the failure rate declines as age increases and fertility and frequency of intercourse decrease.

3. **Motivation**
   Every method depends on the determination of the woman to use it correctly. Thus pills may be forgotten, diaphragm users 'take a chance', even with IUDs a suspicion that the device is out of place may be ignored. Social class affects motivation.

4. **Duration of Use**
   The failure rate, especially with occlusive methods, declines as duration of use and therefore habit, increase. This observation is also true of IUDs, perhaps because the IUD becomes more effective the longer it is in place. Prolonged use is itself an indication of good motivation.

TABLE OF FAILURE RATES

The following table is taken from Vessey et al (1982) and their figures are based on the prolonged observation of over 17000 women, all 25 and over, and about 40% of whom were in social class I or II.

Method	Number of accidental Pregnancies	Number of woman-years of observation	Failure rate per 100 woman-years
OC			
50 μg oestrogen	61	37412	0.16
Progestogen only	21	1756	1.2
IUDs			
Saf-T-Coil	85	6791	1.3
Copper-7	34	2200	1.5
Diaphragm	485	25146	1.9
Condom	449	12492	3.6
Coitus Interruptus	45	674	6.7
Chemicals alone	36	303	11.9
Rhythm Method	25	161	15.5

CONTRACEPTION IN THE MALE

COITUS INTERRUPTUS

This means withdrawal of the penis just before ejaculation. It is widely practised and probably adequate for couples of low fertility, but some sperms must enter the vagina, and withdrawal at the point of orgasm is unnatural.

SHEATH (Condom, 'French Letter')

A thin rubber sheath fits over the penis. It interferes with sensation and is liable to come off as the penis is withdrawn after the act but it is a very efficient method if used correctly.

Beware of using coital lubricants, such as 'baby oil', which may weaken sheaths.

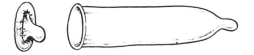

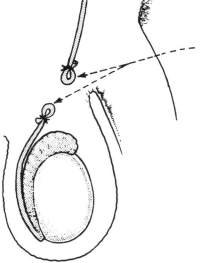

VASECTOMY

The vasa deferentia can be divided by a simple operation done under local anaesthesia.

1. It takes several months for the storage system to become clear of sperms and a few non-motile ones may persist whose significance is uncertain. It may take a year before the ejaculate is completely sperm free.

2. About 5% of patients demonstrate minor complications, including vaso-vagal reactions, haematoma and mild infection. There are occasional reports of severe infection.

3. Possible long-term complications include the development of sperm autoantibodies and there is often great difficulty in reversing the operation if this should be required.

CHAPTER 18

INFERTILITY

INFERTILITY

Percentage of couples pregnant after varying time periods of unprotected intercourse (after Gutmacher, 1956)

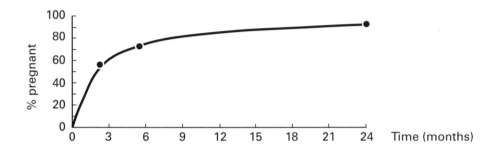

DEFINITIONS

Primary infertility is the inability to conceive in a couple who have had no previous pregnancies.

Secondary infertility is the inability to conceive in a couple who have had at least one previous pregnancy, which may have ended in a livebirth, stillbirth, miscarriage, ectopic pregnancy or induced abortion.

Prevalence

Up to 25% of couples will have difficulty in conceiving at some point during their lives. In the majority of couples this difficulty will resolve following conservative management or active treatment. Some couples will remain infertile ('unresolved infertility'). The prevalence rates for unresolved infertility are around 3-6% for both primary and secondary infertility.

Aetiology of infertility

Unexplained infertility	28%
Male factor infertility	21%
Ovulatory disorders	18%
Tubal disease	14%
Endometriosis	6%
Coital problems	5%
Cervical factors	3%

INVESTIGATIONS

INVESTIGATION OF INFERTILITY

Couples with failure to conceive may present either to the general practitioner or to a gynaecologist. Traditionally, investigations were only performed when conception had not occurred after a year of unprotected intercourse but such an approach is inappropriate in older couples and may cause anxiety in others. The decision as to when, and how far to investigate infertility should therefore be made together with the infertile couple.

Although the management of infertility may involve referral to a specialised unit offering assisted reproductive technologies, basic investigations can be initiated by the general practitioner. As with other conditions, a careful history and physical examination should be performed before initiating laboratory tests. For the purposes of simplicity, investigation of the female and male partner will be described separately. In practice however, the couple should be investigated together.

Female partner

A full history should be taken and examination performed. The following are particularly relevant:

Features in the history/examination	Possible pathology
oligo/amenorrhoea	ovulatory disorder
pelvic infection	tubal disease
STD	tubal disease
pelvic surgery	tubal disease
appendicitis	tubal disease
galactorrheoa	ovulatory disorder
postpartum infection	tubal disease
smoking	possible ovulatory disorder
cervical surgery	cervical cause
advanced age	ovulatory disorder
pelvic pain	endometriosis
lack of secondary sexual characteristics	ovulatory disorder
	intersex
sexual dysfunction	coital problems

History and examination of the male partner

Features in the history/examination	Possible pathology
genito-urinary infection	disordered spermatogenesis
exposure to toxic chemicals	disordered spermatogenesis
testicular injury/surgery	disordered spermatogenesis
smoking	disordered spermatogenesis
recreational drug use (e.g. cannabis)	disordered spermatogenesis
prescription drug use (e.g. cimetidine)	disordered spermatogenesis
testicular malformation	disordered spermatogenesis
mumps	disordered spermatogenesis
genital malformation	coital problems
sexual dysfunction	coital problems

EVIDENCE OF OVULATION

FEATURES SUGGESTIVE OF OVULATION

1. **Clinical symptoms and signs**

   No clinical symptoms or signs are sufficiently reliable to confirm ovulation. Supportive laboratory tests are always required. However, regular menstruation is usually associated with ovulation.

2. **Changes in basal body temperature**

   The secretion of progesterone by the corpus luteum induces a rise of around 0.5°C in basal body temperature (BBT). If BBT is recorded throughout the menstrual cycle, a fall in temperature is often observed at the time of the LH surge. Charts typical of those generated by A: a woman with an normal ovulatory cycle, and B: a woman with an anovulatory cycle are shown below. The differences in BBT between ovulatory and anovulatory women are not sufficiently consistent for a diagnosis of ovulation to be made without further tests.

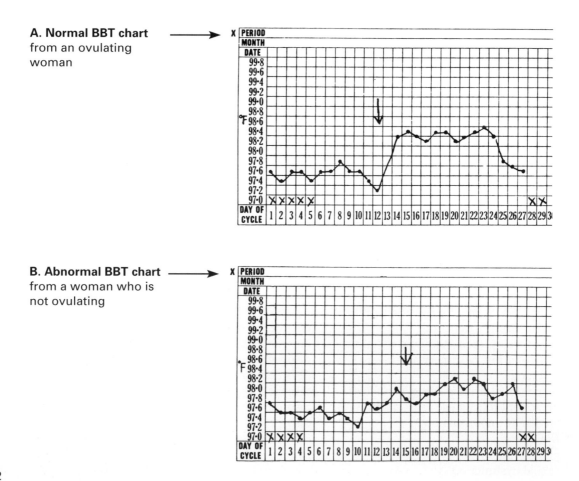

A. Normal BBT chart from an ovulating woman

B. Abnormal BBT chart from a woman who is not ovulating

EVIDENCE OF OVULATION

TESTS WHICH CONFIRM OVULATION IS OCCURRING

1. **Hormone tests**

   Progesterone

   Estimation of serum progesterone is one of the most commonly used methods for confirming ovulation. Progesterone is produced by the corpus luteum and elevated levels are seen in the luteal phase. A serum progesterone level of ≥10 nmol/l is a reliable indication that ovulation has occurred. Progesterone levels peak in the midluteal phase (i.e. 7 days prior to menstruation). If measured serum progesterone levels are low, this may indicate either that the patient is not ovulating, or that blood was withdrawn at an inappropriate time in the cycle. Information about the time of the subsequent menstrual period is required to interpret serum progesterone levels accurately. Progesterone levels should be checked seven days before the next menstrual period.

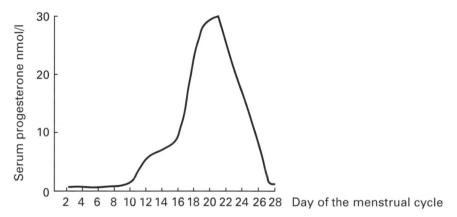

2. **Endometrial biopsy**

   The presence of secretory endometrium confirms that ovulation has taken place. Under the influence of progesterone, the endometrial glands dilate, and secretory vacuoles may be observed within the glandular cells. If an endometrial biopsy is taken in the luteal phase and examined histologically, secretory changes can be observed. Biopsy of the endometrium is a relatively invasive process, but gives useful information if sensitive progesterone assays are unavailable.

Proliferative phase endometrium showing oestrogen stimulation. Note the narrow non-secreting glands. The epithelial and stromal cells show proliferative activity.

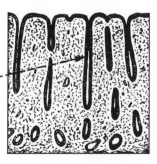

Secretory endometrium showing the effects of progesterone. Note the dilated secretory glands.

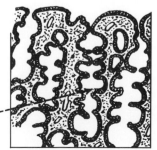

EVIDENCE OF OVULATION

3. **Serial ovarian ultrasound.**
   Over the course of the menstrual cycle, an ovarian follicle develops, grows to 20 mm and the oöcyte is then released at ovulation. This process can be visualised by ultrasound if an examination is performed at frequent intervals (every 2–3 days) during the follicular, ovulatory and early luteal phases. This procedure is too invasive and expensive to be used in an unselected population of women complaining of infertility. However, it is often used to monitor the number and size of developing ovarian follicles in women undergoing ovulation induction. Serial ultrasound is the only method of detecting the luteinised unruptured follicle syndrome (LUF).

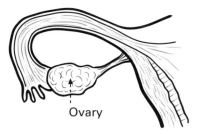

Early follicular phase (no ovarian follicle visible on ultrasound).

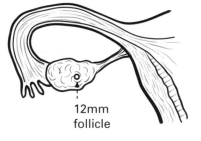

Mid follicular phase (12 mm follicle visible on ultrasound)

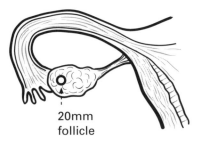

Immediate pre-ovulatory phase (ovarian follicle on 20 mm diameter)

SPERM PRODUCTION TESTS

TESTS WHICH CONFIRM NORMAL SPERM PRODUCTION

Semen analysis

A basic semen analysis assesses the number, morphology and motility of spermatozoa. The patient is asked to provide a sample (usually by masturbation), which should be analysed within two hours of production. The sample should be kept warm (15–38°C) during the interval from production to analysis. A period of 2–3 days abstinence from sexual activity is required before submitting a sample for analysis, otherwise an abnormally low count may be recorded. The patient should also be advised to keep the sample away from spermicidal agents, such as those in condoms.

The criteria for normal spermatogenesis may vary from laboratory to laboratory. The WHO criteria are shown below:

1. Volume: ≥ 2 ml
2. Concentration: ≥ 20 million/ml
3. Motility: ≥ 50% with forward motility (within 60 mins of ejaculation)
4. Morphology: ≥ 30% normal forms
5. White blood cells: <1 million/ml

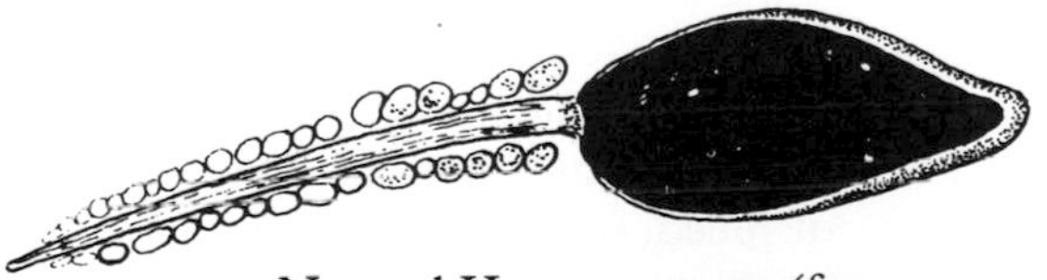

Normal Human sperm (from transmission electron micrograph).

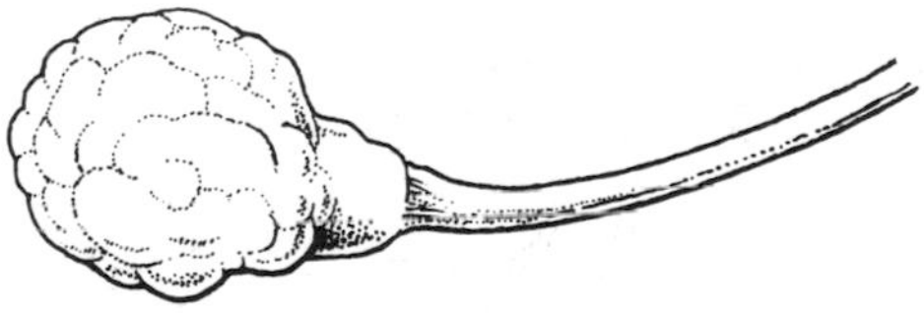

Abnormal sperm (from scanning electron micrograph).

SPERM PRODUCTION TESTS

For completeness, two samples should be analysed, each taken at least three months apart. It should be borne in mind that spermatogenesis takes at least 72 days, so that events such as a viral infection at any time in the preceding three months might adversely influence the result.

Semen analysis is conventionally performed by a trained technician using a microscope with a heated stage. More recently, computerised forms of semen analysis have become available which have the advantages of speed, reproducibility and cost.

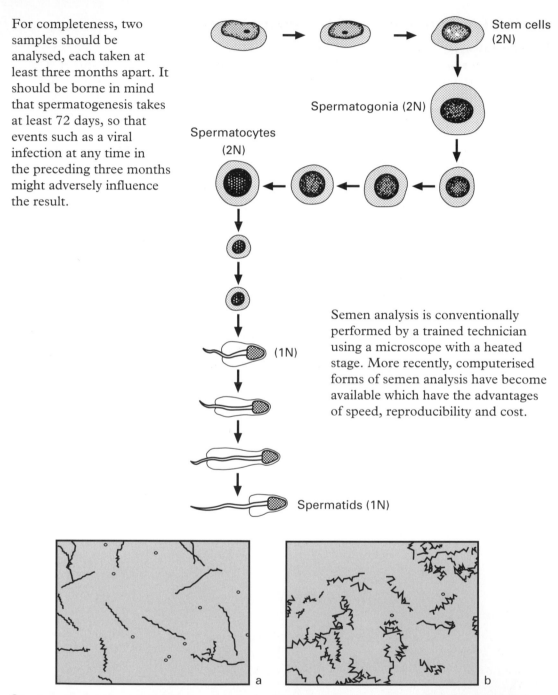

Sperm movement analysed by a computerised image analysis system: **a** linear progressive tracks of a non-capacitated sperm population; **b** high amplitude, non-progressive tracks of a hyperactivated, capacitated sperm population.

ABNORMALITIES IN SPERM PRODUCTION

The causes of abnormalities in sperm production include:

1. **Acute and chronic infection** of the male genital tract. Gonococcal and coliform infections respond to antibiotics but chronic prostatitis can be difficult to treat. Spermatozoa are reduced in number and tend to be malformed and non-motile.

   Chlamydial infection may be found in both partners. Sperm motility is reduced, causing infertility. Both partners should be treated and follow-up examinations of ejaculate carried out.

   Viral infections can be important, especially mumps. Testicular atrophy may follow this infection and systematic immunoglobulin prophylaxis and corticosteroid treatment should be given as soon as there is the slightest hint of this infection.

2. **Immunological reactions** in the form of auto-antibodies occur in a variable number of men (3–12%). Formation of these anti-sperm antibodies may be stimulated by infection or injury but in most cases the cause is obscure. Steroids in short courses may be helpful.

3. **Environmental factors**

   These are a compound of social habits — smoking, alcohol and drugs.

   Included under this heading are occupational hazards such as working with heavy metals, welding processes, exposure to high temperatures, pesticides and radioactive materials.

   The list of occupations involving substances toxic to sperm is remarkably long:
   Agriculture and gardening — pesticides, weed killers.
   Car industry, painters, battery workers, domestic decorators, smelters
      — all using lead products.
   Textile industry — carbon disulphide.
   Plastic manufacture — chlorinated biphenyls.
   Grain storage — benzine hexachloride.

A large number of therapeutic agents also affect spermatogenesis.

1. Chemotherapeutic agents — these depress sperm production and cause germinal epithelial aplasia. Rising FSH levels are an indication of these changes. Mustargen, cyclophosphamide and chlorambucil have been incriminated.

2. Sulfasalazine is used in the treatment of ulcerative colitis. Sperm motility is reduced, as is the number. These effects are reversed if treatment is stopped.

3. Cimetidine — used to reduce gastric acidity, spironolactone — used in oedema and ascites in renal and hepatic disease, and ketoconazole — used in treating micotic infections of skin. These substances interfere with androgen action and may affect spermatogenesis.

4. Anabolic steroids depress spermatogenesis profoundly but the effect is reversible when the drug is withdrawn.

5. Anti-hypertensive drugs, anti-depressants and some sedatives cause impotence and may depress sperm count or motility.

6. Furadantin, anti-malarial drugs, corticosteroids, phenacitin and salicylic acid derivatives can depress spermatogenesis.

SPERM FUNCTION TESTS

Other tests which may be used to assess sperm function

Hamster egg penetration test

The hamster egg penetration test assesses the ability of the human spermatozoa to penetrate a hamster egg. Since there is a species difference, the hamster egg should be stripped of its zona pellucida before the test is performed, otherwise a negative result will be obtained. The hamster egg penetration test is not widely used because of the high incidence of false negative results.

Post coital test

The post coital test assesses the ability of sperm to penetrate human cervical mucus. Healthy sperm are able to swim through cervical mucus obtained at mid-cycle. To perform the test, the couple are advised to have intercourse mid-cycle and a sample of cervical mucus is obtained 9–24 hours later. The presence of ≥ 20 motile sperm per high powered field ($\times 400$ magnification) is a positive result.

Athough the post coital test is still widely used, the requirement for careful timing of intercourse and cervical mucus recovery means that the test can be difficult to perform. An alternative is to assess the distance travelled by sperm through an 'artificial mucus', normally a hyaluronic acid polymer. This latter test is more easily quantified, and when used in combination with antisperm antibodies gives similar information.

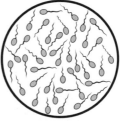

'Positive' post coital test showing presence of ≥ 20 motile sperm in one high power fluid.

Measurement of antisperm antibodies

Antisperm antibodies may be found in the serum, seminal fluid or cervical mucus. Each of these may adversely affect fertility. Many tests have been devised to assess antisperm antibodies. The immunobead test (IBT) detects both IgA and IgG antibody. In the presence of antisperm antibodies, polyacrylamide beads covered with bound antibody react with spermatozoa. The test has good sensitivity and specificity, and can also be used to indicate the antisperm antibody binding site — antibodies bound to the head of the sperm have the most serious effect on fertility.

In vitro assessment of fertilisation ability of sperm

In practice, many couples with male factor infertility are treated with in vitro fertilisation. Some sperm are sufficiently abnormal that they are unable to fertilise the egg in vitro, and this will be detected during the course of conventional IVF. More specialised treatment such as ICSI may then be required.

Abnormal sperm function

Spermatogenesis may be adversely affected by conditions such as a viral illness, hence it is important to obtain two samples of sperm more than 3 months apart for complete analysis. Persisting abnormalities of spermatogenesis are rarely treated successfully without recourse to assisted reproductive technologies. Further investigation and treatment of such men is outwith the scope of this book, but should be considered before ART is embarked upon.

TESTS OF TUBAL PATENCY

1. **Laparoscopic hydrotubation**
    Tubal patency can be assessed at laparoscopy. The cervix is instrumented with a cannula, and 5–20 ml of methylene blue dye is injected into the cavity of the uterus. If the fallopian tubes are patent, dye can be seen spilling out of the end of each tube. Laparoscopic hydrotubation has the advantage that the pelvic organs can be inspected during the procedure. Conditions such as pelvic adhesions and endometriosis, both of which may reduce fertility, can be noted. The major disadvantage of laparoscopy is that it is an operative procedure and that a general anaesthetic is required.

2. **Hysterosalpingography**
    Hysterosalpingography is radiological visualisation of the genital tract by the injection of radio-opaque contrast medium through the cervix. It has largely been replaced by laparoscopic hydrotubation, but may be useful in women wishing to avoid a general anaesthetic. Hysterosalpingography may be a useful supplementary test in women who have tubal blockage demonstrated at laparoscopy. Hysterosalpingography allows the site of tubal blockage to be demonstrated, which is helpful if surgery is contemplated.

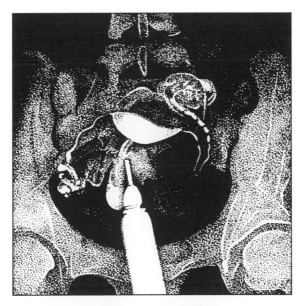

This is a normal salpingogram. Note:
1:   The antevered uterus is foreshortened.
2:   The long thin tubal outline.
3:   The ill-defined shadow of peritoneal spill.
4:   Cervico-vaginal leakage.

TESTS OF TUBAL PATENCY

3. **Ultrasound assessment of tubal patency**

   Tubal patency can now be assessed by ultrasound. A solution containing galactose microparticles visible on ultrasound is injected though the cervix. If the Fallopian tubes are patent, the solution can be observed passing along the tubes and out through the fimbrial end. This techique is sometimes called hysterosalpingo-contrast sonography, (HyCoSy).

4. **Falloposcopy**

   Advances in imaging techniques have allowed the manufacture of hysteroscopes small enough to be passed into the Fallopian tube. Internal tubal morphology can be assessed directly. This procedure is only available in specialised centres, but may be combined with operative treatments to relieve Fallopian tube blockage.

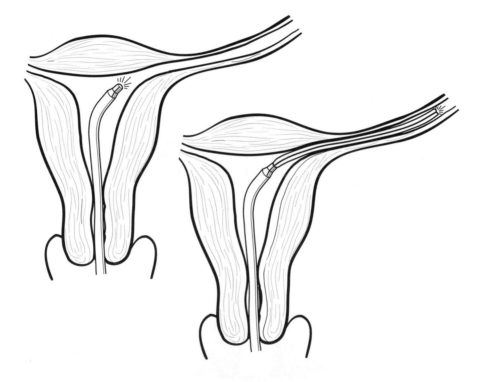

Requirements for the assessment of tubal patency

1. The patient should have a clear understanding of the procedure which is to be performed.
2. To avoid inadvertently performing the procedure when the patient is pregnant, the procedure should be done in the first half of the menstrual cycle, or at any phase of a cycle when adequate contraceptive precautions have been taken.

Contraindications to assessment of tubal patency

1. Pregnancy or possible pregnancy
2. Active pelvic or vaginal infection.

TREATMENT OF INFERTILITY

PRE-PREGNANCY ADVICE

Couples attending infertility clinics are clearly hoping to become pregnant at some point in the future and the opportunity for pre-pregnancy counselling should not be lost. The following should be considered:

Check rubella antibodies

Women who are not immune to rubella should be vaccinated, and advised to avoid pregnancy for three months.

Folic acid administration

Folic acid in doses of 4 mg/day is thought to reduce the risk of neural tube defects in the offspring of pregnant women. All women planning a pregnancy should be advised to commence folic acid.

MALE FACTOR INFERTILITY

There are few effective treatments for male factor infertility other than donor insemination (DI) or IVF.

OVULATORY DISORDERS

1. **Treat cause if known** — e.g. hyperprolactinaemia

2. **Clomiphene**
   Clomiphene is a non-steroidal anti-oestrogen. It has complex actions, including those of oestrogen agonistic activity at the endometrium. The major effect of clomiphene is at the hypothalamus, and its mechanism of action in inducing ovulation is to increase pituitary gonadotrophin production.

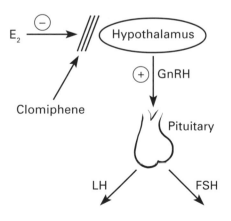

TREATMENT OF INFERTILITY

Administration of clomiphene

Clomiphene is given for five consecutive days in the early part of the menstrual cycle. Treatment can be started on day 2 or day 5 after menstruation has begun. In oligomenorrhoeic women, menstruation can be induced by progesterone (e.g medroxyprogesterone acetate, 10 mg daily for 5 days). A negative pregnancy test should be obtained prior to initiating therapy in oligomenorrhoeic women.

In view of the risk of multiple pregnancy, it is wise to commence with a low dose (25 mg or 50 mg daily) and increase at 50 mg intervals every three cycles. If the patient fails to ovulate on 100 mg clomiphene daily, further increases are rarely of benefit.

Ovulation should be confirmed by estimation of serum progesterone on day 21. Once ovulation has been achieved, most authorities would continue treatment for up to 12 months. In the UK, the product licence for clomiphene allows treatment for six months only. In women with unexplained infertility, an association between ovarian cancer and prolonged (more than 12 months) treatment with clomiphene has been demonstrated. The risks and benefits of clomiphene should therefore be discussed carefully with the patient if treatment of more than six months duration is contemplated.

Efficacy

Clomiphene is effective in inducing ovulation in around 80% of women. Around half these women will conceive. The multiple pregnancy rate is around 10%. Clomiphene is of no benefit in women with unexplained infertility.

Side effects of clomiphene:
    flushing (10%)
    abdominal distension or pain (5%)
    breast discomfort (2%)
    visual symptoms (2%)
    headache (1%)
    possible increased risk of ovarian cancer with prolonged treatment.

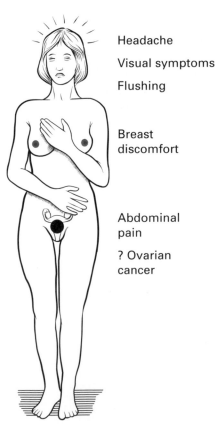

Headache

Visual symptoms

Flushing

Breast discomfort

Abdominal pain

? Ovarian cancer

TREATMENT OF INFERTILITY

3. Gonadotrophin therapy

Gonadotrophin therapy may be required in women with polycystic ovarian disease, who fail to respond to clomiphene. The aim of treatment is to ripen a follicle with repeated doses of FSH and then to stimulate ovulation with an injection of LH or hCG.

The following drugs are commonly in use:
HMG (human menopausal gonadotrophin) — contains 75 iu FSH and 25–75 iu LH
Urofollitrophin — contains 75 iu FSH and almost no LH
Recombinant FSH — contains 75 iu FSH
hCG — contains 1000–5000 iu hCG (this hormone is biologically similar to LH and is cheaper to prepare).

The use of gonadotrophins to induce ovulation should only be carried out in specialised centres. The patient should be monitored by ovarian ultrasound (to determine the number of follicles and their diameter) and by serum or urinary oestrogen assays. The dose of gonadotrophin should be carefully titrated to the patient's response. If the patient fails to respond to a small dose of gonadotrophin the dose should be increased at no less than 4–7 day intervals. The response of the ovary will vary from patient to patient and even from cycle to cycle.

Once a follicle of 17 mm diameter has been achieved by an FSH containing preparation, ovulation is induced by hCG (5000–10 000 iu). To reduce the risks of multiple pregnancy, hCG should be withheld if there are more than three follicles of 16 mm or greater in diameter. In case spontaneous ovulation inadvertently occurs, the couple should be advised to avoid sexual intercourse.

Efficacy
In women with polycystic ovarian syndrome, the conception rate with gonadotrophins is around 70%. The multiple pregnancy rate is 20% even when treatment is closely monitored.

Side effects
The major side effect of gonadotrophin administration is ovarian hyperstimulation syndrome. In carefully monitored cycles, the incidence of moderate to severe hyperstimulation syndrome is around 3%.

TREATMENT OF INFERTILITY

Ovarian Hyperstimulation Syndrome

The ovarian hyperstimulation syndrome is characterised by a sudden increase in vascular permeability with a massive extravascular exudate. The condition is categorised into mild, moderate and severe disease. In severe disease there is evidence of intravascular loss, with ascites and hydrothorax, and haemoconcentration leading to hepatorenal failure and thrombosis. The condition can be fatal and should be managed carefully by colloid support and, where necessary, dialysis and paracentesis. The mainstay of management is prevention, which involves careful monitoring of ovarian stimulation and witholding of hCG in women at risk.

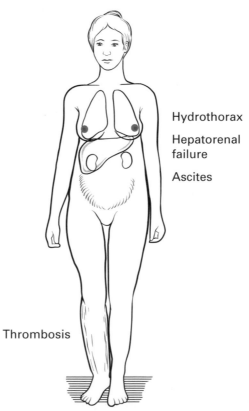

Hydrothorax

Hepatorenal failure

Ascites

Thrombosis

4.   Gonadotrophin releasing hormone (GnRH)

Women with anovulation due to hypogonadotrophic hypogonadism should be treated with GnRH. Natural GnRH is administered either subcutaneously (15 µg) or intravenously (5–10 µg) every 90 mins via a pump. The patient's own pituitary – ovarian feedback mechanism should operate and therefore the risk of multiple pregnancy and ovarian hyperstimulation is minimal.

TUBAL DISEASE

Tubal surgery

When tubal disease has been confirmed, tubal patency may be improved by surgery. The best results are obtained when surgery is performed by an operator trained in these techniques, using an operating microscope. Surgery may be performed laparoscopically, or at an open procedure. The aim of surgery is to restore tubal patency and mobility. However, restoration of tubal patency does not guarantee pregnancy, since tubal function (e.g. the movement of cilia) may have been permanently destroyed or impaired.

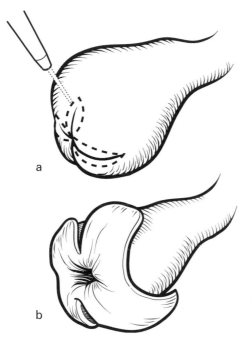

Laparoscopic salpingostomy with laser or diathermy to (a) incise the tube and scar the serosa to cause (b) eversion of the mucosa.

Efficacy

The efficacy of tubal surgery depends on the extent of pre-existing disease and on the particular procedure which is carried out. The best results are achieved after surgery for sterilisation reversal, when pregnancy rates as high as 60% have been reported. However, with severe disease, the cumulative pregnancy rate 24 months after surgery is as low as 10%, little greater than could have been expected after no treatment.

Side effects
— complications of surgery
— increased risk of ectopic pregnancy in a future pregnancy.

ASSISTED FERTILISATION TECHNIQUES

In vitro fertilisation

In vitro fertilisation ('test tube babies') involves the fertilisation of human oöcytes 'in vitro'. Eggs are harvested from ovarian follicles approximately 20 mm in diameter (i.e. immediately before ovulation). The eggs are then placed in a culture medium in an incubator and fertilised several hours later. Gonadotrophins are commonly employed to increase the number of preovulatory oocytes available for collection. The use of a GnRH analogue allows the timing of egg collection to be more tightly controlled.

Indications for in vitro fertilization:

1. In cases of unexplained infertility when anatomy and function appear to be normal, and treatable causes of infertility have been eliminated
2. For patients with endometriosis
3. Tubal disease
4. When the sperm count is low but not so low that fertilisation is impossible (see ICSI)
5. Patients showing evidence of cervical hostility to sperm.

EXAMPLE OF A TREATMENT SCHEDULE

Day 20 of menstrual cycle

The patient starts to take intranasal doses of an LHRH analogue, 100 µg five times a day. (Buserelin is one example of these analogues.) This blocks the LHRH receptors in the pituitary and stops the normal production of LHRH. FSH/LH levels rise suddenly, thus exhausting the pituitary content of FSH and LH, and then return to normal luteal levels. Menstruation occurs. Dosage of the LHRH analogue is continued. LH and FSH levels do not rise again.

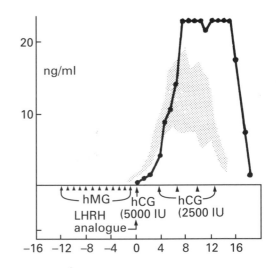

The diagram shows the sequence of hormone treatments, and the much improved luteal progesterone profile (●) compared with the normal (shaded).

Day 10 of the succeeding cycle

Daily injections of human menopausal gonadotrophin are started. LHRH analogue treatment is stopped. Follicular growth is monitored by daily ultrasound.

When follicles reach 20 mm in diameter, ovulation is imminent. An injection of hCG is given at this point. The timing of the injection is important. If given too early it may upset maturation processes. Some observers repeat this injection at 3-day intervals.

During hCG treatment regular ultrasound examination and hormone estimations are needed to monitor follicle development.

ASSISTED FERTILISATION TECHNIQUES

Collection of eggs

Transvaginal egg collection using ultrasound guided aspiration of follicles has now replaced egg collection at laparoscopy. Light sedation is required.

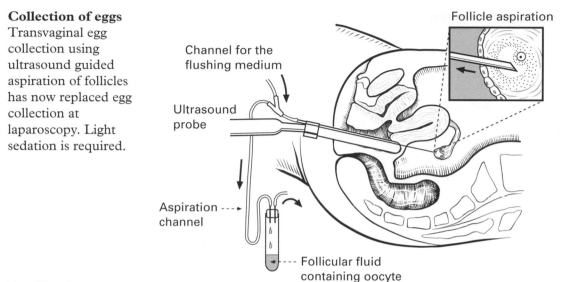

Follicle aspiration

Channel for the flushing medium

Ultrasound probe

Aspiration channel

Follicular fluid containing oocyte

Fertilisation

Eggs and sperm are cultured in vitro so that fertilisation may occur. The fertilised egg (embryo) is then grown to the 4 to 8 cell stage when it may be replaced into the uterus.

Human egg, 18 hours after fertilisation

Two pronuclear bodies (one from the sperm and one from the egg itself)

Normal human embryo at the 4 cell stage 48 hours after fertilisation (ready for transplant to the uterus)

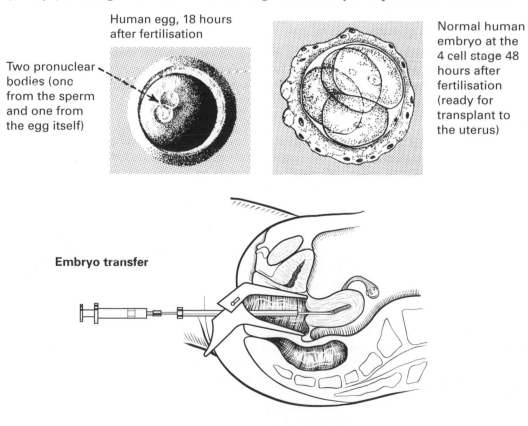

Embryo transfer

ASSISTED FERTILISATION TECHNIQUES

In vitro fertilisation *(contd)*

Efficacy

The success of IVF is dependent on the age of the female partner, the indication for treatment, the number of embryos replaced and the skill of the IVF treatment centre. The cumulative conception rate after three treatment cycles varies from over 40% (in women aged 20–24) to 20% (in women aged 40–45). The livebirth rate is considerably lower at around 30% (in women aged 20–24) to less than 15% (in women aged 40–45).

Side effects

The major complication of IVF is multiple pregnancy. At first sight this may not seem to be an adverse effect, but there is a considerable increase in the fetal mortality and morbidity associated with multiple pregnancy, mainly related to prematurity.

Variations on conventional IVF

1. **Embryo freezing**

   Embryo freezing allows embryos which have not been replaced during the first IVF cycle to be frozen and then defrosted and replaced in a subsequent cycle. Oestrogens and progesterones are administered prior to replacement of the (frozen) embryo in order to generate a secretory endometrium suitable for implantation. The advantage of this technique is that the administration of gonadotrophins, with the consequent risk of ovarian hyperstimulation syndrome, can be minimised.

2. **Use of donor oocytes**

   Since embryos can be frozen, oocytes can be aspirated from one woman (the donor), fertilized in vitro, frozen, and replaced in a recipient who has been treated with oestrogens and progesterones as described above. Such treatment may be useful in women with a premature menopause.

3. **ICSI**

   Intracytoplasmic sperm injection involves the injection of a single sperm into an egg. This technique is useful for men whose sperm count is so low, or whose sperm function is so abnormal, that they would not normally be able to fertilise an egg, either in vitro or in vivo. There are concerns that there may be an increased risk of male infertility in babies born following such a technique, and it is likely that further follow up information will be available in the future.

   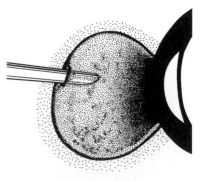

4. **GIFT**

   GIFT (Gamete intrafallopian transfer) involves the replacement of harvested sperm and eggs into the fallopian tube before fertilisation occurs. The advantage of this technique is that the expertise of an embryologist is not required. Clearly GIFT is unsuitable for women with tubal disease. Pregnancy rates are similar to those achieved by conventional IVF.

ASSISTED FERTILISATION

HFEA

The Human Fertilisation and Embrology Authority (HFEA) was created by an act of the UK parliament in 1990. Its function is to license and monitor clinics which carry out ART (e.g. IVF, donor insemination etc). The HFEA inspects each clinic on an annual basis. It also lays down criteria on what is considered acceptable treatment (e.g. it allows only three embryos to be replaced in each treatment cycle, it requires clinics to make counselling facilities available to patients, it forbids the payment of donors, etc). In other countries (e.g. the USA) there are no legal restraints on treatment, however clinics have an ethical obligation to treat their patients with clinical rather than commercial principals in mind.

Counselling

Infertility is not just a medical condition, but also affects the couple's perceptions of themselves as individuals, their relationship, and their functioning in society. The use of assisted reproductive technologies, such as IVF, has allowed many couples to bear children when they would not previously have been able to conceive. However, these technologies may be a mixed blessing — they are stressful to undergo and are by no means completely effective.

It is important in dealing with subfertile couples to give them an accurate description of the cause of their infertility and the prognosis with and without treatment. The efficacy and the side effects of the various treatment options should be discussed. In addition to this detailed medical information, the couple should be encouraged to explore their feelings about their situation. The use of professionals with counselling skills is invaluable and indeed the provision of counselling facilities is required by HFEA as a condition of their licensing of ART providers.

CHAPTER 19

THE MENOPAUSE

THE MENOPAUSE

The word menopause means the cessation of menstruation, but is commonly used instead of 'climacteric', a wider term for events leading up to and following the menopause, the pre-, peri- and post-menopause. The terms menarche and puberty bear a similar relationship.

Menstruation may gradually decrease, suddenly cease or become irregular.

Oestrogen levels fall over the 5 years preceding ovarian failure, which occurs usually between 45 and 55 years of age, with an average around 50 years. The fall in oestradiol has a positive feedback on the pituitary, increasing production of FSH and LH.

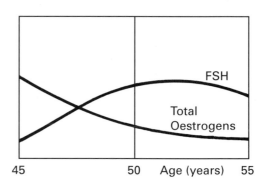

The ovary eventually produces only androstenedione, which is also produced by the adrenals and is converted in peripheral fat to the weak oestrogen oestrone.

Causes of Menopause
Ovarian failure occurs when only a few thousand primordial follicles remain — insufficient to stimulate cyclical activity. Now that women's life expectancy is about 80 years, one third of a woman's life is spent in the post-reproductive 'menopausal' phase.

Premature menopause may occur due to surgical removal of both ovaries, radiotherapy, chemotherapy or an unusually small number of primordial follicles present at birth. Conserved ovaries may fail following hysterectomy. The menopause occurs 6 to 18 months earlier in smokers.

Differential Diagnosis
Before the days of immunological pregnancy tests and effective contraception, pregnancy and menopause could easily be confused.

Polycystic ovary syndrome may produce amenorrhoea in this group. Prolactinoma should be borne in mind, especially in younger women.

Confirmation is by measurement of LH (raised disproportionately in PCO syndrome), FSH and oestradiol, ideally on 2 occasions 2 weeks apart to avoid a mid-cycle FSH peak. Prolactin assay and pregnancy testing are appropriate if clinically indicated.

		FSH (U/litre)	LH (U/litre)	Oestradiol ($p$mol/l)
Principal changes in serum hormone levels:	Pre-menopausal	2–20	5–25	100–600
	Post-menopausal	40–70	50–70	60

THE MENOPAUSE

Signs and Symptoms
These are related to changes in circulating oestrogen levels, and subjective symptoms may occur some years before menstruation ceases, while physical changes are more long-term.

Climacteric Signs and Symptoms

ACUTE ⟶ CHRONIC
and/or early onset   and/or later onset

Vasomotor Symptoms	Psychological Symptoms	Urogenital Tract Symptoms	Skeletal Disease	Cardiovascular Disease
Hot flushes. Sweats — often associated with Palpitation. Panic attacks. Insomnia.	Emotional lability. Anxiety. Depressed mood. Poor memory and concentration. Irritability. Decreased libido.	Breast atrophy. Genital tract atrophy. Dyspareunia. Urethral syndrome. Trigonitis. Urinary urgency and frequency.	Osteoporosis. Vertebral crush fractures with pain, deformity and loss of height. Femoral neck fractures.	Ischaemic heart disease. Cerebro-vascular disease.

Changes in the Genital Tract
These changes are of atrophic type and affect the external genitalia as well as the internal organs. They take time to occur — over a number of years.

Not only are the main pelvic structures reduced in size but, more importantly, the fascial framework and intra-pelvic ligaments supporting the bladder and genitalia are weakened; this may lead to complications.

Vulva: This shows flattening of the labia majora, the minor labia becoming more evident. Sexual hair becomes grey and sparse. The clitoris shrinks.

Uterus: The uterus becomes small with a relatively large cervix — a return to infantile proportions.

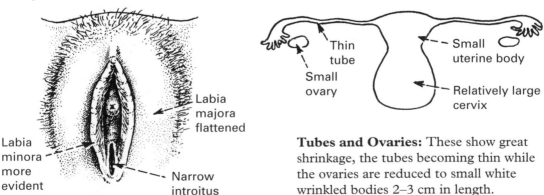

Tubes and Ovaries: These show great shrinkage, the tubes becoming thin while the ovaries are reduced to small white wrinkled bodies 2–3 cm in length.

413

THE MENOPAUSE

Changes in the Genital Tract *(contd)*
In addition to shrinkage of the vaginal introitus, the vagina diminishes in length and its secretions are limited, leading to sexual problems. Changes in the vaginal epithelium increase these problems. There is loss of rugosity and the epithelium becomes atrophic, with petechial haemorrhages in some cases and loss of glycogen.

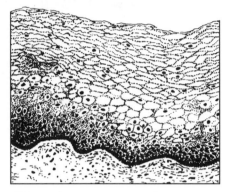

Normal pre-menopausal vaginal epithelium. Note the thick cornified layer.

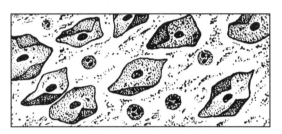

Smear of pre-menopausal vaginal epithelium. The cells are large with small nuclei and characteristic folded edges. Polymorphs are few in number.

Severity and duration of symptoms

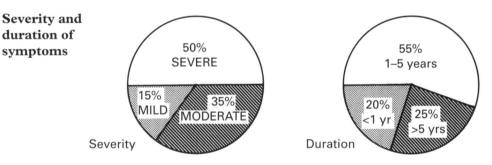

Severity

50% SEVERE
15% MILD
35% MODERATE

Duration

55% 1–5 years
20% <1 yr
25% >5 yrs

Menopausal Symptoms merit treatment
Vascular symptoms can be very distressing especially where night sweats prevent adequate sleep, and are the commonest reason for requests for treatment (65%). Psychological symptoms may cause problems coping with a job or running a home and often cause friction with relatives, friends or work mates. Approximately 45% of requests for treatment are related to such problems.

Of 424 Glasgow women aged between 40 and 60 years, the number and percentage by age groups who had ever felt a need for treatment for the menopause were as follows:

Age	No.	%
40–45	105	38.1
46–50	120	49.2
51–55	114	65.2
56–60	85	40.0

The mean age of onset of need for treatment was 44.3 ± 5.1 years.

Those who suffer symptoms and succeed in obtaining hormone replacement are in fact the fortunate ones, since appropriate treatment for symptoms may reduce skeletal and cardiovascular disease, Alzheimer's disease and colon cancer.

THE GREENE CLIMACTERIC SCALE

Please indicate the extent to which you are troubled at the moment by any of these symptoms by placing a tick in the appropriate box.

SYMPTOMS	Not at all	A little	Quite a bit	Extremely	Score 0-3
1. Heart beating quickly or strongly					
2. Feeling tense or nervous					
3. Difficulty in sleeping					
4. Excitable					
5. Attacks of panic					
6. Difficulty in concentrating					
7. Feeling tired or lacking in energy					
8. Loss of interest in most things					
9. Feeling unhappy or depressed					
10. Crying spells					
11. Irritability					
12. Feeling dizzy or faint					
13. Pressure or tightness in head or body					
14. Parts of body feel numb or tingling					
15. Headaches					
16. Muscle and joint pains					
17. Loss of feeling in hands or feet					
18. Breathing difficulties					
19. Hot flushes					
20. Sweating at night					
21. Loss of interest in sex					

Psychological (1–11) = ☐ Somatic (12–18) = ☐ Vasomotor (19–20) = ☐

Anxiety (1–6) = ☐ Depression (7–11) = ☐ Sexual dysfunction (21) = ☐

[Greene, J.G. (1991), *Guide to the Greene Climacteric Scale.* University of Glasgow.]

This scale may be used to measure climacteric symptoms and the response to treatment or to compare different treatment regimes.

An Anxiety score of 10 or more indicates severe, possibly clinical, anxiety. A Depression score of 10 or more indicates severe, possibly clinical, depression.

HORMONE REPLACEMENT THERAPY (HRT)

Do not confuse HRT with oral contraception.

Do not extrapolate real or imagined side-effects of oral contraception to apply to HRT. HRT is very effective in treating menopausal symptoms, as proved by many placebo-controlled cross-over studies looking at vasomotor, psychological and sexual symptoms, giving an 80–90% success rate. Despite this, less than 10% of women receive HRT and, even after hysterectomy and bilateral oophorectomy, not all women receive oestrogen, although failure to prescribe in these circumstances could lead to litigation. HRT reduces the cardiovascular and skeletal effects of ovarian failure.

Factors Influencing Prescription of HRT

Indications for Therapy: Symptoms — shorter term } Often both.
Prophylaxis — longer term. }

Personal and Family History: Osteoporosis — higher dose, longer term.
Cardiovascular disease — see Cardiovascular Disease and the Menopause (page 425).
Breast cancer — see HRT and the Breast (page 426).

Hysterectomy or not: Usually no progestogen after hysterectomy.

Patient's Preferences: Tablets, Implants, Transdermal patches, Gels, Local preparations.

Avoidance of Fluid Retention: Low dose HRT and low calorie diet may help to minimise fluid retention (bloating and breast discomfort) which occurs quite commonly during HRT. For some women, however, it is impossible to find a dose low enough to avoid fluid retention yet high enough to relieve other symptoms.

Concurrent Medication: With anti-epileptic or other liver enzyme inducing therapy, avoid oral HRT.

Duration of Therapy depends on:

Reason for therapy: Prophylaxis — long-term — 5 years plus.
Symptoms — could stop at intervals and recommence if symptoms recur.

Acceptability of therapy: If side-effects are unacceptable, or worse than symptoms, discontinue. Withdrawal bleeds, fluid retention and fear of breast cancer are common reasons for stopping.

History: No relative contraindications — longer therapy — perhaps till 65 years of age.
Family or personal risk of ischaemic heart disease — longer therapy.
Osteoporosis risk factors — longer therapy.
Family breast cancer history — shorter therapy — 5–10 years counting from age 50 yrs. Possibly an indication for raloxifene.

Screening

Screening before and on HRT is basically well-woman screening.

When a woman has had hysterectomy with conservation of one or both ovaries, it is sensible to measure FSH and oestradiol before commencing oestrogen as symptoms may occur in the presence of normal ovarian function — sometimes due to clinical anxiety.

HORMONE REPLACEMENT THERAPY (HRT)

Screening *(contd)*

Pre-treatment	*On treatment*
FBC Biochemical screen (principally for liver function).	Breast examination regularly.
Breast examination. Mammography if over 50 or if otherwise indicated.	Mammography every 2 years, 50–65 years.
Pelvic examination. Papanicolaou smear. Endometrial sampling if indicated by abnormal bleeding.	Papanicolaou smear every 3 years. Endometrial sampling only if abnormal bleeding occurs (before 10th day of progestogen).
Blood pressure.	Blood pressure 6-monthly.
Weight.	

Contraindications to HRT

These are more theoretical and medico-legal than real. Contraindications have been extrapolated from the old high-dose oral contraceptive formulations to HRT and many contraindications appearing on UK data sheets are not significant. Some, however, such as elevated cholesterol and ischaemic heart disease are actually indications. Not all gynaecologists are aware of the change in attitude to contraindications which has developed in menopause clinics.

Hepatic: Acute Porphyria.

Cardiovascular: Uncontrolled or uncontrollable hypertension. (Controlled hypertension or hypertension not requiring treatment are not contraindications.)

Deep vein thrombosis or pulmonary thrombo-embolism which occurred during pregnancy or when on the oral contraceptive pill or HRT, with anti-thrombin III deficiency, presence of factor V Leiden or other thrombophilia defects. (A past history of thrombo-embolic phenomena without such defect is not a genuine contraindication, but transdermal, percutaneous or implant therapy is preferred, to minimise oestrogen dose to the liver.)

Myocardial infarction and cerebrovascular accident. Once the patient is mobilised, these are indications, not contraindications.

Malignant Disease: Breast cancer is regarded by many surgeons as a contraindication, though there is no proof of adverse effect and breast cancer diagnosed during HRT has a higher cure rate. (Harding. C. 1996 *B.M.J.* 312: 1646-1647.) Caution is sensible and progestogens should be employed first.

Endometrial cancer is oestrogen sensitive and progestogens are usually employed first. Combined oestrogen–progestogen therapy has been shown to be safe in early stage disease. (Wren, B. 1994 *International Journal of Gynecological Cancer* 4: 217-224.)

Melanoma is not now thought to be a contraindication.

HORMONE REPLACEMENT THERAPY (HRT)

Contraindications *(contd)*

Acute porphyria is a contraindication to HRT. There is no significant evidence that multiple sclerosis or otosclerosis are adversely affected by HRT, though anecdotal stories exist, based on extrapolation from effects of pregnancy.

Prolactinoma might be adversely affected and pregnancy is a contraindication, hence the need to exclude pregnancy before commencing HRT should any doubt exist.

Migraine can be adversely or beneficially affected by HRT and is not a reason for refusing to prescribe. Individuals may tolerate one preparation better than another.

Choice of Treatment

This involves the following considerations:
1. Presence or absence of uterus — usually, no uterus no progestogen.
2. Effectiveness.
3. Convenience — convenience aids compliance.
4. Cost.
5. Patient preference — often related to the experience of friends.
6. Medical considerations — parenteral therapy has least effect on and is least affected by the liver.
7. Side effects — see below.

Routes of administration
1. Oral — tablets.
2. Transdermal — patches.
3. Percutaneous — gel.
4. Subcutaneous — implants.
5. Vaginal — Cream
   — Pessary
   — Tablet
   — Ring (silastic)

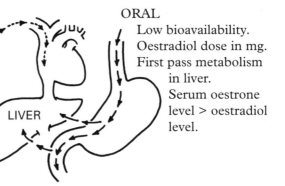

ORAL
Low bioavailability.
Oestradiol dose in mg.
First pass metabolism
in liver.
Serum oestrone
level > oestradiol
level.

LIVER

PARENTERAL
High bioavailability.
Oestradiol dose absorbed in μg per day.
No first pass liver metabolism.
Serum oestradiol level > oestrone level.

HORMONE REPLACEMENT THERAPY (HRT)

Pros and cons of different routes

Oral

1. Economical.
2. Wide choice of preparations and doses.
3. Only route available for progestogens in some countries.
4. Absorbed into portal system and passes through liver before reaching systemic circulation with metabolism to oestrone and liver enzyme induction. More effect on lipids and coagulation.
5. May cause nausea.
6. Majority of data on prevention of osteoporosis and cardiovascular disease relate to oral therapy.

Transdermal and Percutaneous

1. More physiological, with absorption into and distribution by systemic circulation, not hepatic portal system.
2. Minimum effect on liver. 'Coagulation-friendly.'
3. More lipid-friendly route for progestogens.
4. Effective against osteoporosis.
5. High patient acceptability (if no skin irritation).
6. More costly.

Subcutaneous implants (25 mg or 50 mg pure crystalline oestradiol).

1. Effective where other routes fail.
2. Possibly best therapy for decreased libido. Testosterone 100 mg may be added for this.
3. Good skeletal effect.
4. Little effect on lipids.
5. Risk of escalation of oestradiol levels, so strict control of dose and frequency of implants is necessary.
6. Long-term effects on endometrium after stopping treatment, so best used after hysterectomy.

Vaginal preparations

Oestriol preparations and low dose oestradiol tablets (0.025 mg) do not have systemic effects, so do not induce uterine bleeding and can give local benefit in women with contraindications to systemic therapy.

Potent oestrogens given vaginally have systemic effects.

Vaginal preparations relieve atrophic vaginitis, trigonitis, vaginal dryness and dyspareunia.

Vaginal silastic ring pessaries can be low dose for local effect or higher dose oestradiol to get parenteral systemic effect, each pessary lasting for 3 months.

HORMONE REPLACEMENT THERAPY (HRT)

Recommended Regimes

After Hysterectomy

Oral oestradiol, oestradiol esters or conjugated equine oestrogens.

Transdermal oestradiol. Oestradiol implants. Vaginal systemic ring pessary.

Combined oestrogen and progestogen (cyclical or continuous combined) may be employed when the hysterectomy was performed for extensive endometriosis. Norethisterone 5 or 10 mg daily or medroxyprogesterone acetate 10 or 20 mg daily or megestrol acetate 40 or 80 mg daily may be employed after endometrial or breast carcinoma, deep vein thrombosis or pulmonary thrombo-embolism. Norethisterone is effective against osteoporosis in these doses. About 60% of patients obtain vasomotor symptom relief from these progestogens.

With Intact Uterus

Oral oestradiol, oestradiol esters or conjugated equine oestrogens daily with norethisterone, norgestrel, medroxyprogesterone acetate or dydrogesterone added for at least 10 or 12 days per month. This will avoid endometrial hyperplasia and irregular, unpredictable bleeding and reduce the risk of the rare endometrial cancer. Combined continuous oestrogen–progestogen therapy is suitable for genuinely post menopausal women (at least a year since last period) and avoids withdrawal bleeding in a high percentage. Tibolone (Livial) is a single molecule formulation with similar indications and effect.

Transdermal oestradiol and transdermal or oral norethisterone, as above. Norethisterone, megestrol acetate or medroxyprogesterone acetate may be employed after oestrogen-dependent tumours or thrombo-embolic phenomena as in hysterectomy patients.

Proprietary names and dosages are listed in MIMS and the National Formulary.

Alternatives to oestrogen

When systemic oestrogen is contraindicated, not tolerated or declined, the following may be useful:
1. Unopposed progestogens (norethisterone, megestrol acetate, medroxyprogesterone acetate).
2. Oestriol vaginal preparations.
3. Low dose oestradiol vaginal preparations.
4. Clinical psychology.
5. Hypnosis.
6. Bisphosphonates (for skeletal benefit only).
7. Selective Estrogen Receptor Modulators (SERM's) such as raloxifene (for skeletal and cardiovascular benefits).
8. Dacron fabric night-wear, which is non-wettable and minimises discomfort from excessive sweating.

OSTEOPOROSIS

Osteoporosis is the commonest metabolic bone disease. Post-menopausal osteoporosis results from an excess of bone resorption over bone formation associated with loss of oestrogen. Women have 20% less bone than men at peak skeletal development, so women have less bone to lose before reaching the fragility threshold. More than 50% of Caucasian women suffer one or more osteoporotic fractures by the age of 70.

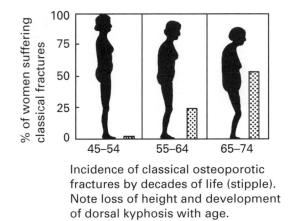

Incidence of classical osteoporotic fractures by decades of life (stipple). Note loss of height and development of dorsal kyphosis with age.

Dual X-ray densitometry is the currently favoured technique for measuring lumbar spine and femoral neck density, though loss of height or radiological demonstration of vertebral crush fractures give clear evidence of osteoporosis. Bone mineral density (BMD) above minus 1 SD below young adult mean is normal, osteopenia lies between minus 1 and minus 2.5 SD and osteoporosis below minus 2.5 SD of young adult mean.

Ultrasonic densitometry of calcaneum is of some value but is not at present a substitute for X-ray densitometry.

OSTEOPOROSIS

BONE DENSITOMETRY

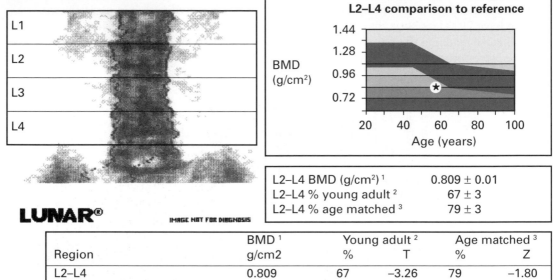

L2–L4 comparison to reference

L2–L4 BMD (g/cm²) [1]	0.809 ± 0.01
L2–L4 % young adult [2]	67 ± 3
L2–L4 % age matched [3]	79 ± 3

Region	BMD [1] g/cm2	Young adult [2] %	T	Age matched [3] %	Z
L2–L4	0.809	67	–3.26	79	–1.80

At –3.26 SD of young adult, there is definite osteoporosis of lumbar spine

Neck comparison to reference

Neck BMD (g/cm²) [1]	0.614 ± 0.02
Neck % young adult [2]	63 ± 3
Neck % age matched [3]	75 ± 3

NECK	:BMC [5] (grams) = 3.06	Area [5] (cm²) = 4.99
WARDS	:BMC [5] (grams) = 1.50	Area [5] (cm²) = 2.76
TROCH	:BMC [5] (grams) = 4.47	Area [5] (cm²) = 9.45

Region	BMD [1] g/cm2	Young adult [2] %	T	Age matched [3] %	Z
NECK	0.614	63	–3.05	75	–1.73
WARDS	0.542	60	–2.83	78	–1.18
TROCH	0.473	60	–2.88	67	–2.07

LUNAR® IMAGE NOT FOR DIAGNOSIS

Osteoporosis at all 3 sites in this hip

OSTEOPOROSIS

Comparative cortical bone thicknesses:

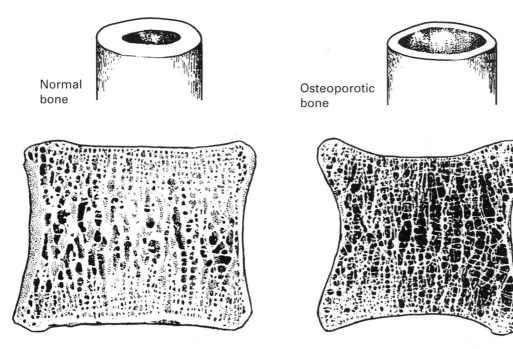

Normal bone

Osteoporotic bone

Normal vertebral body. Note the thick trabeculae of bone.

Vertebrae from post-menopausal woman showing extreme rarefaction of the trabeculae.

OSTEOPOROSIS

Oestrogens have an anti-resorptive effect on bone.

Prevention of osteoporosis is preferable to attempting treatment once osteoporosis is established. It is particularly important after premature menopause, whether natural or surgical, and oestrogen at an appropriate dose (at least 0.625 mg conjugated equine oestrogen orally or equivalent; 50 μg oestradiol patch; oestradiol implants) will prevent development of osteoporosis in the great majority of women. Therapy for 5 years or more may reduce the incidence of Colles' fractures and hip fractures by 50% and vertebral crush fractures by up to 90% in those who take oestrogens. Tibolone (Livial) raloxifene (Evista) norethisterone and bisphosphonates are alternatives.

Bone loss recommences on stopping therapy so that withdrawal of HRT at age 65 results in bone density at 75 or 80 being no better than that of untreated women. Conversely, when treatment is only started at 65 bone density at 75 or 80 is not significantly worse than it would have been with continuous treatment.

Risk factors for osteoporosis are:
1. Female sex.
2. White or oriental race.
3. Family history of osteoporosis.
4. Early menopause (natural or oophorectomy).
5. Sedentary life-style.
6. Low weight for height.
7. Tobacco and alcohol abuse.
8. Low calcium intake.

CARDIOVASCULAR DISEASE AND THE MENOPAUSE

In European countries, 40 to 45% of deaths are due to cardiovascular causes with a relative increase in risk in females after the menopause. (The actual risk is greater in males even after 75 years.)

Mortality rate for selected causes per 100,000 population in Scotland, 1988.
(Source: Registrar General for Scotland.)

	Endometrial cancer	Cervical cancer	Breast cancer	Lung cancer	Fractured femur (estimated)	Ischaemic heart disease	Cerebro-vascular disease
All ages	4	7	48	52	<20	316	196
45–64	6	14	88	114	<10	170	62
65–74	12	22	130	206	<25	854	325

The risk of coronary heart disease is increased sevenfold by bilateral oophorectomy before 35 years of age or premature menopause at 35 years. Oestrogen replacement reduces ischaemic heart disease to less than 50% of the untreated incidence. The greatest reduction in deaths is in women with cardiovascular disease. It is probable that there is no decrease (but no increase) in deaths from cerebrovascular disease. Henderson et al., Arch. Int. Med. (1991), 151, 74, detail the decreased mortality on HRT which may amount to a 20% reduction in all causes of mortality after 15 years of HRT.

It has been feared that addition of a progestogen might reduce the cardiovascular protection afforded by oestrogens, but androgen derived progestogens lower the level of lipoprotein 'a' (LP_a) in women and animal work suggests that progestogens may not be harmful. Epidemiological studies in women increasingly indicate no adverse effects of progestogens on the cardioprotective effects of oestrogens. Raloxifene appears to be cardioprotective.

HRT may influence cardiovascular risk factors through effects on:

Lipid metabolism .... oestrogen increases HDL cholesterol and lowers LDL cholesterol.
Carbohydrate metabolism .... reduced insulin resistance.
Body fat distribution .... oestrogen promotes gynaecoid fat distribution.
Coagulation and fibrinolysis.
Blood flow .... oestrogen increases arterial flow.
Blood pressure .... non-significant fall in blood pressure.

A number of studies have shown no hypertensive effect of HRT. Blood pressure rises with age and may reach levels requiring therapy in the early post-menopausal years, incorrectly attributed to HRT. The occasional idiosyncratic rise in BP may occur.

The H.E.R.S study showed increased mortality in the first year of HRT and no excess in mortality thereafter, in women with severe pre-existing coronary disease.

HRT AND THE BREAST

Fear of an increased risk of breast cancer is the main cause of concern about HRT in patients and doctors.

Breast cancer is increasing in incidence and may affect one woman in 9 in a lifetime.

Alcohol use in young women may increase the risk, and obesity, high socio-economic status and delayed first pregnancy are risk factors. Early menarche, late menopause and nulliparity are also risk factors. Only 20% of subjects have a positive family history. A woman's risk of developing breast cancer is significantly increased when mother, sister or daughter developed the disease before 50 years. The Lynch family syndrome involves familial breast, ovarian and colon cancer.

Early menopause decreases breast cancer risk (70% reduction with menopause before 35 years).

The excellent review by the Collaborative Group on Hormonal Factors in Breast Cancer, principal author Professor V. Beral, in the Lancet of 11/10/97 is strongly recommended reading.

Between the ages of 50 and 70 years, when most HRT is prescribed, 45 women per thousand *not taking HRT*, will develop breast cancer. Using HRT for 5 years between 50 and 70 adds only 2 per thousand, 10 years use adds 6 per thousand and 15 years adds 12 per thousand. This may be counter balanced by a reduction in fatal colon cancer, with a highly significant trend (p = 0.0001) of decreasing risk with increasing years of use and relative risk of 0.55 (0.40–0.76) with current use (Calle et al 1995 *Journal of the National Cancer Institute* Vol 87 7: 517–523).

Oestrogen may be promotive rather than causative. There is insufficient evidence to recommend adding a progestogen to decrease the risk of breast cancer. It is difficult to find evidence that orthodox HRT is harmful to treated breast cancer patients but one must err on the side of caution and unopposed progestogens are preferred for this reason. References such as Di Saia PJ 1996 *Amer J Obstet Gynae* 174: 1494–1498, suggest no harmful effects.

Breast cancer diagnosed while on HRT has a higher survival rate (Harding C 1996 *British Medical Journal* 312: 1646-1647), and it must be remembered that there are 9 times as many deaths from heart disease as from breast cancer, with more than 50% of the cardiovascular deaths potentially preventable by HRT. Perspective and patient choice are important.

HRT: MISCELLANEOUS

Contraception in the Climacteric
Ovulation may occur after 6 months of amenorrhoea.

Most HRT preparations are not contraceptive.

Effective contraception is recommended until one year after menstruation ceases, in the absence of vasectomy or female sterilisation. Cyclical HRT makes it difficult to assess the one year criterion and some family planning doctors add a progesterone only oral contraceptive to cyclical formulations on the days when no progestogen is present.

After the age of 45, it is considered that IUCD's do not require to be renewed regularly and can be left in situ till there is no risk of pregnancy. Levonorgestrel releasing IUDs serve a double purpose, giving excellent contraceptive protection and also countering the effects of oestrogen on the endometrium.

Barrier contraception has a low failure rate in climacteric women.

Future Developments
New progestogens may have more favourable metabolic effects.
Withdrawal bleeding may be avoided in a high percentage of genuinely post-menopausal (1 year or more) women by using a single molecule with oestrogen and progestogen effect (Tibolone), or continuous, rather than cyclical, combined oestrogen and progestogen. Raloxifene appears to be actively breast protective; hopefully similar compounds will become available which will also control vasomotor symptoms.

Benefits and Risks of HRT
Appropriate hormone treatment:
    reduces Alzheimer's disease.
    relieves vasomotor symptoms.
    relieves psychological symptoms.
    protects and restores collagen.
    prevents and improves osteoporosis.
    reduces cardiovascular disease.
    reduces fatal colon cancer
    reduces all-cause mortality.
but
    may increase breast cancer.
    may cause fluid retention.
    may cause 'premenstrual' syndrome.
    may cause unwanted uterine bleeding.
    may increase gallbladder disease.
    may increase thrombo-embolism during the first year of use.

In terms of both symptom relief and mortality statistics, the benefits greatly outweigh the adverse effects.

PROFILE OF AN IDEAL HRT

Once the ideal HRT is formulated, perhaps we can start on one for men — at present there is no convincing evidence for male HRT benefits, but who knows what the future may bring?

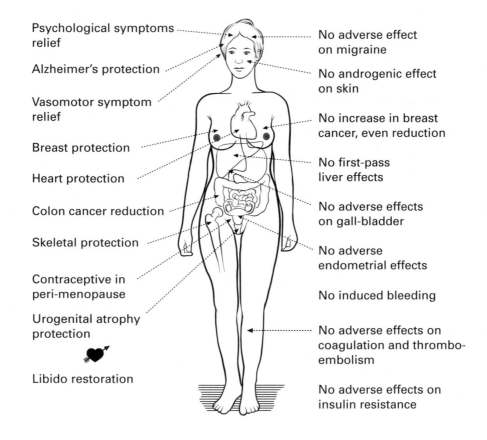

Psychological symptoms relief

Alzheimer's protection

Vasomotor symptom relief

Breast protection

Heart protection

Colon cancer reduction

Skeletal protection

Contraceptive in peri-menopause

Urogenital atrophy protection

Libido restoration

No adverse effect on migraine

No androgenic effect on skin

No increase in breast cancer, even reduction

No first-pass liver effects

No adverse effects on gall-bladder

No adverse endometrial effects

No induced bleeding

No adverse effects on coagulation and thrombo-embolism

No adverse effects on insulin resistance